Care in Nursing

Care in Nursing
Principles, values, and skills

EDITED BY

Professor Wilfred McSherry

Staffordshire University

Staffordshire, UK

The Shrewsbury and Telford Hospital NHS Trust,

Shropshire UK

Haraldsplass Deaconess University College,

Bergen, Norway

Professor Robert McSherry

Teesside University

Middlesbrough, UK

Professor Roger Watson

University of Western Sydney

New South Wales, Australia

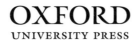

OXFORD

UNIVERSITY PRESS

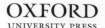

UNIVERSITY PRESS

Great Clarendon Street, Oxford OX2 6DP

Oxford University Press is a department of the University of Oxford.
It furthers the University's objective of excellence in research, scholarship,
and education by publishing worldwide in

Oxford New York

Auckland   Cape Town   Dar es Salaam   Hong Kong   Karachi
Kuala Lumpur   Madrid   Melbourne   Mexico City   Nairobi
New Delhi   Shanghai   Taipei   Toronto

With offices in

Argentina   Austria   Brazil   Chile   Czech Republic   France   Greece
Guatemala   Hungary   Italy   Japan   Poland   Portugal   Singapore
South Korea   Switzerland   Thailand   Turkey   Ukraine   Vietnam

Oxford is a registered trade mark of Oxford University Press in the
UK and in certain other countries

Published in the United States
by Oxford University Press Inc., New York

British Library Cataloguing in Publication Data
Data available

Library of Congress Cataloguing in Publication
Data available

Typeset by TNQ Books and Journals Pvt. Ltd.
Printed in Italy
on acid-free paper by
L.E.G.O. S.p.A.—Lavis TN

ISBN 978-0-19-958385-0

1 3 5 7 9 10 8 6 4 2

Foreword

Ask any seasoned nurse about what healthcare was like when they first joined the profession and they will probably start by saying 'things were different in my day'. And indeed things were different forty, thirty, twenty, and even ten years ago. The number of people needing healthcare services has steadily increased, and people are living longer and with more complex care needs.

What hasn't changed is that patients, no matter where they are being cared for, maintain an almost idealistic expectation of what being cared for by a nurse means in terms of their emotional response to the experience. This ideal continues to be wedged against the 21st Century healthcare backdrop, one where the role of the nurse often involves making complex analytical decisions, diagnosing, prescribing, delegating, mentoring, and leading.

The challenge is to make sure that we as nurses don't lose sight of our responsibility to maintain the principles of care in the code *Standards of conduct, performance and ethics for nurses and midwives* (Nursing and Midwifery Council 2008) and treat our patients in a way that allows them to feel cared for even if we only see them once and for a brief moment. We also must make certain through effective mentoring that every newly qualified nurse is instilled with the high standards of compassion and hands on delivery of care that patients deserve.

Being a caring nurse within the context of today's conveyor belt culture which is focussed on getting people in, and then out, of hospital as quickly as possible challenges us to think differently about how we provide care in a way that is individual, therapeutic, culturally sensitive and is centred on the important partnership between the nurse, patient and their loved ones.

Medical advancements such as keyhole surgery mean that recovery periods are much shorter. While this is good for patients and supports the business efficiency requirements that hospitals are under pressure to deliver, the offshoot is that many patients are in and out so quickly that the time available to build that important nurse patient partnership in care has been truncated into the merest moment in time.

Gone are the days when a new mother could expect to remain in hospital for several days, especially if she had other small children at home as this gave her time to rest, recuperate and bond in peace with her new baby. Today, if a woman has had a straightforward, uncomplicated birth, she could give birth in the morning and home with baby in time to do the washing up before bed.

This book will support nurses at any stage in their career to make the most of that time, by making every second count towards ensuring their patients feel they are being cared for in a way that is appropriate to their needs.

Professor Dickon Weir-Hughes
Chief Executive and Registrar, Nursing and
Midwifery Council, United Kingdon

Foreword

Putting the principles of care into practice...

Nurses are trained to deliver care with a dedication, passion, and selflessness that is the hallmark of a profession than spans centuries; from the battlefields of the Crimea to the modern day frontline in A&E. Time and again, I see nursing staff delivering exceptional, inspirational, and remarkable levels of patient care, often in the toughest of circumstances.

However, how do we ensure that in a fast-moving and ever-changing world, good care is delivered to all that need it?

Firstly, the workforce needs to ensure that the essentials of nursing remain constant, while at the same time adopting new practices and embracing the latest developments in care. This can often seem like a difficult, if not impossible, equation to solve.

However, it *can* be done and *is* being done right across the UK. Take, for example, the introduction of tele-health, systems with which patients can monitor their own conditions electronically, without having to leave their home. Despite the addition of this technology, the fundamentals of the care patients receive remain unchanged. If a patient's symptoms mean that they require nursing care, staff are alerted and the patient receives the type of care that they would on a ward. However, the system means that the patient doesn't have to visit hospital unless they need to, allowing them to feel more comfortable and relieving the pressure on frontline services.

Secondly, we must empower nurses to change how they deliver care. Too often, nursing staff feel under-qualified to lead, but the truth is that up and down the country, thousands of them are doing just that. Nearly 60 per cent of Directors of Nursing already have lead responsibility for clinical governance and just over half lead on quality or performance.

It is not just nurses in senior positions that are able to revolutionize the way things work. By improving the training delivered to Healthcare Assistants in Bradford, one nurse-led initiative cut pressure ulcers by around 25 per cent.

Nurses have a unique insight into the delivery of care, from admission to discharge, specialist appointment to home visit—a patient is never far from a member of the nursing team. This enables nursing staff to push the boundaries, bringing about real changes that genuinely improve the patient experience.

In a time of extraordinary challenges, this book provides an important insight into what it means to deliver patient care. From theory to practice, high quality care must be at the heart of all that we do.

Whether this is by improving communication with patients, making advancements in the treatments on offer or meeting their spiritual needs, this book will give you everything you need to consider what excellent care really looks like and how you can put it into practice.

Nursing staff face numerous significant challenges in today's health service; an increasing number of patients, a drive for deep efficiencies and budget cuts and unrelenting attacks on their hard earned employment rights. However, I am in no doubt that if nursing staff are empowered to lead the care they provide, embrace new technology, and given the resources they require, they will continue to go above and beyond for those in need.

I hope you enjoy this excellent book.

Dr Peter Carter
Chief Executive & General Secretary,
Royal College of Nursing

Preface

Nursing has always been synonymous with the concepts of care and caring, which must be safeguarded and celebrated. However, continued media and press reports highlight significant failings in the ability of some nurses to provide safe, compassionate, and dignified care—a fact that cannot be disputed. Yet the reality is that the majority of nurses do provide and want to provide excellent nursing care in what can often be challenging and complex health and social care environments.

Care in Nursing: Principles, Values, and Skills is written with the intention of restoring nurses' and the public's confidence in the ability of nurses to provide care that is safe and of the highest quality. The book has been written by contributors drawn from a wide variety of educational and clinical settings with the sole purpose of reinstating those core nursing principles, values, and skills that seem to have been lost or misplaced in contemporary nursing practice. This textbook has been developed as a resource for students, staff, and managers, to raise awareness of—as well as explore and debate—what is fundamental and crucial to the delivery of safe, compassionate, and dignified care.

The book is structured around five parts, 1. Defining Care, 2. Human Dimensions of Care, 3. Contexts of care, 4. Evaluating Care and 5. The Cost of Care. The chapters within each part introduce the reader to key concepts allowing them to engage with the core principles, values, and skills that are prerequisite to providing high quality nursing care. It is important to emphasise that while the five parts and chapters do stand alone, they are all interconnected incrementally adding to a broader understanding of care. Together, they provide the reader with a deeper knowledge and awareness of the core principles, values and skills that underpin fundamental nursing care, for example, one may be able to define care (Chapter 1) but without caring for oneself (Chapter 2) nurses may be ineffective in their nursing role and duties. Therefore, collectively the book provides the reader with an introduction and comprehensive overview to care in nursing with the purpose of raising awareness of the knowledge and skills required to provide safe, effective and high quality nursing care in ever changing and challenging environments.

Caring and compassion are the bedrocks of nursing and must be the primary components of all care delivery. They can be achieved only if nurses are professional, accountable, knowledgeable, and skilled; adopting appropriate attitudes and behaviours at all times. This book will enable and support nurses working across all fields of nursing to reflect in and on practice, with the aim of enhancing and promoting essential knowledge and skills. This is imperative if the public's trust and the profession's confidence are to be restored and if nurses are, once again, to be recognized as rightful custodians of care and caring.

Wilfred McSherry
Robert McSherry
Roger Watson

Acknowledgements

Artwork acknowledgements

We would like to thank the following for permission to use their artwork in this textbook:

- Figure 2.1, Burnham suggests we can move from problems to possibilities, is the copyright of John Burnham and was first presented at the following conferences:
  - 2009 UK, AFT National Training Conference, Key note plenary presentation, 'Problems and possibilities—resources and restraints';
  - 2011 Australia, Key note speaker at the 30th Australian and New Zealand Family Therapy Association, Sydney 2011, 'Problems and possibilities—resources and restraints';
  - 2011 Singapore, National Council for Social Service: Family Service Centres, Key note speaker at National Conference, *Community Responses to Families in the 21st Century: Methods that Work*, 'Problems and possibilities — resources and restraints';
  - 2011 UK, The Tenth London International Eating Disorders Conference, Plenary speaker, 'Family and relational resilience: Problems and possibilities—resources and restraints', organized by *British Journal of Hospital Medicine* in association with MA Healthcare.

- Figure 5.1, Consider how you perceive this lady: is her disability her defining characteristic?, © iceteastock–Fotolia.com.
- Fig 6.2, Age Standardised mortality rate by NS-SEC: Men aged 25–64 , England and Wales 2001–03, Crown copyright.
- Figure 7.1, Aaron Beck, © Beck Institute for Cognitive Therapy and Research.
- Figure 9.1, Explanatory model of communication in nursing practice, is adapted from Figures 8.1 and 10.4, in C. McCabe and F. Timmins (2006) *Communication Skills for Nursing Practice*, London: Palgrave Macmillan, with permission of Palgrave Macmillan.
- Figure 14.1, The Court Structure of Her Majesty's Courts Service. Crown copyright.
- Figure 16.1, A definition of quality from Lord Darzi's review of the NHS 'High Quality Care for All' (Department of Health, 2008). Crown copyright.

Contents

Detailed contents   xv

About the editors   xxi

About the contributors   xxiii

How to use this book   xxvii

Part 1 Defining care

Chapter 1 So you think you care?   3

Chapter 2 Caring for oneself   16

Chapter 3 Quality of nursing care   33

Chapter 4 Respecting the individual   47

Chapter 5 Diversity in caring   61

Part 2 Human dimensions of care

Chapter 6 Caring for communities   81

Chapter 7 Psychological aspects of caring   96

Chapter 8 Spiritual care   117

Part 3 Contexts of care

Chapter 9 Communicating care   135

Chapter 10 Pathways of care   150

Chapter 11 Partnerships of care   159

Chapter 12 Caring in challenging circumstances   172

Part 4 Evaluating care

Chapter 13 Leading, managing, and celebrating care   191

Chapter 14 When care is absent   207

Chapter 15 Care to complain   219

Chapter 16 So you think you've cared   234

Part 5 The cost of care

Chapter 17 Cost of care and resource allocation   249

Index   259

Detailed contents

About the editors   xxi
About the contributors   xxiii
How to use this book   xxvii

Part 1 Defining care

Chapter 1 So you think you care? *Roger Watson*   3

Introduction   3
Has caring left nursing?   3
Basic care   4
Nursing education   4
What are 'care' and 'caring'?   5
Affective and instrumental aspects of care and caring   6
What makes a suitable nurse?   7
Theoretical perspectives on caring   7
The place of caring in nursing   8
Caring theories   8
Investigating caring   9
Dimensions of caring   10
Students   11
Patients' perceptions of caring   12
What about care assistants?   13
What is caring in nursing?   14

Chapter 2 Caring for oneself *Anthony Schwartz and Barbara Wren*   16

Introduction   16
Why is self-care relevant in health care?   16
The impact of work on nurses' health   17
Elements of self-care, and self-care skills and attributes   18
Pressure, stress, and performance: how to manage them well   20
Stress and performance: theory, rationale, and evidence base   20
Who is responsible for self-care and managing stress at work?   25
Putting it all together: planning your own self-care   27
Focusing on self-care and thought-traps   28
Cognitive-behavioural strategies   29
Physical health aspects   29
Taking it further   29
Developing resilience   30

Chapter 3 Quality of nursing care *Robert McSherry*   33

Introduction   33
Drivers for quality nursing care   34
Defining 'quality nursing care'   34
Quality care systems and processes   38
Measuring and documenting the provision of quality nursing care   43
Highlighting and accessing support in the provision of quality care   44

Chapter 4 Respecting the individual *Milika Ruth Matiti and Lesley Baillie*   47

Introduction   47
Definitions of 'respect' and 'dignity'   47
Respecting individuals in nursing practice   51
The nature and key dimensions of individualized and holistic care   52
Holistic care   54
Models of nursing care   56
Taking it further   57

Chapter 5 Diversity in caring *Aru Narayanasamy and Gavin Narayanasamy*   61

Introduction   61
Theory, research, and evidence base   61
Caring for disabled people   63
Social model of disability   65
Ethnic and cultural diversity   66
Putting diversity and inclusivity in action   68
The ACCESS model   69

Part 2 Human dimensions of care

Chapter 6 Caring for communities *Sue Thornton*   81

Introduction   81
Professional requirements   81
Defining 'communities'   82
The social context of health care   82
The contributions of sociology and social policy   84
Sociology and social change   85
Application to nursing practice   88
Structure and social action   88
Social factors and health   89
Inequalities and health care   91

Chapter 7 **Psychological aspects of caring** *Glenn Marland and Annette Thomson*   96

Introduction   96
Overview of some major psychological approaches   97
Key theories in psychology   97
Behaviourism and beyond   101
Cognitive-behavioural approaches   103
Humanistic psychology   104
The psychology of emotions   105
How do you feel? The 'self' and emotions   106
Coping with pain and stress   109
Dealing with loss   110
Resilience and social support   112
Why do we care?   113

Chapter 8 **Spiritual care** *Wilfred McSherry and Joanna Smith*   117

Introduction   117
'Spirituality' and 'spiritual care' defined   118
What is spirituality?   121
Historical aspects of spirituality   123
Providing holistic and spiritual care   124
Reductionism   125
Integrated care   126
Spiritual needs   126
Challenges to promoting spiritual care   127
Relationship between the personal and professional   128

Part 3 **Contexts of care**

Chapter 9 **Communicating care** *Catherine McCabe and Fiona Timmins*   135

Introduction   135
Theorists and the nature of care and caring   136
Defining caring and communication   137
Theory, rationale, and evidence base   140
Communicating care with patients   143
Taking it further   146

Chapter 10 **Pathways of care** *Sharon D. Bateman and Jane A. Gibson*   150

Introduction   150
'Care pathways' defined   150
The origins of care pathways   152

The benefits of care pathways   153
Evaluation   155

Chapter 11 Partnerships of care *Eleanor Bradley and Tim Lewington*   159

Introduction   159
Partnerships: between the public and the private   159
Partnership working: a 'third way'?   160
Defining 'partnerships of care'   161
Governance of partnerships of care   162
Do care partnerships work for service users and carers?   163
Building better partnerships with service users and carers   165
Making partnerships of care work   167
Developing the evidence base for partnership working   168

Chapter 12 Caring in challenging circumstances *Karen Breese and Helen Hampson*   172

Introduction   172
Working in challenging situations   173
Definition of 'safeguarding'   174
Dementia   177
Communication in difficult circumstances   178
The dying process   181
Bereavement   182
Care of people with a learning disability today   183

Part 4   Evaluating care

Chapter 13 Leading, managing, and celebrating care *Sam Foster*   191

Introduction   191
Recent developments   192
Political and professional drivers   193
Why leadership is important   193
Modern matrons   193
Potential benefit of nurse-led services   199
The *Next Stage Review*   201
Skills for leadership   203

Chapter 14 When care is absent *John Tingle and Jean McHale*   207

Introduction   207
Clinical negligence litigation   209

A just compensation system?   212

Patient safety   216

Chapter 15 Care to complain *Susan Hamer and Steve Page*   219

Introduction   219

Why is learning from complaints important?   219

The benefits of complaints   224

Ensuring a good service to all patients   225

Major inquiries into poor standards of care   226

How can we ensure effective learning and improvement in organizations?   228

Chapter 16 So you think you've cared *Sally Brearley and Peter Griffiths*   234

Introduction   234

What do we mean by 'quality of care'?   235

What do we mean by 'measurement' and 'evaluation'?   237

Theory, rationale, and evidence base   237

Part 5   The cost of care

Chapter 17 Cost of care and resource allocation *Joanne Gray*   249

Introduction   249

The fundamental economic problem in health care   249

Efficiency and resource allocation   251

Contemporary methods for evaluation of efficiency: economic evaluation   252

The National Institute for Health and Clinical Excellence
   (NICE), economic evaluation, and the impact for nursing care   253

Index   259

About the editors

Wilfred McSherry

Wilfred is professor in Dignity of Care for Older People, Centre for Practice and Service Improvement at the Faculty of Health, Staffordshire University, and The Shrewsbury and Telford Hospital NHS Trust UK. He is also a part-time professor at Haraldsplass Deaconess University College, Bergen, Norway. He has a background in nursing sciences and expertise in general adult nursing. His special interest is in core nursing values, with a specific focus upon spirituality, spiritual care, and dignity. He has written several books on spiritual aspects of care and has published in a wide range of journals. Wilfred is a vice president of The British Association for the Study of Spirituality.

Robert McSherry

Rob has recently completed a full-time secondment (March–July 2011) has Deputy Director of Nursing/Professor of Nursing and Practice Development with Mid Staffordshire National Health Service Foundation Trust. Rob also completed a part-time secondment (October 2009–September 2010) with the North East Strategic Health Authority as Senior Nurse Advisor. He was appointed Clinical Associate Professor with the Australian Catholic University, Brisbane Australia (March 2007–March 2010). Rob's work has focused on promoting patient safety, people-centred care, and quality nursing, and his main aim is seeing research being used at a front-line clinical level, at which nurses and other health professionals are equipped with the essential skills and knowledge to aid with the delivery of evidence-based practice. Rob has shared and disseminated his work around practice development, healthcare governance, and evidence-informed practice internationally through publications, conferences, consultancy, and workshops.

Roger Watson FRCN FAAN

Roger is professor of Nursing, University of Western Sydney. He has a background in biological sciences and in nursing older people. His special interest is the assessment of feeding difficulty in older people with dementia. He has written several books on biology in nursing and has published in a wide range of journals. Roger Watson is editor-in-chief of the *Journal of Advanced Nursing,* and holds several visiting positions in China and Australia.

About the contributors

Lesley Baillie

Lesley is a reader in the Faculty of Health and Social Sciences at the University of Bedfordshire. She has conducted research about dignity of patients and has published widely in this area. She edits the textbook *Developing Practical Adult Nursing Skills*, published in its third edition in 2009, which emphasizes a caring approach to nursing practice. Her edited book *Dignity in Healthcare: A Practical Approach for Nurses and Midwives* (with Milika Matiti) was published in March 2011.

Sharon D. Bateman

Sharon is clinical matron wound care, with the Healthcare Governance Directorate, South Tees Hospitals NHS Foundation Trust, The James Cook University Hospital, Middlesbrough. Sharon has extensive clinical medical skills and knowledge that are applied across all specialities within a large regional teaching environment. She has worked in wound care for three years, setting up a trust wound care service that includes clinical review and education programmes for all disciplines, and has a large corporate agenda. Sharon has published in various wound care journals and poster presentations for local, national, and European conferences. Her research has explored the patient experience in chronic wound care.

Eleanor Bradley

Eleanor is currently employed in a joint post as professor of mental healthcare research and evaluation and director of the Centre for Practice and Service Improvement, Faculty of Health, Staffordshire University, and as head of research and development at South Staffordshire and Shropshire Healthcare NHS Foundation Trust. She is a chartered health psychologist. Eleanor has conducted a large body of research in the area of advanced nursing roles, focusing in particular on non-medical prescribing, which culminated in the publication in 2008 of the edited *Non-Medical Prescribing* (with Peter Nolan). More recently, she has conducted a number of research and evaluation projects focused on practice and service developments in acute mental health care, including projects that look at the role and uptake of service user involvement.

Sally Brearley

Sally is visiting senior research fellow in patient and public involvement at the National Nursing Research Unit, King's College London. She is also a lay member on the NHS National Quality Board.

Karen Breese

Karen is a team leader with the Shropshire Community Learning Disability Service, South Staffordshire & Shropshire Healthcare NHS Foundation Trust.

Sam Foster

Sam is deputy chief nurse at the Heart of England NHS Foundation Trust. Her background is in critical care nursing, and she has a particular interest in nursing leadership, and also in patient experience and fundamental care.

Jane A. Gibson

Jane is a specialist nurse in HIV viral hepatitis. Jane has extensive experience both clinically and academically of the patient remit of blood-borne viruses; she also has an active role in both audit and research within this arena. Jane has a keen interest and is an active participant in Garna initiatives, undertaking a fifth term. She has recently carried out research in the arena of global health and hepatitis B. Jane is hoping to achieve nurse consultant status in the short term and to expand service provision.

Joanne Gray

Joanne is an academic at the School of Health and Social Care, University of Teesside.

Peter Griffiths

Peter is professor of health services research at the University of Southampton. He is also executive editor of the International Journal of Nursing Studies.

Susan Hamer

Susan is a nurse at the University of Leeds, where she is director of enterprise and knowledge transfer for the Faculty of Medicine and Health. Susan's current work promotes knowledge transfer and innovation activities. She is an experienced researcher, who enjoys working at the interface between theory and practice. As a practitioner, Susan currently works in the field of health informatics and develops leadership capacity in organizations. Susan has published widely and is the co-author of two books: *Achieving Evidence-Based Practice* and *Leadership and Management: A Three-Dimensional Approach*. She is a fellow of the Queens Nursing Institute.

Helen Hampson

Helen is adult protection lead at the Shrewsbury and Telford Hospital NHS Trust.

Tim Lewington

Tim is currently employed as a research associate at the South Staffordshire and Shropshire Healthcare NHS Foundation Trust. He completed his graduate work in the USA in economic geography, and has experience of NHS mental health care as both a patient and a service user. Tim contributes to ongoing service evaluation projects and facilitates broader service user involvement in research and development activities.

Glenn Marland

Glenn has a mental health nursing background and is Senior Lecturer and Vice Chair Mental Health Subject Development Group, University of the West of Scotland, University Campus Dumfries.

Milika Ruth Matiti

Milika is a lecturer in the Faculty of Medicine and Health Sciences, School of Nursing, Midwifery and Physiotherapy (Boston Centre) at the University of Nottingham. She has a particular interest in dignity and diversity issues, and has carried out research on patient dignity and diversity. Milika's focus now is on dignity education. She has worked and continues to work with clinical practice to develop practice on dignity issues. She has published in peer-reviewed journals and acts as a reviewer for a number of international journals. Milika also co-edited the 2011 book *Dignity in Healthcare: A Practical Approach for Nurses and Midwives* (with Lesley Baillie). Milika has presented at conferences nationally and internationally.

Catherine McCabe

Catherine is an assistant professor in the School of Nursing and Midwifery, Trinity College Dublin. Her research interests include the use of technology to communicate and improve care, and action research to encourage and support collaborative interdisciplinary practice in achieving high standards of care. She has published widely on issues such as communication and quality of life, and is a reviewer for several peer-reviewed journals.

Jean McHale

Jean is professor of health care law and director of the Centre for Health Law, Science and Policy, Birmingham Law School, University of Birmingham. She is the author of monographs, textbooks, and edited collections in the area of healthcare law, including *Law and Nursing* (3rd edn, 2007, with John Tingle), *Health Law and the EU* (2004, with Tamara Hervey), and *Nursing and Human Rights* (2004, with Ann Gallagher).

Aru Narayanasamy

Aru is associate professor in diversity and spiritual health in the School of Nursing, Midwifery and Physiotherapy, University of Nottingham. In 2008, he was awarded the prestigious National Teaching Fellowship by the UK Higher Education Academy for his outstanding work on spirituality and diversity. His pioneering research in learning and teaching culminated in teaching innovations such as the ASSET (Actioning Spirituality and Spiritual Care Education and Training) and ACCESS (Transcultural) models.

Gavin Narayanasamy

Gavin is a sociologist with an academic background in the sociology of diversity, ethnicity, and social justice. He is undertaking voluntary work as a research assistant at the Ethnicity, Diversity and Spirituality (EDS) Hub of the University of Nottingham. His research interest is in the lived experiences of people with autistic spectrum disorder (ASD). Gavin has co-authored several book chapters.

Steve Page

Steve is the nurse on the Board of Yorkshire Ambulance Service NHS Trust, where he is Executive Director of Standards and Compliance. In his current work, he is responsible for leadership of quality, governance, and risk management issues. This work includes a specific focus on the quality of service user experience. Prior to his current role, Steve worked as a senior nurse in a number of acute hospitals in the north of England and, most recently, as deputy director of nursing at the North East Strategic Health Authority.

Anthony Schwartz

Anthony is a Consultant Psychologist working within the NHS and independently in the field of Corporate Health Psychology Consultancy. Registered as both a Clinical Psychologist and a Health Psychologist, he is a visiting Professor at Staffordshire University (Centre for Practice and Service Improvement). His special interest and experience is in clinical input, consultancy work, coaching, training, and professional development. He is involved in the supervision of allied health professionals, and delivering a wide range of training to nurses, directors, managers and medical consultants. His work focuses on enhancing well-being and performance at work through coaching and the use of Mindfulness as well as helping teams to cope with pressure, conflict, or troubled communications.

Joanna Smith

Joanna has over 15 years experience nursing children with complex needs including neurological conditions and has worked in higher education for 12 years. Joanna is now able to combine her clinical experiences with undergraduate and postgraduate nurse education and research. Although she has used a range of research methods, both quantitative and qualitative, she is particularly skilled in the application of thematic analysis and framework approach. Joanna is a member of the Centre for Nursing and Midwifery Research, and is developing a programme of research that is focussing parent-professional engagement and collaboration in the context of children with long-term conditions, in particular neurological conditions, as part of the Children, Young People and Families (CYP@Salford) research programme. Joanna has written several nursing chapters relating to neurological conditions in children and children's surgery, and assesses articles for a range of peer-review journals.

Annette Thomson

Annette is a lecturer in psychology and sociology at the University of the West of Scotland. She has wide interests in the areas of social and developmental psychology, and has recently published a book on Erich Fromm as part of the Palgrave Macmillan Mindshapers series.

Sue Thornton

Sue is a senior lecturer in the Faculty of Health at Staffordshire University. She has a clinical background in the care of the older person and current teaching responsibilities within the professional nursing practice modules of the pre-qualifying nursing curriculum. She also has extensive teaching experience in the social science disciplines at both pre-qualifying and post-qualifying levels. Sue's areas of special interest relate to issues of diversity, discrimination, and empowerment, with specific reference to the older individual.

Fiona Timmins

Fiona is an associate professor in the School of Nursing and Midwifery, Trinity College Dublin. She has more than sixty publications in peer-reviewed journals and has written and co-authored six nursing text books. Fiona has delivered more than sixty international conference presentations. She is a reviewer for several peer-reviewed journals and sits on several editorial boards. Research interests include professional nursing issues, nurse education, spirituality, and reflection.

John Tingle

John is a reader in health law at the Nottingham Law School, Nottingham Trent University, UK. John teaches the clinical negligence and clinical risk management components in the Nottingham Law School's LLM Health Law Programme, launched in 2001. John also teaches tort and medical law on the LLB. He developed and now directs all of the Law School International Summer School programmes and is part of the Law School Internationalisation, Strategy and Business Development team. John is joint editor of a fortnightly law and nursing series in the *British Journal of Nursing*. His current research interests include the legal aspects of risk management, clinical governance, and patient safety, and he has also widely researched the area of the expanded role of the nurse.

Barbara Wren

Barbara is Consultant Lead Psychologist in Health and Work at the Royal Free Hampstead NHS Trust in London where she established the first in-house occupational health psychology service for staff in the UK. The service provides therapy, consultancy and coaching, team and organizational interventions. In this role she led on the successful implementation of Schwartz Rounds for all hospital staff. The Royal Free was one of the first two UK pilot sites. She has also worked for the Kings Fund as a Consultant on staff experience and supporting the UK roll-out of Schwartz Rounds. She is a founder member and the chair of the UK National Network of Practitioner Occupational Health Psychologists and has worked nationally and internationally to develop theory and practice in this area.

How to use this book

Care in Nursing is designed specifically to help readers debate what caring really means, explore ideas, principles and research in care as well as examine how high quality care can best be delivered. This brief tour of the book shows you how to get the best out of the following features:

Essential knowledge and skills for care

- You will deliver safe, confident, competent, compassionate quality care, whilst maintaining dignity and respect of people at all times.
- You must ensure individualized, personalized, people-centred care by engaging with individuals and empowering them to make informed decisions and choices.

Essential knowledge and skills for care box

In each chapter a box identifies the core knowledge and skills that nurses require to deliver care. These boxes are mapped against the NMC standards for pre-registration 2010 in the United Kingdom and reflect the aims of nursing degrees in other countries.

Stop and consider

Throughout the book readers are encouraged to consider issues in light of their own experience, values, and beliefs.

How do nurses provide holistic care in practice?
Reflect on a recent practice learning experience; what care was given to meet physical, psychological, social, and spiritual needs? Focus on one particular patient in whose care you were involved and identify

---

PRACTICE EXAMPLE 12.3

Communication in difficult circumstances

James is a 25-year-old man living with his parents and two younger siblings. James was born deaf and uses British sign language, Makaton, and gesture to make

Practice Example

Care is at the heart of all nursing practice so it is essential to explore the theory, principles, and skills of care in light of real world nursing practice. These boxes put ideas into context and relate them to everyday practice.

Practical tips

Practice tip boxes outline clear helpful strategies to ensure patients receive sound care and to help nurses meet the challenges of practice.

PRACTICE TIP

- Take a step back and look at what is happening with a fresh set of eyes. Try to imagine yourself as someone different, such as a patient, relative, or new employee.
- Just sit and watch: what is *really* happening?

Part 1: Defining care

1 So you think you care?

ROGER WATSON

Learning outcomes

This chapter will enable you to:

- understand that there are different definitions of 'care' and 'caring';
- understand that caring has affective and instrumental dimensions;
- appreciate the arguments over whether nurses should be trained or educated to care;
- identify some of the key theorists in the field of caring in nursing; and
- reflect on your own values and practice in relation to care and caring outcomes.

Introduction

The purpose of this book is to explore the concept of care—principally in nursing—and to return it to the centre of nursing where, most would agree, it belongs. The problem with returning care to the centre of nursing is made difficult, however, by the assumption that it has left the centre of nursing. And even if it remains at the heart of nursing, just exactly what *is* it? The terms 'care' and 'nursing' are, if not the same, at least close, but the term 'care' is used frequently in everyday use to express a wide variety of emotions, actions, and attachments. And, surely, nurses are not the only ones who care: parents care for their children and for each other; lovers care; friends care; and even organizations claim to care. The issue is complex and definitely worth exploring—so let's begin.

Has caring left nursing?

The initial conversations that took place between the editors of this book were based on the premise that nursing was 'losing its grip' on *caring*. With a focus on the UK, where the editors and authors of this book work, recent years have seen many scandals associated with nursing care; the individual stories are heartrending, infuriating, and embarrassing to those of us in the profession (The Patients Association, 2009). Without meaning to be facile, but to avoid repetition and reporting of what can easily be read almost any day of the week in national newspapers, the stories all have a common theme: neglect verging on abuse. The stories have familiar details and usually involve lack of food, prolonged contact with excreta, and actual physical harm, such as pressure sores or falls.

Essential knowledge and skills for care

- The practice of nursing care must be holistic and non-judgemental, and the nurse must demonstrate attitudes and behaviours that are caring, compassionate, and sensitive to the needs of the individual.

- The nurse, when providing care, must avoid making unnecessary assumptions, supporting individuals by recognizing and respecting individual choice, and acknowledging diversity.

- All nurses must use therapeutic principles to engage, maintain, and (where appropriate) disengage from professional caring relationships, and must always respect professional boundaries.

Frequent reports have emerged from government organizations and charities cataloguing the poor care that people—mainly older people—have received in hospitals and homes where nursing care is part of the provision (Social Care Institute for Excellence, 2009; The Patients Association, 2009). This is followed by copious opinion in the press from columnists and the general public exemplifying further such poor care and, inevitably, blaming nurses and the preparation of nurses, and reflecting on 'better days' when only good care was administered and nurses were 'paradigms of virtue'. This last view has been challenged (McKenna et al., 2006) as being viewed through the lenses of 'rose-tinted spectacles'. There is frank public and political prejudice against university-educated nurses, and while it can be joked that they are 'too posh to wash', the unspoken agenda is one that begins with the view that a university education is not necessary for nurses and ends with the view that, in fact, a university education for nurses is a bad thing, because it detracts from caring; nurses should only be *trained*. Therefore, depending on who has the government ear at the time or on what the latest scandals are, nursing is perpetually a political football, while nurse education becomes a ping-pong ball being perpetually batted back and forth between the education and training camps. Nevertheless, a major challenge for nursing remains: to be able to identify, define, and describe what 'care' or 'caring' in nursing is. Failing that, we will only ever be able to recognize when care or caring is *not* present; this is perplexing for those of us with an interest in care in nursing, because it suggests, perhaps, that caring is simply an absence of something—that is, neglect and abuse.

Basic care

The issue, however, seems to be emphasized in the reporting of such incidents of poor care because, almost inevitably, the failure seems to have been in a lack of 'basic care' (**http://news.bbc.co.uk/1/hi/8223710. stm** [accessed 15 June 2011]) and the solution seems to lie in the application of such 'basic care'. It is not merely playing with words to express the need for an alternative expression to 'basic care' and many of us

often ask for this to be described as 'essential care'. There are several problems with the expression 'basic care': it relegates care that should be seen as essential to being basic, despite the fact that one of the synonyms of 'basic' is 'essential'; others include 'fundamental', 'vital', and 'crucial'. Nevertheless, these synonyms are rarely, if ever, used—especially by the press—and we seem stuck with 'basic'. The implication of 'basic' is that it is easy and that anyone can do it. However, clearly, it is not easy: if it were, then it would not be overlooked. And even if anyone *can* do it, often nobody does: it remains overlooked, undermined, and low priority—often with fatal consequences.

Nursing education

Usually held up to the public as 'angels' by the press (**http://www.nursesareangels.com/** [accessed 15 June 2011]), nurses quickly become 'demons' when anything goes wrong, and the analysis—a topic to be picked up below—usually leads to the current mode of delivery and content of nursing education programmes. The mode is university and there is a view that the content is 'stuffing their heads' with useless—even damaging—subjects such as psychology and sociology (**http://www.truthaboutnursing. org/news/2009/nov/15_marrin.html** [accessed 15 June 2011]). There is a view that nurses are no longer learning to care and that they do not spend enough time in clinical practice—in other words, that nurses no longer know how to administer 'basic care'.

History of nursing education

If we trace the history of policy regarding nursing education since the 1970s in the UK, we see the beginnings of a move away from the old apprenticeship style of training towards an educational model being urged in the Briggs Report (1972). However, the recommendations of the Briggs Report were slow to be taken up and it was not really until the end of the 1980s that we saw the inception of Project 2000 (UKCC, 1986), which clearly moved the preparation of nurses into the educational camp and away from the training camp, with an emphasis on generic theory in the first half (18 months) of the programme followed by specialization into four branches: adult; mental health; children; and learning disability. However, while research into the effectiveness of Project 2000 was ambiguous about its efficacy in the preparation of nurses, publicity was negative; the government, as usual, reacted to the publicity and ignored the research, bringing in, at the end of the 1990s, *Making a Difference* (Department of Health, 1999), which moved the preparation of nurses fully back into the training camp—albeit in universities.

What is not answered in all of this is what exactly the best way *is* to produce a caring nurse. The answer must lie somewhere amongst the following:

- 'caring cannot be taught, it is innate';
- 'caring cannot be taught, but can be learned';
- 'caring can be taught and learned'; or
- some combination of all of the above.

Again, the implications for nursing education are clear: if caring cannot be learned and is innate, then nursing education is a complete waste of time (as is much of training). The key step lies, therefore, in the selection process: there is something that can be gauged about people before they come into nursing and that something is not related to educational qualifications (beyond a bare minimum whereby the ability to count and communicate are demonstrated). This 'something' can be seen only prior to training in an interview and thereafter observed in practice. This extreme view is not far from the present situation in UK nursing whereby the government insist that all candidates for nurse education programmes are interviewed and that the interviews must include National Health Service (NHS) staff. The premise is that it is possible to select a 'good nurse' (definition lacking!) if you can see him or her and speak to him or her. The educational aspect plays some part, but is not, of itself, sufficient. Nursing is not alone in this: medicine routinely interviews candidates in an effort to select people from a pool, all of whom have top educational grades before being invited for interview; similarly, Oxford and Cambridge universities interview candidates for precisely the same reason—demand for places is huge and the pool comprises the highest qualified school leavers in the UK.

Selecting candidates for nursing education

However, this is most certainly not the case in nursing and the author has first-hand evidence of candidates who are more than adequately qualified for the job being turned down for entry, while people with lower qualifications were admitted to a nursing programme. Just exactly what was going on in the interviewers' minds? What was it that they were looking for, and what did they think they could find that would make someone make, in the first instance, a good nursing student and, ultimately, a good nurse? The author has been party to the questions that candidates are asked at interview and they are neither challenging nor probing—but at least they get the candidate talking and provide something for the prejudices of the interview panel to work on.

Clearly, those of us in employment and seeking further employment expect to be interviewed, but in such cases, we are expected to demonstrate what we have learned in our previous job(s) and how we fit the very precise criteria of the advertised position. This is not the case with entry to nursing: while an increasing number of candidates will have had previous life experience, some will not; some will be school leavers and may not have done anything relevant to nursing. And unlike applying for a job, we do not have clear criteria for what a nursing student should be like and what the nurse that is produced should be like—so, again, what is the point in interviewing? Ironically, at precisely the same time as the UK introduced interviewing for selection, Ireland abandoned it on the basis that there was no evidence that it was an effective way of selecting nursing students.

What are 'care' and 'caring'?

The various meanings of 'caring' have been covered elsewhere. Nevertheless, it is probably worth spending a short time looking at the meanings of 'care' and 'caring'. Clearly, the two words are related, but it is their common and widespread use—without much thought being given to their meaning—that leads to problems. Care is apparently an entity, a noun, something that purports to exist and, as we have already seen, it may be more evident by its absence than its presence.

As a *noun*, 'care' can denote attention or protection (**http://dictionary.cambridge.org/results.asp?searchword=care&x=35&y=7** [accessed 15 June 2011]). It also means giving someone attention or providing treatment—which is possibly related to nursing; indeed, we also refer to 'medical care'.

Care is also a *verb*, as in the act of providing attention to someone or providing treatment: 'I care for him' (that is, 'I am providing care for him', in which care is now a noun). However, in this usage the meaning can become confused between providing care for someone and saying that you care about them or worry about them (**http://dictionary.cambridge.org/results.asp?searchword=care&x=35&y=7** [accessed 15 June 2011]). Care for someone usually denotes something instrumental (that is, doing something, such as looking after an older relative or parent), whereas if you care about someone, while that might be expressed instrumentally, it does not necessarily have to be, because you can care about someone—which is an emotional reaction—without being the person providing care: you can care about someone from a great distance.

Caring also shows this confusion between being different types of word. It too can be a noun denoting what people do or feel: what a mother provides for a newborn is caring. However, caring is also used as a verb in the sense that someone is looking after someone else (in whatever sense) and also, possibly most relevant to this chapter, caring is used as an adjective—that is, 'you are a caring person' (**http://dictionary.cambridge.org/results.asp?searchword=caring** [accessed 15 June 2011]).

Affective and instrumental aspects of care and caring

Therefore, with reference to nursing, it appears that we administer an entity called 'nursing care' (that is, a noun) and that we are caring for someone (that is, a

Table 1.1 Caring attributes and abilities

	Good affective care	Bad affective care
Instrumentally good care	A	B
Instrumentally poor care	C	D

verb) in the process, and that we should be described as 'caring' people (that is, an adjective). Hopefully, the complications have been minimized here, but it is important to consider this, because it is crucial to distinguish between the instrumental (that is, what is done in the process of caring for someone) and the affective (the demeanour or attitude of the person—the nurse) when that care is being delivered.

Moreover, we notice the absence of care/caring when things go wrong and we immediately ascribe this to a lack of care in the person not providing sufficient care—that is, he or she is not a caring person. But is this true and does it matter? **Table 1.1** shows four possible combinations of instrumental and affective caring. For example, in A, a nurse administers excellent care to a patient and also is well disposed towards the patient—that is, cares about the patient—and this would be considered to be an example of where care is present. In D, a nurse does not care about the patient and administers very poor care, and this would not be considered to be good care. However, what about B, in which a nurse does not care about a patient—and possibly shows it—but administers excellent care to the patient: is this good care? How different is the outcome for the patient if his or her needs are met and no harm comes to him or her? Finally, in C, a nurse does care about the patient, but is technically incompetent and administers bad care: would this be considered to be good care?

Education or training?

Is the above important? The answer is 'possibly': some nursing theorists see care in nursing as being largely, if not wholly, affective or consider that it is impossible to administer good nursing care without the affective dimensions. Therefore, while the outcome of care is not irrelevant, the process is of prime importance and they would consider that good care cannot be administered without the nurses caring about the patient. On the other hand, if we see the outcome of care as dominating the interaction between nurses and patients, we minimize and possibly eliminate the necessity of any particular qualities in those who nurse and obviate the need for anything other than training in a set of skills for those who wish to become nurses. This does matter—fundamentally—because the resolution to this dilemma surely dictates the philosophy that frames nursing education and the place of nurses and nursing in the delivery of health care.

Some theories about care and caring in nursing will be reviewed below.

What makes a suitable nurse?

Before reading this section, try the following activity.

What makes a caring nurse?
Can you list the attributes that you think make a caring nurse?

There is a continuing tension that is evident in the delivery of nursing education in the UK both at pre-registration and post-registration levels. This tension was evident at the inception of British nurse education—the model mostly adopted across the world—when Florence Nightingale made it clear that nursing—which was assumed to be a female profession—was for a particular type of woman: middle class (Woodham Smith, 1951). Nightingale was, however, referring to the type of woman who should enter nursing and not what entering nurse training would make her become. Clearly, in addition to this affective aspect, a great deal of skill had to be taught and learned. Nevertheless, the view promulgated by Nightingale emphasized the type of person that a nurse should be. At the other end of the spectrum, if we deny the affective aspects of nursing, we consider that anyone can do the job—that there are

no attributes by which a nurse can be described, defined, and recognized. This is a perfectly reasonable view: it is a utilitarian one, whereby the end amply justifies the means; the question is whether or not it works. As already stated, it is unlikely that either extreme is represented to the full in modern nursing education or that either extreme is useful, but the extremes do seem to dictate policy—especially with regard to nursing education, a topic to which we will return below.

Theoretical perspectives on caring

Theories of caring have a history of some thirty years and the majority of writing in this area stems, with some exceptions, from North America. It is interesting to note that while 'caring' and 'nursing' currently seem almost the same—especially in North America—a review of nursing education by Olson (1993), in which nursing training programme documents from 1915–37 were reviewed, showed that the terms 'caring' and nursing care' were completely absent. It is hard to see precisely where and when 'care' and 'caring' as concepts found their place in the lexicon of nursing. However, a frequently cited work entitled *On Caring* (Mayeroff, 1971) is considered to be seminal in theorizing about the concept of caring. Mayeroff was not a nurse and his treatise was about human caring such as that between friends, and by parents for children. Mayeroff's conception of caring was largely affective as opposed to instrumental, because he viewed the ingredients of caring as including:

● knowing;
● patience;
● honesty;
● trust;
● humility;
● hope; and
● courage.

There was therefore nothing in Mayeroff's conception of caring that indicated anything that should or could be done for another; rather it encapsulated a philosophy on life and relationships between people. Nevertheless, Mayeroff's work has been highly influential and frequently referred to in the nursing literature on caring.

The place of caring in nursing

Since Mayeroff's work and its adoption by nursing, there have been debates about the place of caring in nursing and, indeed, whether it has any place in nursing. A key nursing theorist of the last century was Benner: writing with Wrubel (1986), she cast doubt not on the place of caring in nursing, but on its uniqueness within nursing. However, Leininger (1981), a leading proponent of the study of caring in nursing, views caring as being a unique concept in nursing and we will return to her theories below. Alternatively, Phillips (1993) considers that the focus on caring in nursing actually hampers the development of nursing, because it is unnecessary to speak of 'nursing' and 'caring': they are synonymous. Furthermore, Roper (cited in Kyle, 1995) believes that the use of the term 'caring' within nursing actually detracts from nursing: caring may be part of nursing, but it does not represent everything about nursing.

Caring theories

One very useful view on caring was provided by Morse et al. (1990; 1991) who, drawing on several sources, considered that caring could be conceptualized in five different ways (see **Box 1.1**). With reference to the material preceding this section, it can be seen that the affective and instrumental aspects of caring are included in (iii) and (v), respectively. However, a humanistic and moral dimension, similar to Mayeroff's (1971) conception, is included here. Taking Morse's classification, the issue for nursing is whether any or all of the traits apply to what we call 'caring' in nursing and other nurse theorists have different views on this.

Box 1.1 Caring traits (Morse et al., 1990; 1991)

(i)   Caring can be seen as a human trait—that is, as something that is naturally part of the human condition.

(ii) Caring can be considered a moral imperative—that is, as a fundamental value or virtue.

(iii) Caring can be seen as an affect—that is, as extending oneself towards one's patients beyond one's job description.

(iv) Caring can be viewed as interpersonal interaction—that is, as something that exists between one person and another.

(v)   Caring can be seen to be therapeutic intervention—that is, something that is deliberately planned with a goal in mind.

Jean Watson

At one end of the spectrum between the affective and the instrumental lie the theories of Watson (1988), who considers caring to be unique 'in' nursing. It is noteworthy that none of the nursing care theorists consider caring to be unique 'to' nursing. Watson, who believes that caring cannot simply be reduced to behavioural tasks and that, to care adequately, nursing '*entails a commitment to caring as a moral ideal directed towards the preservation of humanity*'. This is a lofty aspiration for individuals who enter nursing and how applicable it is to everyday nursing is questionable: whether it can guide what nurses actually do for individual patients is doubtful and it probably does not distinguish nursing from any other caring profession. The problem in envisaging the utility of Watson's theory of caring to 'everyday' nursing is further compounded by the language that she uses to describe her ten 'carative' factors, including '*humanistic-altruistic system of values*' and '*existential-phenomenological-spiritual forces*'; such concepts are hard to explain and understand, on their own, without attempting to integrate them into nursing practice. However, it can be seen that Watson is attempting to see what is unique about caring in nursing and her use of the term 'carative' is an attempt to distinguish the caring role of the nurse from, presumably, the *curative* role of the doctor. Such efforts tend to polarize the debate about caring, and possibly even detract from the undoubtedly 'curative' aspects of the caring actions of nurses and the fact that doctors are unlikely to admit to not caring about their patients—either affectively or instrumentally.

Madeleine Leininger

Leininger (1981) probably lies more towards the affective end of the caring theory spectrum. Nevertheless, she believes that some aspects of caring are behavioural tasks and she distinguishes between lay caring, which she describes as '*supportive, facilitative acts towards one another*', from professional nursing care, which she describes as '*cognitively learned humanistic and scientific modes of helping or enabling an individual*'. Both of Leininger's definitions incorporate helping another person—but whether that is by physically doing something for them or by affect, being close to and supporting them psychologically, is not clear. What Leininger does, in her definition of professional nursing care, is introduce two key concepts—education and evidence— by the use of the phrases 'cognitively learned' and 'scientific modes'. In other words, to be caring within nursing involves deliberation in terms of learning what is required to do the job—over and above lay caring—and also the application of methods of caring that are shown to work. Moreover, Leininger's (1981) taxonomy of caring constructs includes specific caring actions such as 'comforting' and 'touching', which are clearly instrumental.

Other theorists

There are many other theories on care and caring, but other key theorists from the same era as Watson and Leininger include Gaut (1983; 1986), who, while not ascribing any uniqueness to caring in nursing, does propose that caring can be reduced to behavioural tasks. Within her work, Gaut tries to exemplify caring situations in which care is being exhibited by nurses. A further layer of complexity in the field of caring theory is the outcome in terms of whom caring affects. It may seem obvious that care affects the patient, and Leininger and Gaut subscribe to that view. Watson believes that caring affects both the patient and the nurse, and this seems credible. However, Forrest (1989) proposes that the caring affects only the nurse—but exactly how is not clear; if this is true, then the question 'what is the point?' is surely raised. Nevertheless, nursing research and specific research into caring in nursing have largely failed to define 'caring' in nursing: without definition, it defies description and identification; without either, it defies measurement. Forrest's view may seem extreme or even illogical, but if there is no way in which to measure care—good or bad—it is surely impossible to see its effect on a patient. Nevertheless, our inability to measure care and caring has not prevented nurse researchers and others from trying to measure it; the following section looks at research into caring—primarily research that has tried to quantify it.

Investigating caring

The varied theoretical perspectives on caring ranging from the affective and existential to the instrumental view on caring are reflected in the range of research methods, from qualitative (that is, finding out what people think and observing what they do) to quantitative (that is, measuring opinions and behaviours) that are applied. Watson (1988) considers qualitative methods to be 'optimal' in the study of caring, and these methods have been usefully applied to identify the dimension of caring and what nurses and patients consider to be good care. In terms of quantitative research, a plethora of questionnaires and inventories have been developed—too many to review in detail here. However, these have been usefully reviewed and gathered in a textbook by Watson (2009) and include the 'Caring Dimensions Inventory' (Watson and Lea, 1997), the 'Caring Behaviours Inventory' (Wolf, 1986) and the 'Care-Q' (Larson and Larson, 1984). If the aim of qualitative research into caring is to investigate what people perceive as constituting caring, the aim of quantitative research is to enable numbers to be ascribed to these perceptions and for comparisons to be made between, for example, nurses and patients, to investigate whether perceptions of caring change over time, and to quantify what people consider to be 'good' care and 'bad' care.

Research into caring indicates that, amongst other things, caring is multidimensional, and that nurses and patients hold different views of caring. This knowledge is helpful in understanding our own approach to caring and its application to patients.

Dimensions of caring

There appear to be two main dimensions to caring, which can be described as being 'psychosocial' and 'professional and technical' (Watson and Lea, 1997; Watson et al., 1998). Such labels are never perfect, but the psychosocial dimensions of caring include the more affective dimensions of caring such as 'being with' and 'listening to' a patient. The technical and professional dimension includes such obvious instrumental aspects of nursing as 'measuring vital signs', but the professional aspects that are not directly involved with doing something for, to, or with a patient seem to be inseparable from the instrumental aspects, and these include 'making records of patient care' and 'reporting to senior nurses/doctors'. Clearly, both of these dimensions are important and while it is possible to see a tendency towards one or other of these dimensions in individuals, both are present.

Some items from the Caring Dimensions Inventory are given in **Box 1.2**; you might like to think how

Box 1.2 Caring Dimensions Inventory (Watson and Lea, 1997)

Stem question: Do you consider the following aspects of nursing practice to be caring?

Response on five-point Likert scale:

Strongly agree 1_____2_____3_____4_____5 Strongly disagree

Circle the number that corresponds to your perception of the intervention as caring.

1 Assisting a patient with an activity of daily living (washing, dressing, etc.)

Strongly agree 1_____2_____3_____4_____5 Strongly disagree

2 Making a nursing record about the patient

Strongly agree 1_____2_____3_____4_____5 Strongly disagree

3 Feeling sorry for a patient

Strongly agree 1_____2_____3_____4_____5 Strongly disagree

4 Getting to know the patient as a person

Strongly agree 1_____2_____3_____4_____5 Strongly disagree

5 Explaining a clinical procedure to a patient

Strongly agree 1_____2_____3_____4_____5 Strongly disagree

6 Being neatly dressed when working with a patient

Strongly agree 1_____2_____3_____4_____5 Strongly disagree

7 Sitting with a patient

Strongly agree 1_____2_____3_____4_____5 Strongly disagree

8 Exploring a patient's lifestyle

Strongly agree 1_____2_____3_____4_____5 Strongly disagree

9 Reporting a patient's condition to a senior nurse

Strongly agree 1_____2_____3_____4_____5 Strongly disagree

10 Being with a patient during a clinical procedure

Strongly agree 1_____2_____3_____4_____5 Strongly disagree

11 Being honest with a patient

Strongly agree 1_____2_____3_____4_____5 Strongly disagree

12 Organizing the work of others for a patient

Strongly agree 1_____2_____3_____4_____5 Strongly disagree

you would respond to these questions and how you perceive caring.

What is apparent is that different types of nurse—by age, speciality, or gender—tend to adopt one dimension more than the other. For example, surgical nurses tend more towards the technical and professional dimension of nursing than do medical nurses; older nurses, likewise, tend more towards the technical and professional dimension of nursing than do younger nurses; and, according to the same strand of research, women tend more towards the technical and professional dimension of nursing than do men—but this last point is not upheld by all researchers. It is not possible to say whether adopting one or other of the above dimensions of nursing is an individual trait or if nurses become socialized (a process whereby people behave more like those around them in order to be accepted by them) after working in one particular area of nursing.

What do the scores mean?

It should be noted that scoring more highly on either technical or psychosocial aspects of caring is not a judgement on a nurse, nor is it clear that one type of caring is better than another. Remember: there is no consensus on whether or not the affective or the instrumental aspects of caring are most important in nursing and, presumably, some combination of both is required.

Nurses also seem to be able to identify what they perceive as being self-giving aspects of care, some appropriate and some inappropriate (Watson et al., 1998). It is interesting to note, for example, that nurses nearly always say that it is inappropriate to keep in contact with a patient after discharge and to work long hours to finish a job. One of these could be deemed unprofessional and the other dangerous. Also, nurses are ambiguous about 'feeling sorry for a patient' and this could seem to be in conflict with the view of the public or the lay view of caring, which, if it is at least partly affective, should involve feeling sorry for a patient. However, in professional terms, this could be deemed to be an unnecessary emotional involvement and one that is irrelevant to the delivery of good nursing care; it takes us back to the point earlier about caring *about* and caring *for*. There is an irony here in that not caring about someone emotionally may be a necessary prerequisite to caring for them in a professional sense: it does not involve being negative or wishing harm, but it does involve a degree of distance that enables the nurse to go home at the end of a shift and come back to care another day, and taking care of oneself—the subject of the next chapter—is essential if we are to care for patients.

Students

Perceptions of caring seem to be flexible, at least in nursing students. It might be expected that nursing students setting out on their programme of study would hold very high ideals (Watson et al., 1999). These may come from misplaced views of what nurses are and what nurses do, and also what is achievable as a nurse. In fact, it is possible to measure the change in idealism indirectly through the measurement of caring. In one study (Watson et al., 1999), when questioned on idealistic aspects of caring such as staying behind after a shift to complete work and self-sacrificing aspects of care, nursing students scored highly at the start of their programme compared with their scores two years into the programme. While it is only possible to speculate on the reasons for this loss of idealism, it could be exposure to the reality of nursing that lets them see that such self-sacrifice is neither worth it nor necessary, or—in pursuit of self-preservation—they may simply not wish to do it any longer. It should be made clear that this loss of idealism does not necessarily represent a decline in caring—although that cannot be ruled out. On the one hand, it may represent a move from the lay view of caring—one that sees caring in nursing as being something to do with being 'nice' and 'going the extra mile', even if it is not remunerated. On the other hand, exposure to nursing, even as a student, does lead to psychological distress, stress, and burnout, and this has been measured frequently. Such psychological effects of exposure to nursing and also the other stresses of being a student—such as being away from home, having little money, and having an educational programme to deal with, as well as all of the difficulties of professional socialization with peers, senior staff, and other professions, and patients and relatives—may lead to less commitment to the job of nursing and less likelihood of self-sacrifice.

Patients' perceptions of caring

It might be asked what the importance of the perceptions of caring by nurses is. Surely, the point about caring is how patients perceive it? However, most of the work on patients' perceptions has been done in relation to nurses' perceptions and this has produced some very interesting results.

The following activity asks you to reflect on how patients and nurses perceive caring.

....

How do patients and nurses perceive caring?
Can you think how nurses and patients think about caring?
Do you think that they will all think about caring in the same way?
Will patients want the same things out of caring as nurses think they should?
How do you think patients will recognize caring in nurses?
Does it matter if nurses and patients have different perceptions of caring?
....

Essentially, patient and nurse perspectives on caring differ, and this has been demonstrated repeatedly. Nurses tend to perceive caring in more psychosocial terms than patients: for example, nurses imagine caring to be more about mopping brows and being alongside (being there for) patients. Patients, on the other hand, want competent technical care and 'knows how to give shots' (that is, injections) is one way in which a patient might describe a good caring nurse. The work of Larson (1984; 1987) and von Essen and Sjödén (1991a; 1991b) demonstrates this very well.

Nurses' and patients' views of caring

This difference between nurses and patients is interesting and important—albeit it is hard to understand—and several explanations are possible. Nurses may be making an assumption about what caring means to patients based on their own images of nursing and their own perceptions of caring. This version of caring, by the nurses, takes for granted the technical aspects of the job and envisages the value of what they do in psychosocial terms: comforting, reassuring, encouraging, etc. Patients, meanwhile, may well be people who envisage the caring role of the nurse in psychosocial terms until they are ill and require nursing care. Once they require nursing care and are in an unfamiliar environment in which the consequences of what they will experience may be life or death, patients may be more concerned with the technical competence of the nurse, and may not necessarily see this as different from the technical skills of the physicians and surgeons who will also be involved during their period of illness. The patient may well receive and benefit from a great deal of psychosocial care from nurses; however, his or her anxieties about the investigations, procedures, and outcomes associated with the period of illness may be such that he or she may take these for granted or simply be unaware of the psychosocial aspects of the care that he or she has received. Thus we see a difference in the notion of caring between the perspectives of the patient and the nurse: care is being given and received, but what is important to the giver and the receiver is different.

It is important that nurses appreciate these differences arising from the relative perspectives of nurse and patient. It emphasizes that, from the patient perspective and to make patients feel safe, nurses require a high degree of technical competence; this is what the patient sees. This does not mean that nurses should ignore the psychosocial aspects of care and all of the things on which it depends, such as the spiritual, religious, cultural, and ethnicity aspects: it is often through these aspects that technical aspects of care can be delivered. It is important that patients receive clear, honest, and reassuring explanations of procedures that they will undergo, and that they are given time to ask questions; the patient may not appreciate this aspect of his or her care and the nurse delivering it may not feel appreciated—but care has been delivered, nevertheless.

What about care assistants?

Care assistants pose a dilemma for nursing, and this dilemma is both practical and philosophical. In the context of this chapter, the term 'care assistants' is used as a general one covering other similar roles, such as healthcare support workers, nursing assistants, and nursing auxiliaries. If you look for definitions of any of these on the Internet, they usually cross-refer and it is not entirely clear where the distinction between the roles lies. The practical dilemma is that care assistants are a fact of modern health care in the UK and they carry out many of procedures that used to be carried out by nurses (McKenna et al., 2008). Care assistants now even have their own professional journal (Watson, 2007). However, they are not nurses and, in fact, are not trained in nursing schools—so the practical question arises as to where is the 'care' in nursing and what is the 'care' that is administered by care assistants? The philosophical question—not without practical implications—is: who are care assistants assisting? Are they assisting patients with their care or are they helping nurses to administer care? This matters because while care assistants may be 'trained' in elements of patient care, they are not educated in the same way as nurses, and this highlights the issue of nursing education and what is unique about nursing care.

History of care assistants

There have always been people in the health service assisting with care, but these were nursing staff, in the sense that they had a nursing term in their title: 'nursing auxiliary' or 'nursing assistant'. Thus they were explicitly part of the nursing hierarchy, and what they did with and for patients was directed by the qualified nursing staff. Historically, nursing auxiliaries could, after several years of experience and with the right recommendations, progress to being enrolled nurses—a level of nursing entry to the register (that is, by enrolment) that was always ambiguous, because it was also possible to train through the pupil nurse (as opposed to the student nurse) route to become an enrolled nurse. The point, however, was

that these were nurses with a specific level of training and then professional accountability. This confusing state of affairs was ended in the 1980s when enrolled nurse training was discontinued and the possibility of nursing auxiliaries entering the nursing register had also long ceased. In fact, nursing auxiliaries are now almost extinct, and it is hard to distinguish between them and care assistants (try checking this on the Internet)—but both require some level of training for their job.

Therefore we have arrived at a situation in health care in the UK in which a great deal of what was once considered 'nursing care' is being carried out by staff who are not, in fact, nurses. The question therefore arises: what is the consequence of this for nursing and caring—and does it matter?

The following activity invites you to consider the work of care assistants and whether or not this is the same as nursing.

....

Do care assistants care?
In your experience, what do care assistants do?
Do you think that what they do can fairly be described as 'care' or 'caring'?
Do you think that what they do can be described as 'nursing'?
Are 'caring' and 'nursing' the same?
Are care assistants nurses?

....

It certainly addresses the question that forms the title to this chapter: 'So you think you care?' If you do think that you care and that caring is integral to nursing, then can it be delegated to unqualified assistants? If the answer is 'yes', then the consequence is that while some aspects of care may be unique to qualified nurses (presumably the more highly technical aspects of the job), not all of it is, and the boundary between what a qualified nurse does and a care assistant does becomes increasingly blurred. Following the demise of enrolled nurses, the work of qualified nurses and nursing assistants was quite distinct—until the introduction of care assistants, who increasingly assume nursing tasks such as the measurement of vital signs. While there are arguments around whether or not such care assistants—who, while presumably trained to do such tasks, may not be sufficiently educated to interpret and report abnormalities—are sufficiently prepared to balance the technical aspects with the psychosocial aspects. There is little empirical work in this area, but in relation to the foregoing on what patients prefer, it would be of interest to investigate how satisfied patients were with identical aspects of care delivered by care assistants or nurses. If the answer were that they were only 'equally satisfied' (or, indeed, 'more satisfied' with care assistants), then our proposition that we, as nurses, care and that there is something unique to caring in nursing would be severely challenged.

What is caring in nursing?

We have not answered the question 'what is care?', but we have identified and exemplified how easy it is to recognize when care and caring are absent. It is also possible to begin to see how caring and nursing might be integral, and if not synonymous, at least associated, and that there is something unique about nurses and nursing that optimizes this relationship. As we have already stated, caring is not and cannot be unique to nurses and nursing: it exists and is administered in a great many other situations and by a great many other people. Parents and children are a prime example of care that is tangible and unrelated to nursing. But if this is the case, then what is caring in nursing? These issues remain unresolved, but the prevailing view on nursing and what constitutes caring in nursing at any time has a profound influence on the education and training of nursing students. Presumably, in turn, this influences nursing and nursing care—but, again, this remains unresolved.

Conclusion

This chapter has demonstrated that:

- there is confusion about the concept of 'caring';
- we think that we care, but we do not know what 'care' is;
- we think that we can recognize care and caring, but we do not actually know how to do so; and
- we think that education and training are important for nurses, but we do not know how much of each is sufficient.

Caring in nursing is a very complex subject and the following chapters will explore the concept from many perspectives. These chapters will show that if you think you care, you probably do—but do you care enough in each of the novel and challenging situations that you are likely to meet as a nurse?

References

Benner, P. and Wrubel, J. (1986) *The Primacy Of Caring*, Menlo Park, CA: Addison-Wesley.

Briggs, A. (1972) *Report of the Committee on Nursing*, Cmnd 5115, London: HMSO ('the Briggs Report').

Department of Health (1999) *Making a Difference: Strengthening the Nursing, Midwifery and Health Visiting Contribution to Health and Healthcare*, London: HMSO.

Forrest, D. (1989) 'The experience of caring', *Journal of Advanced Nursing* 14: 815–23.

Gaut, D.A. (1983) 'Development of a theoretically adequate description of caring', *Western Journal of Nursing Research* 5: 313–24.

Gaut, D.A. (1986) 'Evaluating caring competencies in nursing practice', *Topics in Clinical Nursing* 8(2): 77–83.

Kyle, T.V. (1995) 'The concept of caring: a review of the literature', *Journal of Advanced Nursing* 21: 506–14.

Larson, P.J. (1984) 'Important nursing caring behaviours perceived by patients with cancer', *Oncology Nursing Forum* 11(6): 46–50.

Larson, P.J. (1987) 'Comparison of cancer patients' and professional nurses' perceptions of important nurse caring behaviour', *Heart & Lung* 16: 187–93.

Leininger, M.M. (1981) 'The phenomenon of caring: importance, research questions and theoretical considerations', in M.N. Leininger (ed.) *Caring: An Essential Human Need*, Proceedings from National Caring Conference, University of Utah, NJ: Charles B. Slack, pp. 3–15.

Mayeroff, M. (1971) *On Caring*, New York: Harper Perennial.

McKenna, H.P., Thompson, D.R., Norman, I.J., and Watson, R. (2006) 'The good old days of nurse training: Rose tinted or jaundiced view?' *International Journal of Nursing Studies* 43: 135–7.

McKenna, H.P.,Thompson, D.R., and Watson, R. (2008) 'Health care assistants: An oxymoron', *International Journal of Nursing Studies* 44: 1283–4.

Morse, J.M., Bottorff, J.L., Neander, J.L., and Solberg, S.M. (1991) 'Comparative analysis of conceptualisations and theories of caring', *IMAGE: Journal of Nursing Scholarship* 23: 119–27.

Morse, J.M., Solberg, S.M., Neander, J.L., Bottorff, J.L., and Johnson, J.L. (1990) 'Concepts of caring and caring as a concept', *Advances in Nursing Science* 13: 1–14.

Olson, T.C. (1993) 'Laying claim to caring: Nursing and the language of training, 1915–37', *Nursing Outlook* 41: 69–72.

Patients Association, The (2009) *Patients … not Numbers, People … not Statistics*, London: The Patients Association.

Philips, P. (1993) 'A deconstruction of caring', *Journal of Advanced Nursing* 18: 1554–8.

Social Care Institute for Excellence (2009) *Dignity in Care*, London: SCIE.

UK Central Council for Nursing, Midwifery and Health Visiting (1986) *Project 2000: A New Preparation for Practice*, London: UKCC.

Von Essen, L. and Sjödén, P.-O. (1991a) 'Patient and staff perceptions of caring: Review and replication', *Journal of Advanced Nursing* 16: 1363–74.

Von Essen, L. and Sjödén, P.-O. (1991b) 'The importance of nurse caring behaviours as perceived by Swedish hospital patients and nursing staff', *International Journal of Nursing Studies* 28: 267–81.

Watson, J. (1988) *Nursing: Human Science and Human Care*, New York: National League for Nursing.

Watson, J. (2009) *Assessing and Measuring Caring in Nursing and Health Science*, 2nd edn, New York: Springer Publishing Company.

Watson, R. (2007) 'Do HCAs deskill nurses? Yes', *British Journal of Healthcare Assistants* 1: 58.

Watson, R. and Lea, A. (1997) 'The Caring Dimensions Inventory (CDI): Content validity, reliability and scaling', *Journal of Advanced Nursing* 25: 87–94.

Watson, R., Deary, I.J. and Lea, A. (1999) 'A longitudinal study into the perceptions of caring and nursing among student nurses', *Journal of Advanced Nursing* 29: 1228–37.

Watson, R., Lea, A., and Deary, I.J. (1998) 'Caring in nursing: A multivariate analysis', *Journal of Advanced Nursing* 28: 662–71.

Wolf, Z.R. (1986) 'The caring concept and nurse identified caring behaviours', *Topics in Clinical Nursing* 8: 84–94.

Woodham Smith, C. (1951) *Florence Nightingale*, London: Penguin.

Caring for oneself

ANTHONY SCHWARTZ AND BARBARA WREN

Learning outcomes

This chapter will enable you to:

- develop awareness of the relevance of self-care;
- understand pressure, stress and burnout, and their effect on performance;
- recognize the pressures arising from the context of work;
- promote self-awareness and awareness of others;
- understand what motivates us to care;
- understand the concepts of emotional intelligence and emotional labour;
- know what it is that you need to be more effective and a 'good nurse';
- use support systems for yourself and encourage self-care in others (for example, 'signposting'); and
- develop resilience to become professional and personally enabled to make a difference in a challenging career.

Introduction

The central idea of this chapter is that the ability to care for yourself underpins your ability to care for others. Whilst being a nurse can be exciting, interesting, and rewarding, it can also be challenging, draining, and upsetting. As a person, you need to understand yourself, and your motivations and aspirations, as well as how to relate to those around you. Being a healthcare worker means that you have to balance, or learn to juggle, many different things. In your professional role, you will have to manage various tasks, draw on many abilities and competencies, and yet still be expected to show the human qualities of compassion, respect, and

kindness even when the going is tough and your resources are stretched to the extreme limit. You will have to draw deeply on yourself, both on your professional capabilities and personal skills: on your mental, physical, and emotional resources. Although most needed when under extreme challenges, the ability to care for yourself is important at all times and can ensure that the stress of nursing work does not harm your health.

Essential knowledge and skills for care

- You must be aware of the importance of caring for yourself, adopting attitudes and behaviours that will help to maintain your own physical, mental, psychological, and spiritual well-being.

- You will need to increase your awareness of the stresses and demands in the working and caring environment that may lead to burnout and underperformance.

- You must develop knowledge and understanding of the different strategies that can be used to foster resilience, through which you will become professionally and personally enabled to manage change and make a difference.

Why is self-care relevant in health care?

As a nurse, you work in intense, at times fast-paced, environments, with high levels of responsibility—for life-and-death issues, in some specialties. The long period of training you have undertaken as a nurse (as is also true for doctors and other specialized healthcare staff) and years of 'on-the-job' experience equip you to take up leadership, and bear and manage this responsibility. The ethic of care, central in the practice of nursing, comes under pressure in a health service dominated by more commercial values, with imperatives to meet nationally imposed targets for clinical activity creating additional psychological demands. It is inevitable that this range of pressures on you and other healthcare staff at times gives rise to conflict, both internal and interpersonal. These challenges can often lead to problems at a wider organizational level in addition to personal stress, which, if unrecognized, is personally damaging and impacts the ability to care. In the rest of this chapter, we will bring together information about stress and self-care, and evidence about what can be done at a practical level to protect yourself from stress and help you to enjoy the challenges of your job. Examples of good practice will encourage you to develop and maintain appropriate self-care.

The majority of healthcare occupations, not only nursing, can benefit from recognizing the importance of self-care, because they cope daily with high workloads in the context of the need for few errors, while often working in difficult and chaotic conditions. The problem of ill health in all groups of health service staff has been recognized for several years. These problems persist as organizational change continues in healthcare systems. This is compounded by a limited recognition of the high level of psychological demands created by doing healthcare work in cost-conscious organizations with limited resources.

The impact of work on nurses' health

The idea that nurses are there 'to serve' whilst exercising their professional and vocational role is admirable, but surely not at the expense of the health needs of the nurse doing the 'serving'. There is a strong body of evidence that suggests that working in the health services can harm your health (Williams et al., 1999). In the UK, NHS staff have higher sickness absence rates and levels of psychological ill health than comparable staff groups working in other sectors (Confederation of British Industry, 1997). For example, in one report, it was found that 27 per cent of healthcare staff report psychological problems in comparison with 18 per cent of the population in general (Wall et al., 1997). The nature of the work, the way in which it is structured and managed, and the ongoing pace of organizational change have all been proposed to account for the worrying levels of staff illness and turnover in the NHS (Firth-Cozens and Payne, 1999; Wren and Michie, 2003). Another reason for increased pressure on staff is that patients now have shorter stays in hospitals, and need more intensive care in hospital and at follow-up when they are discharged.

What causes stress and how does stress affect us?
Think back to a difficult, emotionally challenging, or frustrating situation at work with a patient/client. Did you notice feeling under pressure or stress? What does this tell you about the notion of stress? What does it tell you about yourself?

Situations that are likely to cause stress are those that are unpredictable or uncontrollable, uncertain, ambiguous or unfamiliar, or those that involve conflict, loss, or performance expectations. Stress may be caused by time-limited events, such as the pressures of examinations or work deadlines, or by ongoing situations, such as family demands, job insecurity, and long commuting journeys.

Signs of stress can be seen in the areas of feelings (for example, anxiety, depression, irritability, fatigue), behaviour (being withdrawn, aggressive, tearful, unmotivated, numb), thinking (difficulties of concentration and problem-solving), or physical symptoms (palpitations, nausea, headaches). If stress persists, there are changes in neuroendocrine, cardiovascular, autonomic, and immunological functioning, leading to mental and physical ill health (such as anxiety, depression, heart disease).

Resources that help to meet the pressures and demands faced at work include personal characteristics, such as coping skills (problem-solving, assertiveness, time management), and the work situation (a good working environment and social support). These resources can be increased through therapy, training and development, redesigning jobs, good management and employment practices, and improving the way in which work is organized.

Elements of self-care, and self-care skills and attributes

To be effective as a professional nurse, it is helpful to consider your internal motivation to care, what has formed this desire 'to care', and how to sustain this over your career. It is also important to understand your resources, your ability to cope, and the amount of support available to you. Understanding the environment or working context is also relevant. For example, it helps to have some clarity about the way in which the healthcare sector works practically and about the external forces affecting health care (that is, government, regional, and local aspects), such as funding and governance. If you recognize and understand the context, you can more easily see what you can do for yourself, what is up to the organization or system to take care of, and how you can make the most of your own resources and those around you, be they colleagues, managers, or patients and carers.

....

What is self-care in the real world of nursing practice all about and how does it apply to you?

....

'Self-care' defined

'Self-care' is about personal health maintenance on several levels: physical, emotional, mental, social and spiritual. It is about improving or restoring health or treating or preventing disease. This comprises contexts such as personal, community and organizational dimensions, lifestyle and activities, including the cornerstones of well-being such as sleep, diet, and exercise. The following activities all contribute to good self-care:

- good self-awareness, understanding your strengths and vulnerabilities, and how stress affects you cognitively, emotionally, physically, and behaviourally;

- talking about your experiences to someone who is trustworthy (a friend, colleague, relative, mentor, coach, supervisor);
- trying not to bottle up emotions and expressing feelings about what has happened;
- keeping daily routines going when under pressure; and
- eating sensibly, not drinking too much, taking exercise, and undertaking some form of relaxation.

Our hope is that, as a nurse, through acknowledging and developing personal strategies for self-care, by reading and considering information contained in this chapter, you too will be able to ensure that you are not a casualty of healthcare work, but instead find it enriching and fulfilling.

Key elements of self-care

Understanding levels of motivation and pressure

How motivated are we, in the normal course of our working schedule, to engage in self-care? Of course, you may argue that our primary purpose for being a nurse is to care for others by actively and conscientiously doing our job and fulfilling the role expectations on us. We can choose when and how to engage in appropriate self-care. It is not self-indulgence: self-care has an impact on how effective and efficient we are at work. The value that we put on our own health will determine our motivation to make sure that self-care is a priority. However, it is not only about us: self-care makes us more effective at work too. All of us require engagement at work, and a certain amount of pressure to motivate ourselves and do the work that we do. When we have too little pressure, we can find ourselves feeling bored and demotivated; similarly, when we have too much pressure, it can be overwhelming and we can find it difficult to feel in control. Whether we experience pressure as too little or too much is individual and personal. It is related to:

- how much stimulation we need;
- the sequence or frequency of changes;
- our thoughts and beliefs about ourselves and our capability; and
- our emotions.

Levels of stimulation

Whilst some people enjoy doing a certain number of tasks of which they are in control during a working day, others like doing a variety of tasks that are changeable and novel. As we develop in our roles, mature, and encounter different life situations (such as social, family life, organizational issues), the amount of stimulation that we need from our work might vary. For example, an activity that we used to enjoy early on in our career may seem like a burden when we have to juggle a new or challenging situation (such as a domestic difficulty, a new baby, or an ill family member). At that point, the pressure from work may seem to be too much. Our degree of self-awareness is important here: it is useful to recognize and observe our internal signs of pressure, and to decide if we need to do something about this before it becomes stressful.

Pace of change

Sometimes, if we have a number of pressures happening all at once, this too can be overwhelming. Changes often require time to process and we need opportunities to adapt and accommodate to things, to develop new habits and behavioural patterns, which might help us to feel safe. One significant life event may be handled well, but if we have several challenges happening in rapid succession, we may feel that our coping resources are stretched. Therefore, if we have to deal with too many 'crises', we need to recognize that our coping can be compromised and that we should not expect to be able to 'do it all'. Whether and how we recognize this and ask for input from others is crucial to managing our well-being and avoiding stress at work. The ability to ask for others' input (whether it be to do practical things, to provide emotional support, or to help at a more strategic planning level) is influenced by our thoughts and beliefs about ourselves. We may, for example, believe that we have to manage on our own, and will have to confront some assumptions we have about ourselves and what gives us personal worth. We may feel we need to 'be strong', 'be perfect', 'please others', 'try hard', or 'be busy' (Berne, 1964). This links with our level of self-confidence, the degree of assertiveness that we have, and also our emotional intelligence.

Thoughts and beliefs about ourselves

How we think—about ourselves, our work, colleagues, and patients, as well as the tasks that we do—can add to our experience of stress and pressure or can relieve it. Psychological models and theories about what influences how we think, feel, and respond will be revisited in later chapters. In practice, when people are stressed and use psychological support, a number of theoretical approaches can be used and research is equivocal about which one theory is best. However, understanding the early influences as well as the way in which we behave in particular situations and contexts is often helpful. Cognitive behavioural therapies, psychoanalytic, systemic, humanistic approaches, and others are used by practitioners to increase personal awareness of both thoughts and feelings, to develop an understanding of patterns and trigger events, and to seek creative solutions to manage distress.

One might come to work with a particular thought pattern or 'mental video', or a belief about the day that has an impact on the way in which we manage it. We also have choices in terms of how we think about what happens in our lives, which we can perceive as good, bad, or somewhere in between, and which can attribute our achievements to our own personal effort or good luck, or something between the two. Whether we feel that something is under our control or not is also important. The concept of 'locus of control' suggests that people have 'expectancies' that influence their behaviour (Rotter, 1966). These 'expectancies', or mental representations, are based on past experiences and views of the situation that they are likely to confront, and affect our judgement on whether we are going to be successful in getting what we want. This judgement can influence what we decide to do or take on. People who take the credit for success (and blame themselves for failure) are considered to have 'internal locus of control'. Those who blame outside forces, people, or bad luck for their failures and view success as being due to good luck are considered to have 'external locus of control'. Of course, many people would fall somewhere along this continuum and recognize what is within their control and what is not, and so behave accordingly. In general, it is thought that perceiving that you have control over things that you can influence is a more psychologically healthy disposition. This is often called having 'self-determination' or 'personal control'. The literature on 'stress at work' suggests that having control over situations mitigates stress. Appropriate skills and self-care strategies aim to reduce levels of stress in healthcare. Zimbardo (1977) suggests a locus of control orientation is a belief about whether the outcomes of our actions are contingent on what we do (internal control orientation) or on events outside our personal control (external control orientation).

Taking this one step further, Bandura (1995) describes how beliefs about our competence determine how we feel, behave, and think. He views self-efficacy as a person's belief in his or her ability to succeed in a particular situation. Martin Seligman (1974) coined the term 'learned helplessness' as a psychological condition in which people behave helplessly in a particular situation, even when they have the power to overcome the obstacle. He saw this as in part arising from a perceived absence of control over the outcome of a situation: if you focus on the negative, then you are priming yourself to attend selectively to what is happening around you. For example, if you think that people do not like you, then you will look out for signs to prove or indicate that that is 'true', and it will become something of a 'self fulfilling prophecy'. This may happen consciously or unconsciously. For example, a person might see things bleakly and spend a lot of time complaining about work, feeling that they are 'a victim', or they may reframe a situation, break the negative pattern, or challenge the negative viewpoint and think about what they can do to make a difference.

....

Reflect for a moment on someone you know who may constantly complain about how things are 'never right' and about how they feel victimized. What impact does this 'negativity' have on colleagues, patients, and managers?
Could you stand back from the situation and recognize that whilst there are some times when this may be the case, there is a case to be made that it is not always so bleak and that the person should try to look for something positive?

....

Pressure, stress, and performance: how to manage them well

The way in which we deal with pressure is a mixture of our history and personal experience, our 'personality', habits that we have developed, as well as the organizational structures that are in place for managing workplace pressure and stress. Individuals differ in their risk of experiencing stress and in their vulnerability to the adverse effects of stress. People are more likely to experience stress if they lack material resources (for example, financial security) and psychological resources (for example, social support, coping skills, resilience, self-esteem). They are likely to be harmed by this stress if they tend to react emotionally to situations and are highly competitive and pressured (Type A behaviour). The first step in changing our exposure to stress and the impact that it has on us is to raise our awareness of our own personal response style to stressors. When considering yourself and your responses to stress, perhaps you might reflect on the 'reflective questions' in **Box 2.1**.

People who are under constant high levels of pressure, who have symptoms of stress, and who feel overwhelmed and as a result find it difficult to cope, are not in a position to give of their best. It is very useful to learn to stop ourselves descending into the whirlpool of negative emotions.

Stress and performance: theory, rationale, and evidence base

Models, frameworks, and concepts

In this section, we will highlight the main theoretical approaches to understanding the concept of stress. We will deal with this in greater depth later on in the book (Chapter 7).

Box 2.1 Reflective questions about pressure and stress

- Are you able to recognize situations that result in you feeling 'under pressure'?
- How do you deal with pressure?
- How does stress or pressure affect you physically, emotionally, cognitively, and behaviourally?
- Do you respond to people differently when under pressure?
- Can you cope comfortably with demands placed on you?
- How do you know when you are not coping?
- Are you clear about your personal responsibilities and boundaries?
- Do you feel that you can have an influence over how things are done?
- Are you well supported practically, managerially, and emotionally at work?
- Do people around you encourage and affirm you in your role?
- To whom do you talk when you are concerned about your functioning at work?

The transactional model of stress

The transactional model of stress (Lazarus and Folkman, 1984) describes the importance of an individual's perceptions of both the stress to which they are exposed and their own coping resources. The model proposes that the ability of a person to prevent or reduce stress is determined by their appraisal of:

(a) the threat within a situation (primary appraisal); and

(b) their coping skills to deal with that threat (secondary appraisal).

These appraisals have been shaped by past experiences of confronting stress and, in turn, influence future behaviour and appraisals. Thus, the process of appraisal, behaviour, and stress is continuous, and managing stress can result from changing the way in which the situation is appraised (cognitive techniques) or responded to (behavioural or cognitive techniques). This model incorporates several areas for potential intervention, which include addressing the actual level of demands and resources to which an individual is exposed, and the individual's perceptions of the situations in which they find themselves and of their own resources. In the practical section at the end of the chapter, we will highlight practical strategies to deal with stress.

The job strain model

The job strain model (Karasek, 1979; 1990) outlines the conditions of work that are likely to lead to stress and outcomes such as job strain, poor health, and sickness absence. According to this model, work-related strain and risks to health are most likely to arise when high job demands are coupled with low decision latitude (that is, low personal control over work and limited opportunities to develop skills). On the other hand, high job demands with high decision latitude give the possibility of motivation to learn, active learning, and a sense of accomplishment. Of the two, decision latitude has been found to be more important than demand (Johnson et al., 1996). Since its introduction in 1979, the model has been extended to include social support at work as a predictor of job strain (Johnson and Hall, 1988), and now links the dimensions of demands, control, and support. Social support at work, which can include support from managers, supervisors, and colleagues, can help to reduce the effects of stressful job conditions. Karasek's model has received sufficient empirical support for it to provide a useful framework for planning and implementing organizational interventions in healthcare settings (see **box 2.2**).

You may like to write down or discuss with a colleague, supervisor or mentor each of the following.

How do you know that you are experiencing the right amount of pressure?

Do you know when you are experiencing too little or too much pressure?

What are the signs of stress that you are aware of in yourself?

Are there certain situations in which you experience more of these symptoms and can you identify the 'triggers'? For example, what was it about this situation that caused you to feel like that? Which of the signs did you notice first?

What can you do about this, if you are aware of these things?
....

Stress management

The association between pressures and well-being and functioning can be thought of an inverted 'U', with well-being and functioning being low when pressures are high *and* very low (for example, both in times of severe overload at work and circumstances of unemployment). Different people demonstrate different shapes of this inverted 'U', with different thresholds and ranges of pressure for experiencing stress. A successful strategy for preventing stress in the workplace will ensure that the job fits the person and exposes them to their optimum level of stress for effective performance.

The key steps in stress management are as follows.

1 Identify stressors.
2 Assess what change is needed.
3 Clarify whether change is needed at an individual or situational level.

When stress is recognized, it can be dealt with at different levels and through various forms of intervention. According to DeFrank and Cooper (1987), these can be aimed at:

- the individual;
- the organization; or
- the individual–organizational interface.

This suggests either that we change ourselves, change the organization, or adapt to the situation and apply a range of coping mechanisms. However, it is important to involve all three dimensions.

Individual-level change involves therapeutic work, training, and one-to-one psychology services—clinical, occupational, health or counselling. They should aim to change and develop individual skills and resources *and* help the individual to change their situation (Cooper and Cartwright, 2001).

Training and one-to-one input helps to prevent stress by allowing you to:

- become aware of the signs of stress;
- use this awareness to interrupt your behaviour pattern when the stress reaction is just beginning (because stress usually builds up gradually and the more the stress builds up, the more difficult it is to deal with);
- analyse the situation and develop an active plan to minimize the stressors;
- learn skills of active coping and relaxation, developing a lifestyle that creates a buffer against stress;
- practise the above in low-stress situations first, to maximize chances of early success and to boost self-confidence and motivation to continue.

A variety of training courses and input (such as executive coaching, counselling) may help in developing active coping techniques, including assertiveness, communications skills, time management, problem solving, and effective management. Some stressors may be impossible to change and, in these cases, individuals need to be supported to adapt to the stressors with the least amount of harm: resilience training and mindfulness can help with this. Other types of intervention at the individual level include using relaxation techniques, exercise, healthy eating, time management, meditation (mindfulness), and cognitive-behavioural (thinking) strategies.

Box 2.2 Psychological model (Karasek, 1979)

a. **High demands + high control + good support**
Good psychological health and high levels of satisfaction with work   **Active job**

b. **High demands + low control + poor support**
Poor psychological health and reduced satisfaction with work   **High strain**

c. **Low demands + high control + good support**
High levels of satisfaction with work and good psychological health   **Low strain**

d. **Low demands + low control + poor support**
Reduced satisfaction with work, poor psychological health   **Passive job**

Input focusing on the individual–organization interface includes supporting relationships at work (for example, mentoring, 'buddying' schemes, and coaching) and dealing with role ambiguity (that is, unclear roles and expectations). Change at a situational level may also involve redesigning jobs, reassigning roles, restructuring teams, and organizational-level change.

Interventions at the organizational level include working strategically on the organizational environment, structure, and policies, and physical characteristics of the job such as heat, lighting, and noise. For example, the shift patterns and rota or schedule (a structural aspect of work) can cause significant levels of physical and mental discomfort if not carefully planned.

Combining these three approaches will increase the likelihood that occupational stress is minimized.

Interventions may also be classified as being preventative, restorative, or recuperative in focus. These are sometimes known as 'primary', 'secondary' and 'tertiary' interventions to reduce stress and promote self-care skills.

- **Primary interventions**
  Primary interventions aim to remove or reduce stress at work. They target aspects of work known to contribute to job strain. This can include clarifying roles and relationships at work, increasing autonomy, and reducing excessive workload.
- **Secondary interventions**
  Secondary interventions seek to improve workers' resources in tackling sources and consequences of stress, for example improving coping skills, developing strategies for managing time and competing priorities, and developing assertiveness skills.
- **Tertiary interventions**
  Tertiary interventions aim to help workers with stress-related disorders, for example by the provision of counselling and psychotherapy services for work-related problems and the establishment of employee assistance programmes. They may also include the provision of consultancy services aiming to help the organization to address and respond to teams and departments in difficulty.

It is the responsibility of the organization to identify sources of stress in the work environment, which can be achieved by studying records of sickness absence and employee turnover, as well as by listening to employees and completing an organizational or staff stress survey. Likewise, it is the responsibility of the individual to identify their own sources of stress, because these are particular to the individual; they must then inform their employer. The central consideration is not the actual work environment, but how the employee reacts to it. The individual needs to take responsibility for how they react and deal with pressure.

Burnout

One of the consequences of stress may be burnout. This is a syndrome of emotional exhaustion, depersonalization, and reduced accomplishment that can occur among individuals who work with people in some capacity (Maslach, 1982, 2003). Since the term was first coined (Freudenberger, 1974), it has come to be seen as a 'wearing out' from the stress of work (McVicar, 2003; Miller et al., 1990; see also Wright, 2005). Burnout is often seen as the end stage of the stress process for those working in helping professions—a final point in a breakdown of adaptation that results from the long-term imbalance of demands and resources.

Maslach (2003) identified three dimensions of burnout, as follows.

1 Loss of energy and a generalized fatigue.
2 Depersonalization, which involves negative perceptions of others—particularly of clients.
3 Negative attitudes towards oneself and a lessened sense of personal accomplishment.

Certain characteristics of both staff and work conditions increase the likelihood of burnout. It is more likely to be experienced by those who enter their profession with high goals and expectations. Younger employees and those with less 'hardy' personalities are likely to be more vulnerable. 'Hardy' personalities have been defined as those who approach demands with a sense of commitment, control, and challenge (Kobasa, 1979). Situations in which there is role conflict or ambiguity can make staff more susceptible to burnout, and there is strong evidence of a relationship between lack of social support, particularly from supervisors, and burnout.

Three work factors have been shown to be related to burnout:

- lack of feedback;
- poor participation in decision-making; and
- lack of autonomy.

Participation in decision-making, support from a supervisor, and support from co-workers can all serve to reduce the perception of stressors in the workplace, decreasing the experience of burnout and increasing the experience of positive outcomes, such as satisfaction and commitment (Miller et al., 1990). The evidence base on burnout highlights areas to which you can pay attention, thereby preventing burning out from your work. It also shows the action that healthcare managers can take to protect their staff.

Emotional labour

Exploring the field of emotions in the workplace has become an area of research over the past decade. Emotions were previously considered 'personal' and healthcare workers often were encouraged to 'be professional'; in essence, this meant ignoring emotions or putting on a 'professional persona' at work. Recognizing emotions does not mean succumbing to expressing negative emotions or reacting in unprofessional ways; it simply means that if we can recognize how we feel and what the reasons are underlying these feelings, we can then learn to manage them appropriately. Studies of emotional labour focus on the stress of managing emotions when the work role demands certain expressions to be shown to those with whom we work (such as with patients, carers, colleagues) that may be different from the emotions that we feel (for example, fatigue, irritation). Hochschild (1983) showed that the stress of emotional labour results in burnout. Employees in customer service roles often expend effort in managing their own emotions in order to display those required for the role (for example, flight attendants, nurses). It is suggested that, in the role, one may engage in 'surface acting' (that is, changing only the outward display, such as facial expressions or voice tone) or in 'deep acting' (that is, changing your feelings to achieve a required display). Studies (see Grandey, 2000) suggest that there is less dissonance between how one feels and how one acts in the latter case (deep acting). It is, therefore an important concept and, in terms of self-care, simply recognizing or noticing that aspects of work can be emotionally taxing gives an individual a chance to make choices about how to manage himself or herself and the impact of work.

Associated with this is the notion of 'emotional intelligence', which has been brought into common parlance by Daniel Goleman (1995) and is based on the earlier work of Salovey and Mayer (1990), who defined emotional intelligence as the ability to monitor one's own and others' feelings, to discriminate among them, and to use this information to guide one's thinking and action. It emphasizes the personal and social dimensions. It begins with self-awareness of emotions and focuses on managing emotions, as well as noticing emotions in others and responding through interpersonal and relationship management.

One study of emotional intelligence in nurses (Rego et al., 2010) shows that the ability to manage emotions can lead nurses to be more respectful, attentive, and trustful towards patients, and to provide them with more explanations regarding treatments and their respective consequences. Nurses who are emotionally intelligent can make choices about how to respond to different interpersonal situations without being emotionally weighed down. With self-awareness, a nurse will respond more openly and with greater self-control when a patient is threatening or complaining: he or she has more self-control and does not take criticism as a personal attack. It will then be possible to listen to and respond to the patient.

It is evident that emotions and their management are really important—particularly in high-pressure situations and when things go wrong. The consequences for staff involved in medical accidents and mistakes can be serious, and include depression, anger, shame, and loss of confidence (Charles et al., 1985). Increasingly, attention is being paid to ways in which to reduce the likelihood of error and its consequences for patients and healthcare staff. The frequency and impact of medical errors on patients, staff, and healthcare systems has been the subject of major academic studies in the USA and Australia (Kohn et al., 1999; Wilson et al., 1995). There is widespread agreement that we need to support the development of a health service culture that takes a systems approach to responding to, and learning from, error.

Who is responsible for self-care and managing stress at work?

Stress at work is about an interaction of many factors: aspects relating to the job and the individual factors that are from outside of work, but which still affect the individual at work. It might be asked: 'Who is responsible for dealing with stress—the individual or the organization?' Pragmatically, dealing with stress is important for both: for the individual, to influence their well-being at work, job satisfaction, and overall functioning; and for the organization, to increase engagement at work, and reduce sickness levels and associated costs. Recently, research has begun to recognize the issues of psychological well-being at work (Wright and Cropanzano, 2001), and Robertson et al. (2007) and Cooper et al. (2010) contend that, without this psychological well-being, it is not possible to engage staff effectively.

The Health and Safety at Work Act 1999 requires organizations, so far as is reasonably practicable, to ensure the health of employees at work. This incorporates identifying the hazards in the workplace, evaluating the risks arising from those hazards, and deciding whether existing precautions are adequate or more needs to be done. However, case law has established that no job 'is intrinsically dangerous to mental health' and that individuals need to bring problems to the attention of management. The issue is that otherwise they may not be recognized as 'foreseeable'. This means that although managers need to be aware of potentially stressful situations for their employees, it is the responsibility of the individual to let the manager know when they are experiencing levels of pressure with which they are finding it difficult to cope (see **Practice Example 2.1**).

Practice Example 2.1 demonstrates the impact of timely interventions on personal and professional well-being, but also on organizational costs. The nurse was helped to use a crisis to develop his own resources and supported to return to work as quickly as possible. In this way, the NHS retained expertise, the investment already made in training, and saved on locum costs and having to manage the knock-on impact on team morale (of having a team member on long-term sick leave). The member of staff was prevented from entering the negative spiral of depression and longer-term sickness absence, both of which would have had a more serious impact on his psychological well-being, ability to return to work, and confidence in future employment. Occupational health psychologists are well placed to provide timely, accessible, and acceptable psychological interventions with wide-ranging benefits (Quick and Tetrick, 2003). A key to this work is enabling staff to develop an understanding of the emotional impact of their work, the way in which they construe their difficulties, the connections between personal and professional relationships, and the impact of how they relate to themselves and to their own role have an impact on how they function at work. The aim is to help staff to develop flexible and compassionate ways in which to manage life and work pressures, and to use support effectively. This protects staff health while saving the NHS from the loss of skilled staff in both the short and long terms.

For a description of the work and services available in occupational health psychology in the NHS, see Wren et al. (2006).

....

Consider and reflect on the following.
Marilyn is a matron in a regional hospital where she has worked for twenty years. She has been under increasing pressure lately due to major changes in hospital structure and changes in role and responsibility, and she has started to feel upset and emotional, reacting to people in an uncharacteristic manner: being short, expressing anger and feeling out of control, and at times crying for no apparent reason.
What is happening?
What should Marilyn do?

How can you understand this and what questions would you ask in order to help Marilyn?

As a member of her staff, how would you react to her abrupt manner?

How would this affect things?

Try to think about the individual and the system—that is, what is happening to the person and how their behaviour may be a result both of their personal situation, and the system of which they are a part.

···

PRACTICE EXAMPLE 2.1

Distressed professional seeking occupational health psychology input

A 37-year-old nurse was referred to the occupational health psychologist in a very distressed state. He was unable to work, had lost confidence in his skills, felt incompetent, was anxious and guilty about the impact of his absence on his colleagues, and was considering leaving his job.

He was a skilled, specialist clinician who had been working in the National Health Service for sixteen years and had recently gone through a number of changes in his professional and personal life. At work, he had moved from ward-based nursing to a clinic in which his roles and responsibilities were greater and based more on specialist expertise. The expectations of other staff were higher; he had more autonomy, but his level of support had drastically reduced; and he (and the team) had much less clarity about his role. He had developed acute situational anxiety with regard to certain clinical tasks: he was losing confidence and found it difficult to ask for help.

In his personal life, he had recently remarried and was finding this transition in his relationship difficult. His first marriage had ended abruptly. He had recently heard that his ex-wife had remarried and was about to have her first child. He was negotiating a number of issues in his new relationship, including whether or not to have a family, and whether to buy a home or to go travelling. As a result of the stress, he was withdrawing from friends, socializing less, and losing confidence both socially and in his marriage.

The aim of the occupational health psychology assessment was to understand both the nurse's work and his home contexts, his attributional and coping styles, and his help-seeking behaviour in order to be able to decide:

• what factors were influencing this presentation to occupational health;

• what would be amenable to intervention (in the context of brief therapeutic interventions in which the goal is to normalize, develop resources, and improve coping); and

• whether any other help was needed (within and/or outside of the organization).

The intervention drew on a number of approaches. Cognitive behavioural work helped to raise the nurse's awareness of his own attributions for his current difficulties, develop alternatives to negative thinking, and create strategies for managing general and situational anxiety. Systemic work helped him to understand his role in the context of this new system, and how the way in which he and his colleagues were relating to this role was adding to his pressure and limiting his opportunities for support. This work identified training and mentoring opportunities that he could access, and coached him to 'manage up' to increase the support that he was receiving from his manager. The job competence model helped him to understand the influence of his current role transition on his levels of anxiety and normalized this experience for him. This, linked to some career counselling using a developmental framework, helped the nurse to understand his experience in a more process-focused and reflective way. Finally, stress management training helped him to increase his exercise levels and reduced his social withdrawal—all of which helped to lessen his anxiety further.

The nurse returned to work after two weeks and, after six sessions with the psychologist, his anxiety and low mood had lifted. His general health questionnaire (GHQ) score was '12' at the beginning of therapy, '6' after completing therapy, and '1' three months later. His confidence and job satisfaction had increased, he had set up regular meetings with his manager and supervisor, and they had agreed a training and development plan. His communication with his wife had improved and he was more able to confront issues in his relationship.

Before focusing on practical ways of maintaining well-being and reducing stress at work, let us look at the way in which negative cycles can become embedded. Remembering the concept of 'learned helplessness' (Seligman, 1974), as psychologists, we are still keen to understand why people become stressed and depressed, and what impacts on this. However, we also recognize that sometimes we may have dwelt on the negative a little too much. It is important to understand why some people become stressed, disillusioned, and depressed; equally important is understanding why others do not, despite having similar circumstances. The originator of the term 'learned helplessness' has, over the past three decades, recognized this and the field of 'positive psychology' has emerged (Seligman, 2002).

Putting it all together: planning your own self-care

In this section, we will look at ways in which you, as a nurse, can develop your personal 'toolkit' to enhance your self-care and achieve greater well-being at work. We know that humans are creatures of habit: once we have learnt something, it becomes embedded over time and with practice. It can be said that when things become a habit, we actually stop thinking about what we are doing and we do the task automatically. For example, when we are learning to drive, we know that we cannot drive and we have to really concentrate on it; we recognize consciously our 'incompetence'. Then we learn and consciously develop competence. Once we know how to drive, we do it automatically without thinking. We have developed a habit: it becomes an unconscious competence and just part of what we do 'naturally'.

It is similar in terms of developing habits relating to how we think about things. We develop patterns and ways of thinking that are no longer conscious, although the way in which we think has a powerful effect on our behaviour. If we are in a difficult situation and we think

that there are no alternatives or solutions to the situation, then no alternatives will come to mind and we 'close down'. However, if we are able to keep an open mind and think that there is a solution, then we will seek a solution.

There are several ways of thinking that can block us from finding a range of possible solutions to the situations in which we find ourselves.

....

Think about what happens when you are in a tricky situation.

Do you engage in wishful thinking and disengage or deny that there is a problem? Or do you recognize that there is a difficulty and then deal with this? How? Do you find yourself getting 'stuck' in the problem and become focused on this? Or do you say to yourself that there are lots of possible ways out of the dilemma or situation?

Do you get caught up in all of the reasons why things may not work or may not be effective options? Or do you focus on your resources and the skills that you have accumulated in different situations in the past, and think of a way out of the situation?

....

Burnham (2005) suggests that we can easily map the route between 'problems', on the one hand, and 'possibilities', on the other (Figure 2.1). Rather than

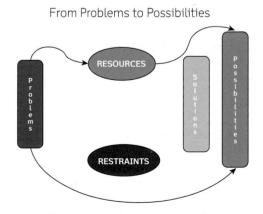

Figure 2.1 Burnham suggests we can move from problems to possibilities. © John Burnham.

speaking of 'solutions', which implies that there is just one correct way in which something may be resolved, he encourages us to think about our use of language and to open up a range of possible actions—hence the idea of 'possibilities'.

When we think in terms of 'possibilities', it also helps us to think more openly and flexibly, and so we can consider what our resources are to help move ahead or what the blocks are that get in the way (see Figure 2.1). We can think about our use of language, instead of using the word 'worrying' when describing our attitude to thinking about a difficulty or problem. Simply using different language and listening to the language that we use can, in itself, reshape or 'reframe' the way in which we think generally.

Using our thoughts and feelings to examine situations or behaviours is often considered under the umbrella term 'cognitive-behavioural' therapy (CBT). This is one of a range of psychological approaches to learning to deal with difficulties or problems. Although very popular—as recognized by the National Institute for Health and Clinical Excellence (NICE)—and seen to be effective in the management of a number of psychological conditions, it is not the only useful framework when considering psychological health. Research on therapies suggests that almost all therapeutic approaches work equally well and that the most important factor is a positive therapeutic alliance (Duncan et al., 2009).

Focusing on self-care and thought-traps

Below, we will consider different blocks to thinking constructively.

....

Read through the list and see if you can relate to some or all of them.
When have you found yourself using this style of thinking? What happened when you used this thinking style? How could you now challenge yourself to think differently about the situation?

....

Let us look at the problem or symptom first, and call it by its name. Then let us think about how it may happen in real life, and, finally, let us look at a possible alternative way—an 'antidote' to that way of behaving.

- **Overgeneralizing (that is, applying one instance to all)**
  For example, if one person in your team lets you down, you then conclude from this that everyone in your team will let you down—but this has not happened in reality: only one person has let you down. You can then begin to recognize the 'fact' or logical explanation, rather than the way in which you have interpreted the information. We may call this more effective response one of 'reflection' or of challenging the thoughts.
- **Catastrophizing (that is, blowing the situation out of proportion)**
  For example, you might not have reached your target or written all of the reports, or you may not have undertaken the audit work that you had hoped to do this month. You might think that not reaching your goal or target means that you are in the wrong job, which means that you have to find another job—and what happens if you do not find another job? You may then begin to ruminate and worry that you'll get sacked, and then you will lose your house, and then… Catastrophizing happens when your thinking spirals downwards negatively. You can jump to conclusions without there being any evidence for your thinking. Again, it is helpful to stand back and examine what is actually going on. You have only struggled to reach one particular goal; it does not mean all your work is poor. However, you will need to reassure, challenge, or refute the negative and self-defeating thinking.
- **Personalizing (that is, relating the situation back to yourself)**
  You may be in a meeting and someone may make an excellent point; you may then begin to wonder why you did not say that, or wish that you had… When you do this, you are automatically viewing yourself negatively and can find yourself in another negative spiral.

- Mind-reading (that is, assuming that you know what someone else is thinking or feeling)

For example, when you are making a point in a discussion and someone is looking away through the window, or is tapping their pencil on the table and not making eye contact with you, you might assume that they are not happy with what you are saying and so you stop, or become more self-conscious and lose confidence. How do you know that your listener is critical of you, or is unhappy or disagrees with what you are saying? Have you asked them? Very often, we make assumptions based on our own psychological baggage and experiences. By making assumptions, we can also easily get caught up in misunderstandings. We then begin to assume that we know what the person thinks or feels, without checking out the situation more fully and asking the person involved. When you notice yourself using these thought processes, you can encourage yourself to 'stand back'—to stop and think. Then you will be in a better position to confront or let go of those internal dialogues—'the mental video' or 'mind-chatter'—and you can begin to make choices: do you wish to continue the negative cycle or can you pull yourself out of it?

Cognitive-behavioural strategies

To manage some of the 'thought traps' highlighted above, there are several simple strategies to encourage self-management. One of the tools that can help to change habits is called 'reframing'. This involves taking an event and presenting it a different way. The key to this strategy is remembering to use it. You will need to consciously practise it, so that it becomes a habit itself, and you can then call on it in stressful situations. Reframing is about how you think about the situation: it is viewing the situation from another perspective. For example, when climbing up a hill, you can only see one part of the view—but when you get to the top of the hill, you can see all around. You are seeing views that you can only see from the top. Reframing is

like this: it is about seeing *more* of the picture. Rather than focusing on one aspect, encourage yourself to think differently.

Physical health aspects

As mentioned before, sleep, exercise, and diet are cornerstones for health and well-being, and self-care should not ignore these aspects—particularly when considering the impact of shift work.

Undisturbed sleep is essential for people who work nights and long hours. It is important to get good sleep, to undertake exercise regularly, and to eat and drink correctly. Developing a sleep routine and establishing as steady a pattern as you can is essential for people working nights. A light snack (such as sandwich, toast, cereal) before going to sleep may help to increase the duration of your sleep. Consider blackout curtains and earplugs if you are sensitive to light and noise. Try to get between six and eight hours of sleep every 24 hours, and watch for the effects of napping both during the day and at night.

Regarding exercise, it is important to get regular physical and active exercise, which promotes better physical, emotional, and mental health: physically, because it impacts on heart, circulation, and energy levels, and affects appearance and weight; emotionally, because it improves motivation, and is calming and relaxing; and psychologically, because it affects concentration and alertness, and helps you to focus more clearly.

Also remember to take diet and eating habits into account, especially when working at night. Try to avoid eating heavy meals (especially rich, spicy, and fatty foods) before and during working hours. Stick to snacks and protein foods, as well as vegetables and fruit. Remember that alcohol, caffeine, and nicotine harm sleep and stimulate the nervous system rather than relax you.

Taking it further

To think about the subject personally and to apply the core principles around self-care, take a few moments to consider what you need to do to enhance your self-care (for example, through internal and external factors, focusing on mental, emotional, social, or spiritual sources of support). You may like to use the questions in **Box 2.3** to promote your own self-care.

Developing resilience

To round off the chapter on well-being and self-care, a final point of focus: resilience. The concept of resilience has been around for a long time: for example, the work of Kobasa (1979) on hardiness and Antonovsky (1979; 1987) on salutogenesis. More recently, Padesky (2009) examined it within a cognitive-behavioural framework. She suggests that there are six categories or dimensions: the cognitive; the physical; the emotional; the social-relational; the environmental; the spiritual; and the moral. These have an impact on an individual's ability to address problems and to develop optimism, based on the degree to which an individual is aware of, and can access, use, and develop these dimensions (see **Box 2.4**).

Psychological flexibility is the key in relation to resilience. McCracken (2005) suggests that the mechanism by which largely verbally based processes (thoughts and beliefs, attributions) mix with direct experiences (what we

Box 2.3 Reframing a challenging situation

Questions that you can ask yourself to encourage this wider thinking include:
- how else can I view this situation?
- how can I balance this perspective?
- if I were [someone else], how would they see the situation? (For this question, choose someone who has a tendency to think differently from you.)
- does this happen regularly? If not, it may be the exception to the rule rather than 'the rule': for example, if your manager cancels a meeting in an unusually abrupt manner, you can reframe that by recognizing that they are under pressure and feel overwhelmed with demands. The manager's postponement of the meeting may then be seen as them being honest with you.

Box 2.4 Promoting your own self-care

- What can you do to further your awareness of self-care?
- When is it self-care and when is it self-indulgence?
- How do you separate out the personal pressures from the work-related challenges?
- Where do you go for help?
- What sources of support are there (informational, skills-based, emotional)?

attend to, often seeking confirmation of our habitual thoughts and beliefs) and exert restricting influences on behaviour (stop us from changing). He proposes that these are contextually determined and result in psychological inflexibility. This is because we pay so much attention to the wrong things (Flaxman, 2009).

To counter this and develop resilience there are a range of interventions possible. These include personal development, therapeutic input, training and education, focusing on the physical, mental, emotional, and spiritual. Resilience is promoted by developing a wide range of possible actions, including the use of mindfulness training (Baer, 2003; Flaxman and Bond, 2006; Hayes et al., 2004; Kabat-Zinn, 1990). Resilience is underpinned by the way in which we make sense of life and create meaning, and this spiritual dimension forms the basis of the work of Frankl (2004). He emphasizes that we have a freedom to choose, even though circumstances may often significantly limit the range of options. (For more on spirituality and care, see McSherry, 2006, and Chapter 8.) Like any other endeavour, improving resilience skills involves learning, and choosing to engage in a process of change, growth, and development. Interventions may focus on recognizing skills and abilities, developing and using supportive relationships, social networks, or physical or community activities, or focusing on effective problem-solving.

Conclusion

Health care is rewarding, but challenging, and as the healthcare context continues to change, thinking about self-care can protect us from harm. Self-care is of pivotal importance in order to manage the tricky balance between the demands that you experience as a nurse and the resources that you have available to you. These are internal, interpersonal, and external, and need to be recognized and dealt with using a variety of tools and techniques at individual, team, and organizational levels. There is a range of creative ways in which to look after ourselves at work that we have described for you in this chapter; a mixture of approaches works best. The role of nurses in nurturing and caring for sick people needs to be supported to ensure that nurses remain effective and well. Self-care means taking individual responsibility for this and making sure that the balance in your life ensures that you gain as much satisfaction from your work as you hoped you might when you first started.

References

Antonovsky, A. (1979) *Health, Stress and Coping*, San Francisco, CA: Jossey-Bass.

Antonovsky, A. (1987) *Unraveling the Mystery of Health: How People Manage Stress and Stay Well*, San Francisco, CA: Jossey-Bass.

Baer, R.A. (2003) 'Mindfulness training as a clinical intervention: A conceptual and empirical review', *Clinical Psychology Science and Practice* 10: 125–43.

Bandura, A. (1995) *Self-Efficacy in Changing Society*, Cambridge: Cambridge University Press.

Berne, E. (1964) *Games People Play: The Psychology of Human Relationships*, New York: Ballantine Books.

Burnham, J. (2005) 'Relational flexibility: A tool for socially constructing therapeutic relationships', in C. Flaskas, B. Mason, and A. Perlerz (eds) *The Space Between*, London: Karnac, pp. 1–17.

Charles, S.C, Wilbert, J.R., and Franke, K.J. (1985) 'Sued and non-sued physicians' self reported reactions to malpractice litigation', *American Journal of Psychiatry* 192(4): 437–40.

Confederation of British Industry (1997) *Managing Absence: In Sickness and in Health*, London: CBI.

Cooper, C.L. and Cartwright, S. (2001) 'A strategic approach to organizational stress management', in P.A. Hancock and P.A. Desmond (eds) *A Strategic Approach to Organizational Stress Management*, Hillsdale, NJ: Lawrence Earlbaum Associates, pp. 235–48.

Cooper, C.L., Field, J., Goswami, U., Jenkins, R., and Sahakian, B.J., (2010) *Mental Capital and Wellbeing*, Oxford: Wiley-Blackwell.

DeFrank, R.S. and Cooper, C.L. (1987) 'Worksite stress management interventions: Their effectiveness and conceptualisation', *Journal of Managerial Psychology* 2: 4–10.

Duncan, B.L., Miller, S., Wampole, B., and Hubble, M. (2009) *Heart and Soul of Change: What Works in Therapy*, Washington DC: American Psychological Association.

Firth-Cozens, J. and Payne, R. (1999) *Stress in Health Professionals*, Chichester: John Wiley & Sons.

Flaxman, P.E. (2009) Promoting Individual Resilience through Psychological Flexibility and Recovery. Conference presentation at Royal Free Hospital London, September 2009.

Flaxman, P.E. and Bond, F.W. (2006) 'Acceptance and commitment therapy in the workplace', in R.A. Baer (ed) *Mindfulness-based Treatment Approaches*, San Diego, CA: Elsevier, pp. 281–306.

Frankl, V.E. (2004) *Man's Search for Meaning. An Introduction to Logotherapy*, London: Random House/Rider.

Freudenberger, H.J. (1974) 'Staff burn-out', *Journal of Social Issues* 30: 159–66.

Goleman, D. (1995) *Emotional Intelligence: Why it can Matter More than IQ*, New York: Bantam Books.

Grandey, A.A. (2000) 'Emotional Regulation in the Work-place: A New Way to Conceptualise Emotional Labor'. *Journal of Occupational Health Psychology* 5(1): 95–110.

Hayes, S.C., Follette, V.M., and Linehan, M. (2004) *Mindfulness, Acceptance, and Relationship: Expanding the Cognitive Behavioral Tradition*, New York: Guilford Press.

Hochschild, A.R. (1983) *The Managed Heart: Commercial-ization of Human Feeling*, Berkeley, CA: University of California Press.

Johnson, J.V. and Hall, E.M. (1988) 'Job strain, workplace social support and cardiovascular disease: A cross-sectional study of a random sample of the Swedish working population', *American Journal of Public Health* 78: 1336–42.

Johnson, J.V., Stewart, W., Hall, E.M., Fredland, P., and Theorell, T. (1996) 'Long-term psychosocial environment and cardiovascular mortality among Swedish women', *American Journal of Public Health* 86: 324–31.

Kabat-Zinn, J. (1990) *Full Catastrophe Living: Using the Wisdom of your Body and Mind to Face Stress, Pain and Illness*, New York: Delta.

Karasek, R.A. (1979) 'Job demands, job decision latitude and mental strain: Implications for job redesign', *Administrative Science Quarterly* 24: 285–306.

Karasek, R.A. (1990) 'Lower health risk with increasing job control among white-collar workers', *Journal of Organisational Behaviour* 11: 171–85.

Kobasa, S.C. (1979) 'Stressful life events, personality, and health: An inquiry into hardiness', *Journal of Personality and Social Psychology* 37(1): 1–11.

Kohn, L., Corrigan, J., and Donaldson, M. (1999) *To Err is Human: Building a Safer Health System*, Washington DC: Institute of Medicine.

Lazarus, R. and Folkman, S. (1984) *Stress, Appraisal and Coping*, New York: Springer.

Maslach, C. (1982) *Burnout: The Cost of Caring*, Englewood Cliffs, NJ: Prentice Hall.

Maslach, C. (2003) 'Job burnout: New directions in research and intervention', *Current Directions in Psychological Science* 12: 189–92.

McCracken, L.M. (2005) *Contextual Cognitive-Behavioral Therapy for Chronic Pain*, Seattle, WA: IASP Press.

McSherry, W. (2006) *Making Sense of Spirituality in Nursing and Health Care Practice: An Interactive Approach*, 2nd edn, London: Jessica Kingsley.

McVicar, A. (2003) 'Workplace Stress in Nursing: A literature review'. *Journal of Advanced Nursing* 44(6): 633–42.

Miller, K.I., Ellis, B.H., Zook, E.G., and Lyles, J.S. (1990) 'An integrated model of communication, stress and burnout in the workplace', *Communication Research* 17(3): 300–26.

Padesky, C. (2009) 'Uncover strengths and build resilience', Workshop presented at Institute of Education, University of London, London, 15–16 June.

Quick, J.C. and Tetrick, L.E. (2003) *Handbook of Occupational Health Psychology*, Washington DC: American Psychological Association.

Rego, A., Godhino, L., McQueen, A., and Pina e Cunha, M. (2010) 'Emotional intelligence and caring behaviour in nursing', *Service Industries Journal*, 30(9): 1419–37.

Robertson, I.T., Tinline, G., and Robertson., S. (2007) 'Enhancing staff well-being for organisational effectiveness', in R.J. Burke and C.L. Cooper (eds) *Building More Effective Organisations*, Cambridge: Cambridge University Press.

Rotter, J. (1966) 'Generalized expectancies for internal versus external control of reinforcements', *Psychological Monographs* 80(609): all.

Salovey, P. and Mayer, J.D. (1990) 'Emotional intelligence', *Imagination, Cognition and Personality* 9: 185–201.

Seligman, M.E. (1974) 'Depression and learned helplessness', in R.J. Friedman and M.M. Katz (eds) *The Psychology of Depression: Contemporary Theory and Research*, New York: Winston-Wiley, pp. 83–113.

Seligman, M.E. (2002) *Authentic Happiness: Using the New Positive Psychology to Realize Your Potential for Lasting Fulfillment*, New York: Free Press/Simon and Schuster.

Wall, T.D., Bolden, R.I., and Borrill, C.S. (1997) 'Minor psychiatric disorder in NHS Trust staff: Occupational and gender differences', *British Journal of Psychiatry* 171: 519–23.

Williams, S., Michie, S., and Pattani, S. (1999) *Improving the Health of the NHS Workforce: Report of the Partnership on the Health of the NHS Workforce*, London: The Nuffield Trust.

Wilson, R.M., Runciman, W.B., Gibbard, R.W., Harrison, B.T., Newby, L., and Hamilton, J.D. (1995) 'The quality in Australian health care study', *Medical Journal of Australia* 163(4): 458–71.

Wren, B. and Michie, S. (2003) 'Staff experience of the healthcare system', in S. Llewelyn and P. Kennedy (eds) *Handbook of Clinical Health Psychology*, Chichester: John Wiley & Sons Ltd, pp. 41–60.

Wren, B., Schwartz, A., Allen, C., Boyd, J., Gething, N., Hill-Tout, J., Jennings, T., Morrison, L., and Pullen, A. (2006) 'Developing occupational health psychology services in healthcare settings', in S. McIntyre and J. Houdmont (eds) *Occupational Health Psychology: European Perspectives on Research, Education and Practice*, Nottingham: Nottingham University Press, pp. 177–204.

Wright, S.G. (2005) *Burnout: A Spiritual Crisis*, Harrow: RCN Publishing/*Nursing Standard*.

Wright, T. and Cropanzano, R. (2001) 'The role of psychological well-being in job performance: A fresh look at an age-old guest', *Organizational Dynamics* 33(4): 338–51.

Zimbardo, P.G. (1977) *Shyness: What it is, What to do about it*, Reading, MA: Addison-Wesley.

3 Quality of nursing care

ROBERT McSHERRY

Learning outcomes

This chapter will enable you to:

- outline the drivers for quality care;
- define what we mean by 'quality nursing care';
- detail quality care systems and processes;
- explore how you measure and document the provision of quality care;
- document the provision of quality care; and
- highlight and access support in the provision of quality care.

Introduction

My mother kept soiling the bed and we had to beg nurses to come and change the bed.
(Mid Staffordshire NHS Foundation Trust Inquiry, 2010)

It is imperative that nurses can appreciate what quality nursing care is and is not. The chapter addresses some fundamental questions: what are the drivers for quality nursing care? How do you know you are delivering quality care? Of what quality systems and processes are you aware? How do you measure nursing care? How are patients and carers involved, and how do their experiences feed back to celebrate when things are going well or to improve nursing care when things are not as good as they could be? What support and resources are available to enable nurses to provide quality nursing care?

The chapter will *not* cover how to measure and present the impact and outcomes of care, because these will be highlighted in Chapters 16 and 17.

Reflective questions and case studies will be used to encourage you to reflect on clinical situations and, in turn, to help you to reflect positively and constructively upon your *own* nursing practice. These reflections will enable you to build up a comprehensive knowledge, understanding, and confidence to support you in the provision of people-centred, quality nursing care.

Essential knowledge and skills for care

- You will deliver safe, confident, competent, compassionate quality care, whilst maintaining dignity and respect of people at all times.

- You must ensure individualized, personalized, people-centred care by engaging with individuals and empowering them to make informed decisions and choices.

- You will demonstrate professional accountable practice in which honesty, openness, and trust ensure that personal attitudes, beliefs, prejudices, judgements, and/or experiences do not compromise the provision of quality care.

- You will communicate effectively and sensitively with individuals and colleagues by listening and by responding to verbal and non verbal cues, along with factually recording information within documentation.

- You will use a variety of strategies and associated frameworks/tools to evaluate the effectiveness of your care, treatments, and or interventions, by taking account of people's and carers' interpretations of the their lived experiences, and of the impact of outcomes on health and well-being.

- You will challenge discriminatory attitudes and behaviours, along with inadequate or unacceptable standards and practices of nursing care and services.

The chapter is designed to support you in delivering safe, confident, competent, compassionate quality care and to help you to evaluate the quality of the care provided. The chapter will also help you to develop the essential knowledge and skills for care identified overleaf.

Drivers for quality nursing care

'Delivering safe, confident, competent, and compassionate quality care' should be the primary goal of every single registered and non-registered nurse, but sadly this is not the case. Unfortunately, the image of the nursing profession has been globally affected through news and mediated reports suggesting that nurses do not care, have lost the ability to care, do not have the knowledge, skills, and confidence to care, and are even too educated to care or 'posh to wash'. Some of the headlines making the news and media include.

- 'Nurses should be more caring to restore public confidence: Report' (Smith, 2010);
- 'Patients "demeaned" by poor-quality nursing care' (Boseley, 2009);
- 'Basic care "lacking" in hospitals' (Mair, 2009);
- 'Patients Association brands NHS nurses "cruel and demeaning"' (Nursing Times, 2009)
- 'Poor dementia care in hospitals costing lives and hundreds of millions' (Alzheimer's Society, 2009).

This unsatisfactory image and growing public perception is surely a misconception originating from a small minority that cannot and should not be allowed to affect the majority of registered and non-registered nurses who deliver safe, confident, competent, and compassionate quality care—a point echoed by Dame Chris Beasley, Chief Nursing Officer, who states:

> **The National Health Service (NHS) treats millions of people every day and the vast majority of patients experience good quality, safe and effective care.**   (Mair, 2009)

Sadly for the majority of conscientious, caring, and compassionate registered and non-registered nurses, the phrase 'poor care' has become a mainstream media headline that has to be dispelled if we are to restore the true image of nursing for the future. The phrase 'poor

care' is highlighted in the report of the Mid Staffordshire NHS Foundation Trust Inquiry (2010), known as the 'Francis Report', which regrettably provides a litany of patient accounts, experiences, and stories to which the phrase 'poor care' is applied. Similarly, the report by the Prime Minister's Commission on the Future of Nursing and Midwifery in England (2010: 26) argues that:

> **poor care is damaging and even deadly to its recipients, and undermines confidence in services and care-givers. Some employers see cost and quality as trade-offs, but we think the best care is provided at the least cost to the organization. 'It is poor care which brings added financial burdens to the health care organization', the RCN told us. 'Money is not saved by reducing nursing numbers and diluting skill mix.**

The challenge facing registered and non-registered nurses globally is to dispel the unfortunate imagery surrounding the provision of quality care in order to reaffirm our status and confidence with the public and professional bodies in having the ability to adhere to our professional codes of practice. The primary basis of this must be a focus on respecting individuals' rights and preserving dignity by delivering safe, confident, competent, and compassionate quality care. The Nursing and Midwifery Council's Code (NMC, 2010) argues that registered nurses and midwives should '*make the care of people your first concern, treating them as individuals and respecting their dignity*'. Similarly, the International Council of Nurses (ICN, 2010: 1) states that '*inherent in nursing is respect for human rights, including cultural rights, the right to life and choice, to dignity and to be treated with respect*'. What exactly do we mean by 'quality nursing care' and why is it imperative that, as a student and or registered nurse, you ensure that this happens in practice?

Defining 'quality nursing care'

Everyone has a right to receive quality nursing care. The provision of quality nursing care according to Lynn et al. (2007: 159) '*is the right of all patients and the responsibility of all nurses*'. Yet the reality of this happening for all patients is not the case. The King's College London National Nursing Research Unit (2008: 1–2) suggests that the failure of nurses to provide quality nursing care might be attributed to the fact that nursing and nurses struggle to articulate what 'quality nursing care' is and how they can best ensure its delivery. Taking into account Lynn et al. (2007), King's College London National Nursing Research Unit (2008), and the Department of Health (2008) *High Quality Care For All: NHS Next Stage Review Final Report* (the 'Lord Darzi Review'), in order to understand what quality nursing care is and involves, it is imperative to develop a definition of 'quality nursing care'.

....

Write down what you understand by the term quality nursing care.
Read on and compare your answers with the definitions that follow.

....

In order to define what quality nursing care is and involves, it is imperative to define what nursing is and what nurses do. Nursing, according to the ICN (2010):

> **encompasses autonomous and collaborative care of individuals of all ages, families, groups and communities, sick or well and in all settings. Nursing includes the promotion of health, prevention of illness, and the care of ill, disabled and dying people. Advocacy, promotion of a safe environment, research, participation in shaping health policy and in patient and health systems management, and education are also key nursing roles.**

The American Nurses Association (ANA, 2004) defines nursing as:

> **the protection, promotion, and optimization of health and abilities, prevention of illness and injury, alleviation of suffering through the diagnosis and treatment of human response, and advocacy in the care of individuals, families, communities, and populations.**

The Royal College of Nursing (RCN, 2003: 14) suggests that:

> **nursing is the use of clinical judgement in the provision of care to enable people to improve, maintain, or recover health, to cope with health problems, and to achieve the best possible quality of life, whatever their disease or disability, until death.**

A review of the above definitions of nursing suggests that the ultimate goal of every nurse should be the delivery of efficient and effective, safe, quality person-centred care through involving the patient/carer/user and other relevant heath and social care professionals in promoting quality life until death.

Having highlighted what nursing is and involves, it is important to distinguish the fact that defining 'nursing' and defining 'quality nursing', while similar because many core themes and elements emerge associated with care, are distinctly different. Put simply and succinctly, defining 'nursing' is about what nursing is and involves. Defining 'quality nursing care' is about demonstrating what nurses do as they go about their daily practice and the impact that this has on the patient, carer, and/or significant others.

Defining quality nursing according to the works of Burhans and Alligood (2010), Lynn et al. (2007), Larrabee and Bolden (2001), and Irurita (1999) is dependent on two important perspectives: what nurses themselves perceive quality nursing care to be and what those who are in receipt of it perceive it to be. McCormack and McCance (2006) suggest that quality nursing is associated with the development of a holistic therapeutic person-centred relationship between the nurse, patient, and significant others. Similarly, the King's College London National Nursing Research Unit (2008) reveals several significant core elements akin to the provision of good quality nursing care (see **Table 3.1**).

Table 3.1 is useful in that it highlights the fact that good quality nursing care is dependent on nurses and students:

- knowing what the core elements are and how these influence their ability to provide quality nursing care;
- being able to identify and articulate what the core elements mean; and
- having the ability to relate and apply the core elements in practice.

Table 3.1 Core elements influencing the provision of quality nursing care (adapted from King's College London National Nursing Research Unit, 2008)

Core element	Core element defined	Relevance to nursing practice
Holistic approach	The provision of a holistic approach to the assessment of the physical, mental, spiritual, and emotional needs of the patient, and in the provision of patient-centred and continuous care	Informs the ongoing nursing assessment and associated care plans/processes
Patient empowerment	Involves ensuring the efficiency and effectiveness of care, combined with ensuring humanity and compassion by engaging and involving the patient, carer, and significant other, including offering choices and options associated with care and services	Essential in communications, and in ensuring engagement and a partnerships approach to the provision of care
Professional accountability	The provision of professional, high-quality evidence-based practice	To ensure that practice complies the NMC Code (NMC, 2010) and your contract of employment, it is imperative that you maintain your knowledge and skills through engaging with best evidence
Patient safety	The delivery, continual maintenance, and monitoring of care and interventions to ensure a safe environment and efficient and effective services	Ensuring safety of patients/carers/public and other professionals is a major part of the role and responsibility a registered nurse/midwife
Integrated teamwork	Working within a multidisciplinary team to provide the patient with seamless care	Promotes optimal team work and an appreciation of roles and responsibilities, thus avoids conflicts within the care provided
Efficiency and effectiveness	Providing the best possible safe patient care and experience for the best costs	Encourages focusing on the provision and evaluation of quality care, and the impact on achieving the best possible outcomes for the patient

The Department of Health (2010b: 2) further exemplifies the core elements for the provision of quality nursing care by indicating that:

> quality is at the heart of everything we do in the modern health service, and frontline nurses play a vital role in achieving the quality of care that people expect. We can only deliver consistently safe and effective patient centred care with the full involvement of those nurses and other health professionals who provide the care.

Based on the works of McCormack and McCance (2006), the King's College London National Nursing Research Unit (2008), and the Department of Health (2010b), quality nursing care could be defined as in **Box 3.1**.

Box 3.1 Defining 'quality nursing care'

... as patients want to be treated well, to know their nurse is knowledgeable, skilled and competent, to have high quality care every time and want nurses to have a humane attitude, make them feel safe and comfortable—'*cared about*' as well as '*cared for*'. The attitude and approach of the nurse is the most important factor in securing this experience for patients, enabling them to be '*treated as a human being not a case*' with compassion, respect, [dignity], empathy and by staff who are 'interested in YOU'.

(Adapted from King's College London National Nursing Research Unit, 2008: 1–2)

The above definition of 'quality nursing care' high-lights that the provision of quality nursing care is not negotiable or optional, but a must. As a registered nurse, midwife, and/or student nurse, quality nursing care is interwoven and entwined within our professional codes of practice, contracts of employment, professional accountability, and roles and responsibilities. Quality nursing care is about assuring, ensuring, and acquiring the information that ensures the dignity of each individual within our contact is uncompromised. Quality nursing care involves the development of a holistic, therapeutic, person-centred relationship acknowledging and respecting the uniqueness of each individual, involving them as equal partners in every aspect of the caring relationship founded on the core elements of a holistic approach, patient empowerment, professional accountability, patient safety, integrated teamwork, and efficiency and effectiveness.

The provision of quality nursing care is associated with the way in which we communicate and interact with our patients, carers, service users, and professional colleagues. Attitudes, behaviours, and the way in which we listen, respond and interact are fundamental to ensuring quality. As reported by the Prime Minister's Commission on the Future of Nursing and Midwifery in England (2010: 58):

Front-line nurses and midwives should be visible guardians of quality and safety, and take control of the supervisions and monitoring of care within and across teams and throughout the care

pathway. All directors of nursing, heads of midwifery and other nurses and midwives in senior management roles should accept individual managerial and professional accountability for ensuring their organisation provides high quality care.

Considering this alongside Department of Health (2008; 2010b) and the Francis Report (Mid Stafford-shire NHS Foundation Trust Inquiry, 2010), it is clearly imperative that quality becomes central to all that we do.

PRACTICE TIP

Remember that, as a registered nurse, midwife, or student nurse, you are professionally accountable for providing safe, quality care, and for ensuring, assuring, and demonstrating that this happens for yourself, your patients, your employer, and professional bodies.

Exercise 3.1 Checking your readiness for the quality challenge and provision of quality nursing care

Having identified what nursing is and involves, and what nurses do, Table 3.2 provides you with a series of statements to complete and the compare to see if you are up to the quality challenge and the provision of quality nursing care. Tick the appropriate box and compare your findings at the end of the activity.

Feedback

If you have ticked 'Agree' to every question, then you are well on your way to knowing and showing the fact that quality nursing care involves all of the statements above.

If you have only agreed with several statements, then it is imperative that you take time to explore and develop your knowledge, understanding, and skills associated with what quality nursing care is and involves, and how this can be demonstrated in practice. Reviewing Table 3.3 may support you in developing your knowledge and understanding surrounding the provision of quality nursing care in the future.

Table 3.2 Quality nursing care checklist

Question no.	Statement	Agree	Disagree
1	Quality nursing care is dependent on knowing what nursing is and what nurses do.		
2	Defining quality nursing care is highly challenging and complicated because it is linked to so many of the core elements of nursing.		
3	Providing quality nursing care is an integral part of every nurse's professional code of practice, contract of employment, professional accountability, and roles and responsibility.		
4	Quality nursing care is dependent on developing an honest, open, transparent person-centred relationship between patients, carers, and significant others.		
5	The provision of quality nursing care is about listening and responding to the experience of people.		
6	Quality nursing care requires leadership, team working, collaboration, and engagement with people.		
7	The best way of establishing the quality of nursing care is through directly asking the patient, carer, and significant others, in conjunction with the nurses providing the care.		
8	Providing quality nursing care is everyone's responsibility and does not happen in isolation.		
9	Ensuring and assuring quality nursing care is dependent on having sufficient support and resources from leaders and managers.		
10	Ensuring dignity with respect is regarded as an integral part of quality nursing care and should be your number one priority.		

In order to achieve the core element 'quality nursing care' identified in Box 3.1, there is a fundamental need to know and understand what care quality systems and processes are available for you to access and apply in practice.

Quality care systems and processes

The Nursing Midwifery Council (2010) *The Code: Standards of Conduct, Performance and Ethics for Nurses and Midwives* argues that, as a practising registered nurse and midwife, a major part of our professional

Table 3.3 Quality nursing care checklist feedback

Question no.	Statement	Rationale and relevance to the provision of quality nursing care
1	Quality nursing care is dependent on knowing what nursing is and what nurses do.	To provide quality nursing care, it is imperative that you are able to articulate and demonstrate what nursing is and involves, and are able to highlight the impact that your caring has on someone's health and well-being.
2	Defining quality nursing care is highly challenging and complicated because it is linked to so many of the core elements of nursing.	The provision of quality nursing care is dependent on having sound leadership and management, effective team working and communication, patient and user/carer participation, and evaluation. It also depends on identifying and dealing with risks and robust systems of information governance for accessing and recording strong information, and record-keeping.
3	Providing quality nursing care is an integral part of every nurse's professional code of practice, contract of employment, professional accountability, and roles and responsibility.	The provision of caring and compassionate quality nursing care is not optional, but an integral part of your contract of employment, roles and responsibility, and code of practice. Ensuring the provision of safe patient care and challenging inadequate standards of care is essential.
4	Quality nursing care is dependent on developing an honest, open, transparent person-centred relationship between patients, carers, and significant others.	The establishment of a holistic people-centred relationship to caring— based on the principles of honesty, openness, and transparency with the patient, carer, users, the public, and professional colleagues—is a major component of assuring patient safety and quality care.
5	The provision of quality nursing care is about listening and responding to the experience of people.	Effective communication is about listening and responding to feedback and informing people of the outcomes.
6	Quality nursing care requires leadership, team working, collaboration, and engagement with people.	Demonstrating sound leadership and developing integrated team working through engaging and involving the patient, carers, users, and various members of the team is a major part of delivering and establishing quality.

(continued)

Table 3.3 (*continued*)

Question no.	Statement	Rationale and relevance to the provision of quality nursing care
7	The best way of establishing the quality of nursing care is through directly asking the patient, carer, and significant others, in conjunction with the nurses providing the care.	Seeking the lived experience of patients, carers, and significant others in conjunction with the nurses' opinions about the provision and standards of care is imperative.
8	Providing quality nursing care is everyone's responsibility and does not happen in isolation.	Quality requires the involvement of the team and is everyone's responsibility.
9	Ensuring and assuring quality nursing care is dependent on having sufficient support and resources from leaders and managers.	Having and seeking the support of leaders and managers is important in ensuring quality care.
10	Ensuring dignity with respect is regarded as an integral part of quality nursing care and should be your number one priority.	Dignity with respect for all should always be provided and maintained.

accountable role and responsibility is to '*provide a high standard of practice and care at all times*' (ibid: 6). The statement is profound, because it implies that providing quality nursing care is a duty, expectation, and non-negotiable regardless of the time of day, complexity of organizational cultures and working environment, or settings in which we deliver and care for our patients, carers, and/or significant others, including fellow colleagues and professionals. Ensuring quality nursing care, according to the NMC (ibid), requires you to '*Use the best available evidence; Keep your skills and knowledge up to date; Keep clear and accurate records.*'

....

Before reading any further, jot down what quality systems and processes are available to support you in your practice.
Now read on and compare your notes with the following.
....

Do not be surprised if, initially, you find it difficult to answer the above reflective question. Several reasons may account for the challenges. You may not be familiar with the terminology and jargon often associated with defining and outlining quality care systems and processes

within health and social care. The terms and phrases may have been incorporated into a broader concept as part of your nurse education and training—for example, clinical governance, evidence-informed nursing, accountability, etc—so that you find it hard to isolate them from the integrated approach to care. You may not have been provided with the necessary information to inform your knowledge, understanding, skills, confidence, and competence. You may have chosen to focus on other important aspects of nursing. Or you may be well informed about quality systems and processes. Whatever your response is to the above reflective question, it is imperative to reiterate the following.

As a registered nurse, midwife, and or student nurse, it is fundamentally important that, as part of your daily practice, your number one priority must be to '*make the care of people your first concern, treating them as individuals and respecting their dignity*' (NMC, 2010: 2) and to ensure that you practise professionally and safely, and have the knowledge, skills, competence, and confidence to continue to work and stay within the NMC Code (ibid: 6) by '*provide[ing a] high standard of practice and care at all times*'.

Quality care systems and processes are designed to improve, monitor, safeguard, protect, assure, evaluate, and evidence outcomes of care. Recently, there has been a shift towards emphasizing quality nursing because '*there is ongoing professional concern that nursing's contribution to quality healthcare is under-recognised, leaving nursing services vulnerable to cost-reducing efforts*' (Maben and Griffiths, 2008: 18). Ultimately, the future of nursing will depend on registered nurses and midwives having the ability to '*adapt how they work and what they do. To demonstrate the benefit and contribution of nursing means having the right information by collecting new evidence in new ways*' (Department of Health, 2010b: 13). Providing quality nursing care is more than just knowing what it means. As a registered nurse, midwife, and/or student nurse, it is imperative that you know and understand what 'quality' means, and how to ascertain and assure that it is delivered, and how to assess the impact that this has on the patient and wider practice setting.

Best and Neuhauser (2010: 472) rightfully position Avedis Donabedian as the 'father of quality assurance'. Through his article 'Evaluating the quality of medical care', Donabedian (1966) provided the health community with a quality framework that is known throughout the world. Donabedian argued that establishing the quality of health care could be undertaken by focusing on measuring structure, process, and outcome. The Nursing Management (2010) 'Quality assurance in nursing: Standards' describe structure, process, and outcomes in the following way.

- **Structure** is associated with the setting up of an organization such as the National Health Service and associated goals in which nursing is implemented. For example, does an NHS trust have a clear vision and how is this cascaded to influence the delivery of care at a divisional, department/directorate, ward, and individual level? The ward may have developed a philosophy of care or a mission statement incorporating the wider organizational goals of which the team are aware, and may have integrated information outlining how quality is to be provided and experienced by the patient, carer, service users, and associated professional colleagues. Establishing the impact, or evaluating a structural standard, of quality nursing care should therefore focus on highlighting what a registered nurse, midwife, student nurse does and the environment in which care is provided.

- **Process** is about the delivery of quality nursing care and the specific nursing actions or omissions of nursing actions akin to the activity, intervention, procedure, and technique performed, and how this is experienced by the patient. Process standards are essentially about observing and measuring the effectiveness of a registered nurse, midwife, and student nurse, and their knowledge, skills, and competence, along with the level of interaction, engagement, and participation of the patient in practice, for example the safe administration of a medicine to the patient.

- **Outcomes** are standards about capturing, measuring, and demonstrating the impact of a registered nurse, midwife, and student nurse's activity, intervention, procedure, and/or technique on changing the patient's health and well-being or social care status. Quality standards identify and reflect the effectiveness and outcomes of the process of providing care, for example the timely management and prevention of pressure ulcers where the registered nurse, midwife, and/or student nurse undertakes a detailed risk assessment of the patient's risk factors of developing pressure ulcers. The care plan involves the use of appropriate pressure-relieving equipment, improved fluid intake, nutrition, and mobilization. The outcome is the avoidable occurrence of pressure ulcers, improved patient care and quality of life, along with the avoided costs of treating a hospital-acquired pressure sore and the associated complications for the organization.

> **PRACTICE TIP**
>
> The importance of familiarizing oneself with what quality nursing care is and involves, and how it can be measured by focusing attention on structure, process, and/or outcomes, is such that it cannot be left to chance. Chapter 10 offers useful insights into how pathways of care can help in designing, implementing, and evaluating standards of care.

Every aspect of nursing and midwifery care could essentially be framed around structure, process, and outcome, as **Practice Example 3.1** illustrates.

The practice example illustrates fundamental issues and concerns about patient safety, safeguarding vulnerable adults, quality, and standards of care for the patient, to name but a few.

By focusing on structure, process, and outcome, it is possible to create a picture of key questions to address the issues and concerns arising in Practice Example 3.1 (see **Box 3.2**). The same can be done for a situation that has gone well and in which an accolade has been received and acknowledged for the quality of nursing care. The fundamental message from Practice Example 3.1 is the fact that patient safety and quality nursing care is about learning from incidents, events, complaints, and accolades, and escalating issues and concerns as they occur, not after the event.

Clinical governance (CG) offers a useful framework for the provision of quality care. This is because CG is defined by McSherry and Pearce (2010) as '*a robust framework that acknowledges the importance of adopting a culture of shared accountability for sustaining and improving the quality of services and outcomes for both patients and staff*'. Similarly, McSherry and Haddock (1998) indicate that CG is:

ultimately an umbrella term for all the issues and concepts that clinicians, non clinicians, mangers and board members know and foster, including standard setting, risk management, patient safety, user involvement, performance management, clinical audit, training, reflection and continuous professional development.

Box 3.2 Structure, process, and outcomes

Structure

This is associated with the purpose and remit of the team and organizations in delivering care.

- What are the vision and goals of the AMAU in Practice Example 3.1?
- What is the mission statement and philosophy of the unit?
- What are the attitudes and behaviours of staff in providing and maintaining care and quality?

Process

Is associated with delivering quality nursing care and the specific nursing actions or omissions of nursing actions akin to the activity, intervention, procedure, technique performed, and how this is experienced by the patient.

- Why didn't the nursing assessment and associated care plan implemented and evaluated detect the patient's problems?
- What about the safe administration of a medicine to the patient?
- And what of the nutritional assessment of the patient?

Outcomes

These involve standards about capturing, measuring, and demonstrating the impact of a registered nurse, midwife, and student nurse's activity, intervention, procedure, and/or technique on changing the patient's health and well-being or social care status.

- Was the nursing assessment and care plan completed and evaluated?
- Was the administration of medication timely?
- Were medications changed to suit the needs of the patient?

PRACTICE EXAMPLE 3.1

Identifying quality nursing care by focusing on a framework of structure, process, and outcome

Mr A, a 78-year-old gentleman, was admitted to the acute medical admissions unit (AMAU) with difficulty mobilizing, and eating and drinking, due to an exacerbation of his Parkinson's disease. The patient informed the nursing and medical staff that he was having difficulty swallowing, and had been unable to take oral medication for the past two days. The patient was assessed and admitted by the nursing and medical staff, and a pathway of care was introduced.

Mr A's condition began to deteriorate over the coming week, during which he was transferred to a critical care unit. On transfer to the unit, the senior nurse noticed that the patient's medication chart had been signed 'unable to swallow'.

Clinical governance supports registered nurse, midwives, and students in providing safe, quality care by drawing together the key concepts associated with patient safety, risk management, information and communication, accountability, and evidence-based nursing, through:

- **The systematic harmonisation of clinical and managerial responsibilities with accountable practice**
- **Team working and interdependency through integrated working with and between health and social care both public and independent [private]**
- **Monitoring, changing, evaluating and improving practice to safeguard standards**
- **The drive for constant quality improvement in all that we do**
- **Nurturing a culture of continuous learning**
- **Placing a duty of care to improve individual, team and organisational performance**
- **Adopting a person-centeredness approach in all that we do is the heart of clinical governance**

(McSherry and Pearce, 2010)

> **PRACTICE TIP**
> Familiarizing yourself with clinical governance is a good way of learning about patient safety and the provision and demonstration of quality nursing care. For further information, see McSherry and Pearce (2010).

Having highlighted the importance of quality systems and processes, the challenge is now to explore how you might measure and document the provision of quality nursing care.

Measuring and documenting the provision of quality nursing care

All registered nurses, midwives, and students should be familiar with how and why you need to measure the impact of nursing care, treatment, and interventions provided to patients. 'Nursing metrics', 'nursing quality indicators', 'patient-related outcomes', and 'patient outcome measures' are all terms used to describe how nursing care can be measured and documented. More detailed information on measuring care is provided in Chapter 16.

Measuring and documenting standards of nursing care is fundamental in assuring quality for patients, carers, users, professional colleagues, and the public, along with registration and regulatory organizations. The introduction of 'comparative benchmarking' and 'independent peer review' offer opportunistic ways in which registered nurses, midwives, and students can focus attention on establishing on how well or otherwise they are performing, and how this compares with other teams and organizations and nationally. Box 3.3 offers some examples of possible standards and frameworks for measuring and documenting the quality and standards of care.

Familiarizing and engaging with the tools and frameworks detailed in Box 3.3 is imperative, and should not be left to chance. Achieving quality for all patients, carers, users, professionals, and the public according to the Department of Health (2010b) *The Nursing Roadmap for Quality: A Signposting Map for Nursing* is about targeting three key areas.

- Safety—how safe will our patients be?
- Effectiveness—how effective will my nursing care and medical treatment be?
- Experience—what will I feel and experience as part of my nursing and medical care?

> **Box 3.3** Standards and frameworks for measuring and documenting the quality and standards of care
>
> - Royal College of Nursing (2010) Principles of Nursing Practice
> - Department of Health (2010a) *Essence of Care*
> - NHS Institute for Innovation and Improvement (2010) *High Impact Actions for Nursing*
> - The Productive Series
> - Pathways of care
> - Storytelling
> - Patient satisfaction surveys

The Department of Health (ibid) argues that there are seven steps to delivering and assuring quality nursing: '*Bring clarity to quality, measure quality, publish quality performance, recognise and reward quality, leadership for quality, safeguard quality and stay ahead.*'

Highlighting and accessing support in the provision of quality care

Highlighting and accessing support in the provision of quality care is available locally, regionally, and nationally. There are numerous resources and sources of information and guidance available to support every stage of the 'seven steps to quality' road map. **Box 3.4** offers some useful information and guidance to begin the seven-step journey.

••

How would you rate yourself and team in achieving the seven steps to quality?
If you are unfamiliar with the seven steps to quality and/or find them difficult to engage with, it is imperative that you seek support and guidance on how to measure and document quality care.

••

Box 3.4 offers some useful tools and frameworks for measuring and documenting the quality of care.

> **The development of a framework of explicit, nationally agreed indicators for nursing, including performance indicators such as patient-related outcomes, should be accelerated.**
>
> (Prime Minister's Commission on the Future of Nursing and Midwifery in England, 2010)

Ensuring that you begin to engage with, apply, and evaluate the impact of your care is imperative for assuring the quality of nursing in the future. Accessing and using the various tools and frameworks offered in Box 3.4 will support you in beginning the journey of assuring and evidencing patient safety and quality nursing in the future. Providing and evidencing that we are all offering quality nursing care that is caring, compassionate, and respectful of individual rights by

Box 3.4 The seven-step journey to quality

Step 1	*Clarify*	NHS Evidence
		RCN Clinical Guidelines
		High Impact Actions for Nursing and Midwifery
Step 2	*Measure*	NHS Choice
		NHS Institute Productive Series
Step 3	*Publish*	Quality Accounts
Step 4	*Reward*	The Commission for Quality and Innovation
		The Quality and Outcomes Framework
Step 5	*Leadership*	Realizing Time to Care Series
Step 6	*Safeguard*	Root Cause Analysis (RCA) toolkit
Step 7	*Stay ahead*	Innovation, Quality, Prevention, and Productivity

affording dignity, through choice and participation, is not optional, but a must. Counteracting damaging media coverage by restoring the image of registered nurses, midwives, and student nurses through ensuring that our every thought, action, and deed encompasses patient safety and quality is the only way forward.

Headlines such as '*None of the staff seemed to care about any of the patients*' and '*My mother told me not to say anything because she would still be there after we had gone home, and was so scared the nurses would be mean to her*' (Mid Staffordshire NHS Foundation Trust Inquiry, 2010) should never need to be written.

Conclusion

The provision of quality care is an integral component of every registered nurse, midwife, and student nurse's contract of employment, role and responsibility, and professional accountability. Challenging inadequate standards of quality care and sharing successful outcomes of care is the foundation to excellence in nursing practice. Developing honest, open, and transparent cultures in which learning with and from each other through adopting the principles of shared working relationships and sustained leadership is essential. Caring, compassion, respectfulness, and maintaining dignity are integral components of patient safety and quality nursing, and are not optional. Defining what 'quality nursing' is and involves, and how to measure and highlight the impact of care, must become the central component of any healthcare organization's integrated governance systems and processes.

People-centredness and patient-centredness have to regain centre stage in the design, implementation, and evaluation of nursing care standards, nursing care indicators, and key performance indicators in order to evidence and assure that 'people'; (patients, public, professionals) are equally as important as 'processes' and 'products'. To attest the latter, all registered nurses, midwives, and student nurses should be delivering safe, confident, competent, and compassionate quality care, and should have the knowledge, skills, attitudes, and behaviours to demonstrate this in their daily practice. The provision of quality nursing should be the primary goal of every single registered and non-registered nurse, and should be the lived experience of every single patient.

Further reading

King's College London National Nursing Research Unit (2008) 'High quality nursing care: What is it and how can we best ensure its delivery?', *Policy Plus Evidence, Issues and Opinions in Healthcare* 13: 1–2
Mair, E. (2009) 'Basic care "lacking" in hospitals', BBC News, 27 August, available online at **http://www.bbc.co.uk/blogs/pm/2009/08/basic_care_lacking_in_hospital.shtml** [accessed 16 June 2011]

References

Alzheimer's Society (2009) 'Poor dementia care in hospitals costing lives and hundreds of millions', 17 November, available online at **http://alzheimers.org.uk/site/scripts/news_article.php?newsID=579** [accessed 16 June 2011].

American Nurses Association, The (2003) *Nursing's Social Policy Statement*, 2nd edn, Washington DC: ANA.

American Nurses Association, The (2004) *Nursing: Scope and Standards of Practice*, Washington DC: ANA.

Best, M. and Neuhauser, D. (2010) 'Heroes and martyrs of quality and safety: Avedis Donabedian—Father of

quality assurance and poet', *Quality Safety Health Care* 13: 472–3.

Boseley, S. (2009) 'Patients "demeaned" by poor-quality nursing care', *The Guardian*, 27 August, available online at **http://www.guardian.co.uk/society/2009/aug/27/patients-association-poor-quality-care** [accessed 16 June 2011].

Burhans, M.L. and Alligood, R.M. (2010) 'Quality nursing care in words of nurses', *Journal of Advanced Nursing* 66(8): 168–97.

Department of Health (2008) *High Quality Care for All: NHS Next Stage Review Final Report*, London: HMSO.

Department of Health (2010a) *The Essence of Care*, London: HMSO.

Department of Health (2010b) *The Nursing Roadmap for Quality: A Signposting Map for Nursing*, London: HMSO.

Donabedian, A. (1966) 'Evaluating the quality of medical care', *Milbank Memorial Fund Quarterly* 44: 166–206.

International Council of Nurses (2010) 'Definition of nursing', available online at **http://www.icn.ch/about-icn/icn-definition-of-nursing/** [accessed 16 June 2011].

Irurita F.V. (1999) 'Factors affecting the quality of nursing care: The patient's perspective', *International Journal of Nursing Practice* 5: 86–94.

King's College London National Nursing Research Unit (2008) 'High quality nursing care: What is it and how can we best ensure its delivery?', *Policy Plus Evidence, Issues and Opinions in Healthcare* 13: 1–2.

Larrabee, H.J. and Bolden, V.L. (2001) 'Defining patient-perceived quality of nursing care', *Journal of Nursing Care Quality* 16(1): 34–60.

Lynn, R.M., McMillen, J.B., and Sidanai, S. (2007) 'Including the provider in the assessment of quality care: Development and testing of the nurses' assessment of quality scale—Acute care version', *Journal of Nursing Care Quality* 22(4): 328–36.

Maben, J. and Griffiths, P. (2008) *Nurses in Society: Starting the Debate*, London: King's College National Nursing Research Unit.

Mair, E. (2009) 'Basic care "lacking" in hospitals', BBC News, 27 August, available online at **http://www.bbc.co.uk/blogs/pm/2009/08/basic_care_lacking_in_hospital.shtml** [accessed 16 June 2011].

McCormack, B. and McCance, V.T. (2006) 'Development of a framework for person-centred nursing', *Journal of Advanced Nursing* 56(5): 472–9.

McSherry, R. and Haddock. J. (1998) 'Evidence-based health care: Its place within clinical governance', *British Journal of Nursing* 8(2): 113–17.

McSherry, R. and Pearce, P. (2010) *Clinical Governance: A Guide to Implementation for Healthcare Professionals*, 3rd edn, Oxford: Wiley Blackwell Publishers.

Mid Staffordshire NHS Foundation Trust Inquiry (2010) *Independent Inquiry into Care Provided by Mid Staffordshire NHS Foundation Trust January 2005–March 2009*, London: HMSO.

NHS Institute for Innovation and Improvement (2010) *High Impact Actions for Nursing and Midwifery: The Essential Collection*, Coventry: NHS Institute for Innovation and Improvement.

Nursing and Midwifery Council (2010) *The Code: Standards of Conduct, Performance and Ethics for Nurses and Midwives*, London: NMC.

Nursing Management (2010) 'Quality assurance in nursing: Standards', available online at **http://currentnursing.com/ nursing_management/quality_standards_nursing.html** [accessed 16 June 2011].

Nursing Times (2009) 'Patients Association brands NHS nurses "cruel and demeaning"', 27 August, available online at **http://www.nursingtimes.net/whats-new-in-nursing/acute-care/patients-association-brands-nhs-nurses-cruel-and-demeaning/5005658.article** [accessed 12 July 2011].

Pollner, J. (2006) 'Defining nursing', available online at **http://www.wepapers.com/Papers/55360/Defining_ Nursing** [accessed 16 June 2011].

Prime Minister's Commission on the Future of Nursing and Midwifery in England (2010) *Front Line Care: the Future of Nursing and Midwifery in England*, London: HMSO.

Royal College of Nursing (2003) *Defining Nursing*, London: RCN.

Royal College of Nursing (2010) 'Principles of Nursing Practice', available online at **http://www.rcn.org.uk/ nursingprinciples** [accessed 12 July 2011].

Smith, R. (2010) 'Nurses should be more caring to restore public confidence: Report', *The Telegraph*, 3 March, available online at **http://www.telegraph.co.uk/health/ healthnews/7351513/Nurses-should-be-more-caring-to-restore-public-confidence-report.html** [accessed 16 June 2011].

Respecting the individual

MILIKA RUTH MATITI AND LESLEY BAILLIE

Learning outcomes

This chapter will enable you to:

- recognize that respecting and preserving people's dignity is fundamental in nursing practice;
- explore the meaning of respect and dignity in order to apply these in practice;
- discuss the nature and key dimensions of holistic and individualized care;
- recognize models of nursing care that promote a holistic approach and dignity in care; and
- appreciate the importance of respecting individual beliefs and values.

Introduction

Respect is important in maintaining the dignity of individuals. This chapter will introduce concepts and values associated with respect; some of these will be developed further in later chapters. Here, we explore the concepts of respect and dignity, and consider what makes us all individuals and the nature of holistic care. The case studies will encourage you to reflect on clinical situations and your own nursing practice, which will enable you to develop understanding of how nursing care can meet the holistic needs of individuals and their families within a diverse society. At the end of this chapter, you should be able to understand the importance of treating people with respect so that their dignity is maintained and promoted regardless of age, colour, creed, culture, disability or illness, gender, nationality, politics, race, or social status. Note that it is also

Essential knowledge and skills for care

- You must be aware of the importance of always practising in a compassionate, respectful manner to maintain and preserve the dignity and well-being of each individual person in your care.

- You must support and promote the health, well-being, rights, and dignity of people, groups, communities, and populations. These include people whose lives are affected by ill health, disability, ageing, death, and dying.

- You will ensure that you preserve the safety, security, and dignity of people when attending to their essential care needs.

- You will use effective communication strategies and negotiation techniques to uphold and safeguard the needs of the individual, while respecting the dignity and human rights of all concerned.

- You must be aware of the systems and strategies that exist for reporting and challenging undignified care and practice.

important that nurses respect themselves, as we saw in Chapter 2.

Definitions of 'respect' and 'dignity'

Nurses and other healthcare professionals need to develop a clear understanding of the nature of respect and dignity so that they can apply these concepts in their practice. However, the concepts 'respect' and 'dignity' are complex and multidimensional, and often ambiguous. Remember that:

- respect is perceived differently by individuals depending on how they have been socialized;
- dignity is better understood by considering the values that constitute it and respect is one of these values.

Before we consider the meanings of 'respect' and 'dignity', we will first explore personal values and beliefs, because these are closely aligned with respect.

Personal beliefs and values

Beliefs and values underpin our attitudes and these can affect our interactions with others. As nurses, it is essential to be non-judgemental in our approach to patients: a judgemental stance portrays a lack of respect for individuals' own beliefs and values. The activity below will help you to explore your beliefs and values.

....

Consider the following questions.
What are beliefs and what are values? How are they different?
What are *your* beliefs and values?
How might these differ from those of people for whom you are caring?

....

Gross and Kinnison (2007) suggest that a *belief* is an opinion—information, knowledge, or thoughts about a particular thing. We sometimes refer to religious beliefs, but people can hold beliefs about many things, which can be influenced by knowledge or arise from within the person and relate to their upbringing, culture, or spirituality. A *value* concerns what is important to us and often relates to worth. Gross and Kinnison (2007) define value as being the person's sense of desirability, worth, or utility of obtaining some outcome. Examples of values are equality, freedom, or respect. Cherry (1997) proposes two terms to describe value.

- The first is 'extrinsic' or 'instrumental', which is assigned to a person on the basis of their features.

This is called 'relative' and is defined by wealth, skills, competence, creativity, and looks, among other features. In this case, one is respected for what one has, which entails a conditional value.

- The second is 'ultimate' or 'absolute', which is determined by whatever one's intrinsic values are; thus one is respected for what one is and not because of what one has.

Whether these definitions are similar or seem to contradict one another, one point is certain: all human beings have self-worth that needs to be recognized in health care. It is this absolute value that nurses and other healthcare professionals should be concerned about.

If we understand our patients' beliefs and values, we can better understand their behaviour and respect them as individuals. In turn, our values and beliefs underpin our attitudes and affect how we behave with others. We must recognize that our own beliefs and values may differ from those for whom we care. For example, jewellery or clothing can relate to religious beliefs; therefore, during personal care, we must demonstrate respect for these items. Some patients have particular beliefs about modesty and being exposed in the presence of people of the opposite sex. Nurses must be sensitive to beliefs and values and respond respectfully. Nurses must also not let their own religious beliefs affect their relationships and practice with patients.

Now that we have considered the nature of values and beliefs, we will explore the meaning of respect and dignity.

What is respect and what is dignity?

Almost everyone has some understanding of the words 'respect' and 'dignity'; we can all provide simple and informal definitions of these words. In **Box.4.1** you are asked to reflect upon the terms 'respect' and 'dignity'. The following sections explore the meaning of these words in more depth by presenting published definitions from a range of resources—that is, in dictionaries, books, and journals.

Box 4.1 Reflective activity: the meaning of respect and dignity

Make notes on the following.

Respect

- What does the word 'respect' mean to you?
- What does it feel like to be respected?
- How do you know that someone has given you respect?
- How do you know that someone has not given you respect?
- What kind of behaviour indicates respect for individuals?

Dignity

- What does the word 'dignity' mean to you?
- If someone says that you have dignity, what do you think the person means?
- How do you know whether the person to whom you are talking is upholding your dignity?
- How do you know whether the person to whom you are talking is not maintaining your dignity?
- What kind of behaviour promotes a sense of dignity for individuals?

Respect and dignity

- Did you find it easy or difficult to define 'respect' and 'dignity'? Why do you think that is?
- Can you come up with other words that describe respect and dignity?
- How precise were these words in describing respect and dignity?
- Ask a family member or a friend what the words 'respect' and 'dignity' mean to them, and compare their views with your own.
  - Did they provide you with the same meaning of respect?
  - Did they provide you with the same meaning of dignity?
- While you were discussing these terms, did it occur to you that the perception of respect and dignity may be influenced by the person's age or social or educational background?
- Did you learn what it means to respect someone?

Respect

The concept of 'respect' is often referred to in everyday life. In a hospital setting, one hears claims such as 'I was treated with respect', or 'the nurse treated me with respect', or (unfortunately) 'the staff showed me no respect at all'. The use of the word 'respect' in these situations may carry different meanings for each speaker. Several authors have acknowledged that the concept of respect is difficult to define (Thomson, 2002; O'Toole, 2008). Thomson (2002) points out that although respect is a complex concept that is difficult to define, it is recognized in interactions with individuals. But according to Baldwin (2008), respect is valuing the person as a whole and relates to attitude, which includes an aspect of behaviour of one person towards another. It is acknowledging the feelings and interests of another party in a relationship. This definition recognizes that respect links to the person's worth and value. Respect is central in dignity, being one of the values through which one feels dignified (Matiti, 2002, Thomson, 2002; Walsh and Kowanko, 2002). This leads us to the concept of dignity.

Dignity

Like the word 'respect', 'dignity' is vague and difficult to define. According to *Collins English Dictionary* (2003), the word comes from the Latin words *dignus*, meaning 'worth', and *dignitas*, meaning 'merit'. After reviewing the literature, Nordenfelt (2003) argued for four categories of dignity:

(a) dignity as *Menschenwürde* (human rights), which claims that all humans have the same value and the same rights independent of gender, age, race, or religion, and assumes that every individual should be treated equally;

(b) dignity as merit, which includes rank in society, earned or inherited, entailing a set of rights and honours installed in this position;

(c) dignity of moral stature, which includes respect of oneself as a moral being and respect from others related to performances and attitudes, and may vary in relation to one's own needs;

(d) dignity of personal identity, which focuses on human beings' self-respect, including notions of integrity and autonomy, and which may be violated when a person is prevented from doing what they want to do or are entitled to do.

These categories attempt to portray a comprehensive understanding of dignity, but Baillie (2009) and Gallagher et al. (2008) question the applicability of 'dignity as merit' and 'dignity as moral stature' in health care, because all patients should be treated with equal dignity. In other words, people are valued regardless of their looks and background. Ridgway (2008) states that dignity refers to care in any setting that supports and promotes, and does not undermine, a person's self-respect regardless of any difference. Fenton and Mitchell (2002) add a spiritual dimension to the definition of the concept of dignity: They define dignity as '*a state of physical, emotional and spiritual comfort, with each individual valued for his or her uniqueness and his or her individuality celebrated*' (ibid: 21). Spirituality is more than having religious beliefs; it is concerned about meaning and purpose in people's lives (Moss, 2008). This demonstrates that spirituality is also an important aspect of dignity of every person.

By completing the reflective questions in Box 4.1 you may have identified a number of factors that individuals associate with respect and dignity—for example, family, culture, education, and work.

Now look at **Practice Example 4.1**, which will help you to explore respect and dignity in practice.

The following are some possible responses to the questions in the practice example, but you may have thought of others too.

1. You might have thought of upbringing (that is, how Mr Fountain was brought up) and his training in the military (the way in which he was trained to respect other people and had others respecting him). Also, Mr Fountain had a rank in the RAF and was a councillor, which might have influenced him in terms of how he perceives himself within society and how people perceive him in terms of respect.

2. Mr Fountain is less mobile due to his fractured hip, so he will be dependent on other people in hospital. He might perceive that he is seen as helpless in the community in which he has been very active.

3. You might have considered how hospitalization can cause loss of identity. People become part of a group of patients, can lose individuality, and are expected to follow hospital routine. These factors could influence how Mr Fountain sees himself in terms of respect and dignity.

Having defined respect and dignity, and explored questions regarding Mr Fountain, the next section applies

---

PRACTICE EXAMPLE 4.1

The Meaning of Respect and Dignity

Mr Fountain is a 70-year-old retired Royal Air Force pilot. He is very independent and he still enjoys gardening and a game of golf. Although he has impaired hearing, this has not affected his daily living activities, because he uses a hearing aid. He is very active in community work and has been a local councillor. He has had a fall and fractured his right hip. The multidisciplinary team do their best to make sure that he is well cared for and prepared for theatre. While in hospital, he tells the nurses:

'I do like respect. I have been a councillor helping people, and I have worked in the air force, therefore I deserve to be respected'.

1 What factors in his life might influence how he perceives his dignity and how he should be respected?

2 How would his fractured hip influence or affect his respect and dignity?

3 How will the hospitalization affect his respect and dignity?

these concepts in practice. It will equip you with the knowledge, skills, and appropriate attitude required for respecting patients and maintaining and promoting their dignity.

Respecting individuals in nursing practice

From Mr Fountain's scenario, you are now aware that hospital admission can lead to a loss of individuality and identity by subsuming the patient within a group. Furthermore, patients' dependency on healthcare-workers may lead to patients feeling less respected. All healthcare workers should therefore develop skills and attitudes to minimize feelings of loss of individuality, identity, and respect. However, this section focuses on nursing practice.

Professional requirements confirm that respect is an important concept in nursing practice. The International Council of Nurses (ICN, 2006: 1) states, that 'Inherent in nursing is respect for human rights, including cultural rights, the right to life and choice, the right to dignity and to be treated with respect'. This idea has been embraced by codes of conduct in different countries. In the UK, the Nursing and Midwifery Council (NMC, 2008) The Code: Standards for Conduct, Performance and Ethics urges nurses to 'make the care of people their first concern, treating them as individuals and respecting their dignity' (ibid: 2). The NMC's Guidance on Professional Conduct for Nursing and Midwifery Students (NMC, 2009a) discusses the application of the NMC's Code for students. The NMC's Standards for Pre-Registration Education (NMC, 2010) states that the public should be confident that all new nurses practise in a respectful way and maintain dignity. Thus, respecting individuals and preserving their dignity are fundamental and inherent in professional nursing practice.

Nurses work in teams with other professionals, and they too are required to treat patients with respect and dignity; thus there should be a whole inter-professional team approach to respect for individuals. The Health Professions Council (2008), which registers non-medical professions such as radiography and physiotherapy, has standards of conduct, performance, and ethics, which require that registrants treat service users with respect and dignity. Likewise, the General Medical Council (2006) requires doctors to respect the dignity of patients. In 2009, the Department of Health published the NHS Constitution, which identified NHS values, the first of which is 'Respect and dignity'. These values relate to everyone working in the National Health Service, whether they are registered professionals or not. In addition, from a legislative viewpoint, the Human Rights Act (HRA) 1998 recognizes that all individuals have minimal and fundamental human rights, and two of the sections of the Act relate to aspects of dignity and are clearly relevant to health care: the absence of inhumane or degrading treatment (s 3) and the right to privacy (s 8). Clearly, the HRA is applicable to the practice of all healthcare professionals, not only nurses.

However, studies have highlighted that patients' dignity is not always maintained to a high standard (Gallagher and Seedhouse, 2000; Turnock and Kelleher, 2001; Matiti, 2002; Baillie, 2009). Reports from varying care settings have also expressed concern that patients are not always treated with respect, leading to compromised dignity (Healthcare Commission, 2007; Help the Aged, 2007; Mencap, 2007; Mental Welfare Commission for Scotland, 2007; Patients' Association, 2009). Due to concerns about diminished dignity in UK health care, dignity campaigns have been launched by the Department of Health (2006) and Royal College of Nursing (2008). Whether such campaigns can be sustained and have a long-term impact on healthcare practice is, however, open to question (Baillie and Gallagher, 2010). It is also interesting and somewhat concerning that a dignity campaign should be needed when promoting dignity is, in fact, a professional and legal requirement of nurses, other healthcare professionals, and NHS trusts.

The essential knowledge and skills for care listed at the beginning of the chapter stress the importance of care, compassion, and respect. To show respect, nurses need to understand the elements that we now examine below.

Self–awareness

To develop self-awareness, you need to identify your values and beliefs in relation to respect and dignity, thus assisting you to make sense of, and understand, them. This is important, because values and beliefs influence behaviour and nurses demonstrate respect for patients through their own behaviour. Self-awareness also entails reflecting on your knowledge and skills for respecting patients, which will make you aware of your own limitations while caring for patients. Therefore self-awareness allows you to know and understand yourself, and helps you not to impose your personal values on patients and to care for patients more effectively.

Meeting patients' needs

Patients' needs may be unique to them; they may be due to the patient's illness, the process of admission, or a result of cultural influences. You should recognize patients' individual needs, pay attention to them, and address them promptly (McGee, 1994). Nurses should be aware of what patients can or cannot do for themselves. Carrying out tasks that patients feel capable of doing can make them feel patronized and not being aware of what they are incapable of may cause loss of dignity. For example, not recognizing that a patient is unable to go to the toilet unassisted may lead to embarrassment and a sense of worthlessness. The patient may soil themselves, leading them to feel embarrassed and believe they have lost respect in the presence of the nurse. Nurses will be confronted with many forms of diversity in health care, with different expectations and needs. It is important to recognize these needs and provide what Rogers (1951) calls 'unconditional positive regard', which implies that the person is respected regardless of the person's actions or what he or she says, or irrespective of any conditions that he or she may have. This is accepting the person without judging him or her.

Knowledge, skills, and attitude

Knowledge of the patient's cultural background, their illness, and its effect promotes respect (Baldwin, 2008). Nurses should be aware of the values and expectations of patients in relation to respect. They should also be aware of the importance of verbal and non-verbal cues, because these may assist them in identifying subtle signs of violation of respect. If patients are unable to communicate due to frailty or illness, nurses should refer to members of their family who may be in a better position to know the patient's needs and what behaviour will enhance respect for them.

It is important to know the resources that are available in health care and which will influence the maintenance of respect. For example, the presence or absence of a private side room on the ward will allow the nurse to make necessary arrangements for the care of patients that will promote respect and dignity.

Nurses need to develop the necessary skills and attitudes to enable them to respect patients, thereby promoting their dignity. These include good interpersonal skills, such as verbal and non-verbal communication, because these are key to treating patients with respect (Price, 2004). Full explanation of the patient's health care and procedures will minimize disorientation and loss of patients' control. It might be necessary to negotiate with patients or their families to avoid misunderstandings and encourage respect. Once nurses have such knowledge and skills, they will start to develop appropriate attitudes for the promotion of respect and dignity. According to Rughani (2008) having appropriate attitudes means taking an active interest in patients, treating them with respect, and avoiding prejudice.

Having appropriate knowledge, skills, and attitudes in relation to respect and dignity will help you to provide holistic patient care. The next sections explore individualized and holistic care in more detail.

The nature and key dimensions of individualized and holistic care

Holistic and individualized care aims to ensure that our patients and clients feel that we respect them as individuals, thus promoting their dignity. First, consider what it is that makes someone an individual by carrying out the reflective activity below.

What makes an individual?

Reflect upon yourself: what makes you an individual? Jot down your ideas. We will return to these later.

One view is that individuals comprise four dimensions: biological; psychological; social; and spiritual. Therefore an individualized approach to care ensures that all of these aspects are included in assessment and care delivery, rather than only one or two aspects. For example, a man with an acute heart problem would have a poor experience of care if only his physical dimension were to be recognized. The patient's accompanying fear and anxiety, if not addressed, will adversely affect physical recovery, as well as psychological status. It is a professional requirement that nurses should be able to conduct a holistic and individualized assessment of patients, including their physical, psychological, social, and spiritual needs. McSherry (2006) provides a brief description of the four dimensions (see **Table 4.1**). By considering each of these areas during assessment and care, patients are more likely to feel that they have been respected as individuals because you are taking a holistic approach to their care.

Now, look back at your notes from the reflective activity: did you include all of the four dimensions listed in Table 4.1? Were some areas more dominant

in the notes that you jotted down? It is likely that you will have included most of these aspects and certainly not only your biological or social characteristics, for example. Therefore, if you were to need health care, perhaps for an injury such as a fractured leg, nurses would need to consider more than only your injury for you to feel respected as an individual. For example, you might be afraid of losing your mobility, thus affecting your career, or you might be worried about your family at home.

One aspect of showing respect for a person's individuality is to use their preferred name. This might seem obvious, but there are many reports of nurses and others not addressing patients in a way that respects their individuality. Use of endearments such as 'sweetheart' are sometimes used, which patients, particularly older people, may consider demeaning (Help the Aged, 2007). Reflecting on the poor care delivered to his mother in a care home, Johns (2009) expressed distress that a staff member referred to her as 'the new lady' rather than by her name and that the door to her bedroom did not have her name on (unlike those of the other residents), and he observed that staff carrying out his mother's care did not address her by her preferred name even when he had corrected them. This example demonstrates that it is also important to relatives to feel that their loved ones are being respected

Table 4.1 The four dimensions of individuals (McSherry, 2006: 72)

Dimension	Explanation
Biological	This refers to the physical and biological process or function of an individual that is essential to maintain life.
Psychological	Usually implies the cognitive, intellectual, and emotional aspects of the individual that may shape personality and mental functioning.
Social	The cultural norms, values, and beliefs that influence and classify individuals into different groups or communities.
Spiritual	A vague term used normally to indicate an individual's inner beliefs, commonly related to religious affiliation or belief in the existence of a god or supreme power.

as individuals. The NMC (2009b) publication *Care and Respect Every Time: New Guidance for the Care of Older People* also highlighted the need to address people by their preferred name and further recommended that:

> **The essence of nursing care for older people is about getting to know and value people as individuals through effective assessment, finding out how they want to be cared for from their perspective, and providing care which ensures that respect, dignity and fairness are maintained.**
>
> (NMC, 2009b: 8)

While the guidance focuses on older people, these principles are relevant to people of any age, including children and families. People feel respected and that their dignity is promoted when their personal identity is recognized by nurses who are caring for them. Nurses can demonstrate that they respect the people for whom they are caring through individualized, person-centred, and holistic care.

It is important to model respectful behaviour and to be prepared to challenge colleagues' behaviour if it is not respectful to patients. Now consider **Practice Example 4.2**.

Unfortunately, you may encounter healthcare workers making disrespectful, and indeed judgemental, comments about patients, particularly during shift handovers. However, as discussed earlier, it is a universal requirement for healthcare workers to treat patients with respect and preserve dignity. In responding to the colleague in **Practice Example 4.2**, for example, you could point out that there are many reasons why people drink alcohol and that healthcare workers must remain non-judgemental, that we have a duty of care to all patients, and that healthcare workers must respect patients and treat them with dignity. It is very important for the woman's dignity and comfort, and indeed for infection control reasons, that the care needed is carried out quickly and with respect and sensitivity. If you witness colleagues being disrespectful to patients directly, then you should ensure that the situation is rectified for the patient by meeting their needs and restoring their dignity, but you must also report such incidents to the nurse in charge. Seek guidance from your personal tutor or other university staff if you need support.

Holistic care

To provide dignity in care, nurses need to approach people in a person-centred way, with respect for each person as an individual with attention to their holistic care needs. Byatt (2008) asserts that holistic care is an approach or value system held by practitioners who provide care that recognizes the patient as a whole person, with physical, psychological, sociological, and spiritual dimensions. A concept analysis of the term 'holistic nursing practice' led to the following working definition for application by nurses in practice:

> **Holistic nursing care embraces the mind, body and spirit of the patient, in a culture that supports a therapeutic nurse/patient relationship, resulting in wholeness, harmony and healing. Holistic care is patient led and patient focused in**

PRACTICE EXAMPLE 4.2

Challenging disrespect

A woman is brought to the accident and emergency (A&E) department by ambulance after a fall while under the influence of alcohol. The ambulance crew report that the patient is 'a known alcoholic'. The patient is very drowsy and, a little while later, you find that she has been incontinent of urine and faeces. You ask a colleague to help you to wash and change her. The colleague makes a tutting noise and comments that it is the patient's 'own fault' and that she is 'disgusting', and complains that 'Now we have to clean her up'.

How might you respond to these disrespectful remarks?

order to provide individualised care, thereby, caring for the patient as a whole person rather than in fragmented parts.

(McEvoy and Duffy, 2008: 418)

The definition emphasizes patients as individuals and as a whole, and highlights the importance of the nurse–patient relationship. Approaching patient care in this holistic way will help you to show respect for each patient as a person and a valued human being, thus promoting their dignity during nursing care. You will also see that the definition of holistic care refers to 'mind, body, and spirit', a concept often referred to in sources exploring holistic practice.

Now read through **Practice Example 4.3** and consider the questions posed.

Practice Example 4.3 illustrates that people who require nursing care may have diverse needs, relating to their physical, psychological, social, and spiritual dimensions. From a biological perspective, as well as Amanda's acute physical problems of chest pain and breathlessness, she is also morbidly obese. Her obesity could be influenced by the medication for her mental health problem, because weight gain is a common side effect; this is an example of how problems can interrelate. Amanda's psychological status will be influenced by her mental health problem and her related medication, but is also affected by her dislike of hospitals (perhaps due to previous experiences), and probably her fear about the cause of her chest pain and breathlessness. From a spiritual perspective, Amanda's religion seems important to her as an individual and also leads to social support. Amanda could otherwise feel lonely because her immediate family are not in close contact. Amanda could also be worried about leaving her dog alone at home.

Your approach to Amanda should show that you care about her as an individual and that you respect her dignity. First, introduce yourself and find out how she wishes to be addressed. You should quickly assess whether she has any immediate needs, using observation skills (for example, does she look frightened?), questioning skills (for example, ask her how she feels now), and measurement skills (including vital signs). You should respond to Amanda's immediate care needs, based on your assessment. This would include ensuring that she is physically comfortable, explaining to Amanda what will happen next, and assuring her that she can ask you anything at any time. By showing concern for Amanda as an individual and meeting any immediate needs, you will start to develop trust and establish a nurse–patient relationship. You will then be able to conduct a more detailed assessment of her physical, psychological, social, and spiritual needs.

This exercise highlights the meaning of holistic care, illustrating that all individuals, irrespective of age,

---

PRACTICE EXAMPLE 4.3

Holistic care and respect

Amanda is 42 years old and has a long history of schizophrenia, for which she is on medication, supervised by the community mental health team. She is divorced and lives alone in a local authority flat with her Jack Russell dog, Toby. She has three teenage children who live with her ex-husband. She sees them infrequently, because they live in a town some distance away. Her father is dead, but she has occasional contact with her mother and one of her brothers. She attends a local Baptist church regularly and gains support from members of the congregation. She is morbidly obese and she smokes approximately thirty cigarettes a day. A friend has called an ambulance because Amanda has developed chest pain and breathlessness. Following assessment and initial investigation in the A&E department, Amanda has been admitted to a medical assessment unit for observation and further tests. Amanda's appearance is rather unkempt and she appears agitated. Her friend says that Amanda 'hates hospitals'.

Identify Amanda's needs relating to the four dimensions in Table 4.1.

How might you approach Amanda with respect for her as an individual in a way that promotes her dignity?

gender, sexuality, race, ethnicity, or religious belief, are made up of the same dimensions. By ensuring that we support each individual with their needs, we can help to promote and preserve the dignity of every patient. Providing 'holistic' nursing care can be complex, because individuals are not only physical beings requiring food, shelter, and warmth; they are all unique, with a distinct personality, and distinct intellectual and emotional needs. Furthermore, individuals are influenced by the environment, society, and culture in which they live and socialize. This means that individuals possess diverse sets of beliefs and values, whether cultural, religious, or spiritual. These beliefs and values can have a profound impact upon the way in which people from different regions of the world, and indeed the UK, view health and well-being.

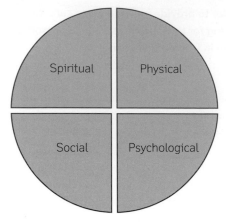

Figure 4.1 A common representation of holistic practice.

> **PRACTICE TIP**
>
> Always treat people with courtesy, respecting that their beliefs and values may be very different from your own.

Models of nursing care

Having identified that individuals are composed of different dimensions and that we are all unique, with varying beliefs and values, we will next explore the practicalities of providing holistic care. Some writers suggest that holistic care emerged to combat the 'medical model of care', whereby people were cared for solely according to their medical diagnosis. For example, in the medical model of care, Amanda's care would focus solely on her physical symptoms and the associated medical diagnosis. From a nursing perspective, such an approach would not meet her individual needs in a holistic way. Nursing models are conceptual, rather than physical, models and are composed of concepts and theories. They are underpinned by beliefs and values about nursing and provide a framework for nurses to follow in their practice.

Figure 4.1 represents one model of holistic care. In the pie chart, the four dimensions appear to be all equal and of the same value. However, in practice, nurses may not always address all dimensions with equal importance.

How do nurses provide holistic care in practice? Reflect on a recent practice learning experience: what care was given to meet physical, psychological, social, and spiritual needs? Focus on one particular patient in whose care you were involved and identify care related to the four dimensions.

Your experiences may reveal that nurses are particularly likely to address needs that are easily identifiable and measurable, for example administering oxygen therapy or assisting with hygiene. Some nursing theorists (Roper et al., 2000) describe this as supporting patients to meet their activities of daily living (ADL). Ellis (1999) reported that using the Roper et al. model can lead to a checklist approach to care and over-emphasize physical care needs. The model does recognize individuality in living and it includes most of the dimensions that we have discussed, referring to these as factors (biological, psychological, socio-cultural, environmental and politico-economic) that influence ADLs. However, spirituality is not included as an influencing factor, even though it can affect all aspects of how individuals live. Depending on how the model is applied, there is a risk that the influencing factors can lead to a fragmented perspective rather than a holistic and integrated approach. For example, as we discussed in relation to Amanda (Practice Example 4.3), the physical and psychological factors affecting her ADLs are closely linked. Ellis (1999) described a 'patient-centred care model' used in a hospice setting, which she argued involved a more holistic care approach. There are various nursing models and all aim to promote holistic care through different representations and frameworks. Humanistic nursing theories particularly emphasize dignity and the person as a holistic and unique individual. Pearson et al. (2005) and Fitzpatrick and Whall (2005) focus on nursing models in detail and are recommended for further reading.

There are some aspects of holistic care that nurses still feel uncomfortable exploring—in particular areas such as sexuality, spirituality, and death and dying. These have been described as the 'last taboos' of nursing because there is still related misconception and anxiety. However, if nurses are to provide truly holistic care, they must engage with these important subjects. As regards sexuality, Magnan et al. (2006) highlighted that nurses often neglect to explore the effect of illness on sexuality due to their own inhibitions about discussing intimate issues. However, there are many health conditions that affect sexuality: for example, diabetes can affect sexual function and breast surgery can affect a woman's feelings about her sexuality because breasts are part of a woman's sexual identity. Furthermore, various medications (including beta-blockers and some anti-psychotics) affect sexual function. Thus sexuality should not be avoided in holistic patient care and is included as an ADL in the Roper et al. (2000) model.

There is growing evidence for links between spirituality and human health, healing, and well-being (Walton, 1999; Sessanna et al., 2007; Koslander et al., 2009). However, Koslander et al. (2009) highlight that while people with mental health problems often have spiritual care needs, these have not always been addressed. They identify reasons why the spiritual dimension may be neglected, including a lack of knowledge about spirituality and that mental health professionals may be unaware of their own spiritual needs, making it difficult for them to be aware of those of their patients. McSherry (2006) suggested reasons why the 'spiritual needs' section in assessment documentation may be left incomplete, including: intrusiveness; discomfort of the nurse; the patient not wanting to answer the question or not identifying any spiritual needs; the patient and/or nurse not understanding the term 'spiritual'; and identified spiritual needs being considered too personal to document. Miner-Williams (2006) suggested that spirituality is the essence of being human, and can include meaning and connectedness, and important values and beliefs. Thus, as you will see from our earlier exploration of the meaning of dignity, 'spirituality' and 'dignity' are closely linked and so, to promote dignity in care, nurses must consider patients' spirituality. Miner-Williams (2006) suggests that a meaningful assessment of spirituality includes asking 'How are your spirits today?' or 'How does this hospitalization affect you and your family?', and, most importantly, showing a genuine interest in the person. Chapter 8 will further help you to understand how you can assess and provide care relating to spirituality.

In individualized care, plans of care should be developed with patients' full consent and involvement, leading to their engagement in decision-making, control, and empowerment. In some situations, this may not be possible, for example with a person with profound learning disability or when nursing unconscious patients. In these situations, nurses act in patients' best interests according to their known preferences and wishes. The person's next of kin or a primary carer who knows the patient should be involved.

Taking it further

In this section, an example from practice will enable you to take this chapter's learning further. The scenario is based on a young woman with a learning disability. The document *Valuing People: A New Strategy for Learning Disability for the 21st Century* (Department of Health, 2001) stressed that people with learning disabilities are people first and that there should be a focus on what they *can* do rather than what they cannot. *Valuing People Now* (Department of Health, 2007) highlighted that progress in good quality health care had been disappointing, with poor access to the NHS and the undermining of personalization, dignity, and safety.

Read through the scenario in **Practice Example 4.4** and answer the questions, looking back through the chapter where necessary.

PRACTICE EXAMPLE 4.4

Applying Dignity and Respect in Holistic Care

Michelle is 25 years old and has a severe learning disability accompanied by profound physical health problems. She lives in a house with one other person with a learning disability and there are full-time, live-in carers. Michelle has her nutritional needs met via a gastrostomy tube (an opening in the abdominal wall through which a tube allows feeds to enter the stomach directly). She wears incontinence pads and she uses an electric wheelchair to mobilize. She has no verbal communication, but she can communicate non-verbally and shows pleasure through smiling and laughing. Michelle has recurrent chest infections for which she is usually cared for at home with community team support. However, today she has been brought to the A&E department by a carer due to deterioration in her breathing. Her carer has brought a 'passport', which details Michelle's likes and dislikes and what is important to her. After initial treatment, Michelle is transferred to your ward.

1 How might Michelle's dignity be affected by her admission into hospital?
2 What skills could you apply to demonstrate respect for Michelle?
3 How could you meet Michelle's individual needs and provide holistic care?
4 How could you use her passport to help you to show respect for her as an individual?

Conclusion

Respecting individuals, promoting their dignity, and providing holistic and individualized care are absolutely central to caring and the practice of nursing. This chapter has encouraged you to explore your own values and beliefs, and to recognize that these may differ from those of the people for whom you care. You should now have an understanding of the meaning of 'dignity', which is complex and multidimensional, but is fundamental to the care of patients and clients in any setting. The chapter has introduced skills that are important for demonstrating respect for individuals, including self-awareness and communication. You have considered that individuals have physical, psychological, social, and spiritual dimensions, which must all be addressed within the context of holistic care. You have also been introduced to the concept of nursing models that aim to promote a holistic approach. Your understanding of how you can demonstrate respect for individuals should lie at the heart of your nursing practice throughout your career, and will demonstrate to patients and clients that you care *about* them as well as *for* them.

Further reading

Baillie, L. (2007) 'A case study of patient dignity in an acute hospital setting', Unpublished PhD thesis, London South Bank University.

Gray, A. (2009) 'Respecting a patient's religious needs is key to holistic care', *Nursing Standard* 23(40): 27.

House of Lords/House of Commons Joint Committee on Human Rights (2007) *The Human Rights of Older People in Healthcare*, London: HMSO.

References

Baillie, L. (2009) 'Patient dignity in an acute hospital setting: a case study', *International Journal of Nursing Studies* 46: 22–36.

Baillie, L. and Gallagher, A. (2010) 'Evaluation of the Royal College of Nursing's "Dignity at the Heart of Everything we do" campaign: Exploring challenges and enablers', *Journal of Research in Nursing* 15(1): 15–28.

Baldwin, M.A. (2008) 'Respect', in A. Mason-Whitehead, B.A. McIntoch, and T. Mason (eds) *Key Concepts in Nursing*, Los Angeles, CA: Sage, pp. 278–84.

Byatt, K. (2008) 'Holistic care', in A. Mason-Whitehead, B.A. McIntoch, and T. Mason (eds) *Key Concepts in Nursing*, Los Angeles, CA: Sage, pp. 168–74.

Cherry, C. (1997) 'Health care, human worth and limits of the particular', *Journal of Medical Ethics* 23(5): 310–14.

Collins (2003) *Collins English Dictionary*, Complete and unabridged edn, Glasgow: Collins.

Department of Health (2001) *Valuing People: A New Strategy for Learning Disability for the 21st Century*, London: HMSO.

Department of Health (2006) 'About the Dignity in Care campaign', available online at **http://www.dh.gov.uk** [accessed 16 June 2011].

Department of Health (2007) *Valuing People Now: From Progress to Transformation*, London: HMSO.

Department of Health (2009) 'NHS Constitution', available online at **http://www.eoe.nhs.uk/nhs_constitution/values. php** [accessed 16 June 2011].

Ellis, S. (1999) 'The patient-centred care model: Holistic multiprofessional/reflective', *British Journal of Nursing* 8(5): 296–301.

Fenton, E. and Mitchell, T. (2002) 'Growing old with dignity: A concept analysis', *Nursing Older People* 14(4): 19–21.

Fitzpatrick, J.J. and Whall, A.L. (2005) *Conceptual Models of Nursing: Analysis and Application*, Upper Saddle River, NJ: Prentice Hall.

Gallagher, A. and Seedhouse, D. (2000) 'The practical implications of teaching philosophy to practitioners: Dignity— A pilot study', Unpublished report held by the authors.

Gallagher, A., Li, S., Wainwright, P., Jones, I.R., and Lee, D. (2008) 'Dignity in the care of older people: A review of theoretical and empirical literature', *BMC Nursing* 7(11): 1–12.

General Medical Council (2006) 'Good medical practice: Duties of a doctor', available online at **http://www. gmc-uk.org/guidance/good_medical_practice.asp** [accessed 16 June 2011].

Gross, R. and Kinnison, N. (2007) *Psychology for Nurses and Allied Health Professionals*, London: Hodder Arnold.

Health Professions Council (2008) *Standards of Conduct, Performance and Ethics*, London: HPC.

Healthcare Commission (2007) *Caring for Dignity: A National Report on Dignity in Care for Older People While in Hospital*, London: HMSO.

Help the Aged (2007) *The Challenge of Dignity in Care: Upholding the Rights of the Individual*, London: Help the Aged.

Human Rights Act (1998) c42. HMSO. Available at **http:// www.legislation.gov.uk/ukpga/1998/42/schedule/** [Accessed 9 January 2012].

International Council for Nurses (2006) *Code of Ethics for Nurses*, Geneva: ICN.

Johns, C. (2009) 'Reflection on my mother dying: A story of crying shame', *Journal of Holistic Nursing* 17(2): 136–40.

Koslander, T., da Silva, A.B., and Roxberg, A. (2009) 'Existential and spiritual needs in mental health care: An ethical and holistic perspective', *Journal of Holistic Nursing* 27: 34–42.

Magnan, M.A., Reynolds, K.E., and Galvin, E.A. (2006) 'Barriers to addressing patient sexuality in nursing practice', *Dermatology Nursing* 18(5): 448–54.

Matiti, M.R. (2002) 'Patient dignity in nursing: A phenomenological study', Unpublished PhD thesis, University of Huddersfield School of Education and Professional Development.

McEvoy, L. and Duffy, A. (2008) 'Holistic practice: A concept analysis', *Nurse Education in Practice* 8: 412–19.

McGee, P. (1994) 'The concept of respect in nursing', *British Journal of Nursing* 3(13): 681–4.

McSherry, W. (2006) *Making Sense of Spirituality in Nursing and Health Care Practice: An Interactive Approach*, 2nd edn, London: Jessica Kingsley.

Mencap (2007) *Death by Indifference: Following up the Treat Me Right! Report*, London: Mencap.

Mental Welfare Commission for Scotland (2007) 'Older and wiser: Findings from our unannounced visits to NHS continuing care wards', available online at **http://www. mwcscot.org.uk/web/FILES/Publications/Older_and_ Wiser_web.pdf** [accessed 16 June 2011].

Miner-Williams, D. (2006) 'Putting a puzzle together: Making spirituality meaningful for nursing using an evolving theoretical framework', *Journal of Clinical Nursing* 15: 811–21.

Moss, B. (2008) *Communication Skills for Health and Social Care*, Los Angeles, CA: Sage.

Nordenfelt, L. (2003) 'Dignity of the elderly: An introduction', *Medicine, Health Care and Philosophy* 6(2): 99–101.

Nursing and Midwifery Council (2008) *The Code: Standards of Conduct, Performance and Ethics for Nurses and Midwives*, London: NMC. Available online at **http://www. nmc-uk.org/Nurses-and-midwives/The-code/** [accessed 3 October 2011].

Nursing and Midwifery Council (2009a) *Guidance on Professional Conduct for Nursing and Midwifery Students*, London: NMC.

Nursing and Midwifery Council (2009b) *Care and Respect Every Time: New Guidance for the Care of Older People*, London: NMC.

Nursing and Midwifery Council (2010) *Standards for Pre-registration Education*, London: NMC.

O'Toole, G. (2008) *Communication: Core Interpersonal Skills for Health Professionals*, Sydney: Churchill Livingstone.

Patients' Association (2009) *Patients … not Numbers, People … not Statistics*, London: Patients' Association.

Pearson, A., Vaughan, B., and Fitzgerald, M. (2005) *Nursing Models for Practice*, 3rd edn, Edinburgh: Butterworth Heinemann.

Price, B. (2004) 'Demonstrating respect for patient dignity', *Nursing Standard* 19(12): 45–51.

Ridgway, V. (2008) 'Dignity', in A. Mason-Whitehead, B.A. McIntoch, and T. Mason (eds) *Key Concepts in Nursing*, Los Angeles, CA: Sage, pp. 103–8.

Rogers, C.R.(1951) *Client-Centred Therapy: Its Current Practices, Implications and Theory*, Boston, MA: Houston.

Roper, N., Logan, W.W., and Tierney, A.J. (2000) *The Roper–Logan–Tierney Model of Nursing: Based on Activities of Living*, Edinburgh: Churchill Livingstone.

Royal College of Nursing (2008) *Defending Dignity: Challenges and Opportunities for Nurses*, London: RCN.

Rughani, A. (2008) 'The clinical skills assessment process', in K. Mohanna and A. Tavabie (eds) *General Practice Speciality Training: Making it Happen—A Practical Guide for Trainers, Clinical And Educational Supervisors*, London: Royal College of General Practitioners.

Sessanna, L., Finnell, D., and Jezewski, M.A. (2007) 'Spirituality in nursing and health-related literature: A concept analysis', *Journal of Holistic Nursing* 25(4): 252–62.

Thomson, J.E. (2002) 'Midwives and human rights: Dream or reality?', *Midwifery* 18: 188–92.

Turnock, C. and Kelleher, M. (2001) 'Maintaining patient dignity in intensive care settings', *Intensive and Critical Care Nursing* 17(3): 144–54.

Walsh, K. and Kowanko, I. (2002) 'Nurses' and patients' perceptions of dignity', *International Journal of Nursing Practice* 8: 143.

Walton, J. (1999) 'Spirituality of patients recovering from an acute myocardial infarction: A grounded theory study', *Journal of Holistic Nursing* 17: 34–53.

5 Diversity in caring

ARU NARAYANASAMY AND GAVIN NARAYANASAMY

Learning outcomes

This chapter will enable you to:

- respond with sensitivity and inclusivity to individuals from diverse backgrounds;
- understand what is meant by 'diversity' in caring;
- reflect on personal values related to inclusivity and diversity in caring;
- explore strategies to promote inclusivity and caring responses to diversity; and
- act as a patient's advocate with regard to inclusivity and caring in diversity.

Essential knowledge and skills for care

- You must have a good knowledge and understanding about diversity, and recognize different forms of discrimination or social exclusion.
- All nurses must practise in a holistic, non-judgemental, caring and sensitive manner that avoids assumptions, supports social inclusion, recognizes and respects individual choice, and acknowledges diversity.
- Where necessary, nurses must be prepared to challenge inequality, discrimination, and exclusion, and any form of prejudice that may prevent people from diverse backgrounds from having equal access to care.

Introduction

This chapter explores and provides guidance on visible and hidden diversity in care. Visible diversity includes 'race', gender, and physical attributes, whereas hidden diversity include political opinion, sexual orientation (lesbian, gay, bisexual and transgender, or LGBT), ethnicity, teaching and learning styles, regionalism, class, family history, and religion, which are not always apparent on first impressions, but nevertheless have an impact on care. Since diversity and inclusivity are important parts of our humanity, a holistic approach is vital when assessing and planning the care of our fellow humans of diverse backgrounds in suffering, health crisis, and need.

Theory, research, and evidence base

Evidence suggests that caring promotes healing when various dimensions of humanity are part of healthcare strategies. Social and healthcare practitioners with competency in diversity and inclusivity are seen as effective. Social and health care and healing require more than a mechanistic and procedural approach to care practice (Narayanasamy, 2006), for example cultural safety and cultural negotiation (Polascheck, 1998). Service users and their families/friends and practitioners derive greater satisfaction when these dimensions of care are addressed (Department of Health, 1999, 2009; Narayanasamy, 2004; Equality Act 2010).

Liberal civil societies acknowledge that visible and hidden diversities have existed since time immemorial. Most liberal societies, including the UK, recognize their diverse populations and have responded in various ways to address their rights and responsibilities. Within health care there is a drive to promote diversity in practice due to social and health policies to bring about greater social justice. Such drives include the NHS Plan (Department of Health, 2008), the *National Service Framework (NSF) for Older People* (Department of Health, 1998; 2001), the Benchmark Statement

(Quality Assurance Agency for Higher Education, 2001), the Equality Act 2010, the *Religion or Belief* resource (Department of Health, 2009), and user groups, which highlight that health care education and service should respond to diversity and inclusivity.

Since 2000, the British government has actively pursued policies influencing organizations to promote diversity and inclusivity (Nzira and Williams, 2007: 83). In this regard, many employers show commitment to diversity by:

- aspiring to be a beacon on equality matters;
- considering equality and diversity to be complementary;
- setting realistic and achievable equality goals that are measurable;
- mentioning the importance of employers and customers for business success; and
- incorporating the notion of social values and communitarianism.

Promoting equality entails responding to diversity in health. Service users reflect diversity in terms of 'race', ethnicity, spirituality or religion, sexuality, disability, age, and many more. There is consensus in the literature that diversity benefits societies in terms of social, psychological, economic, cultural, and biological richness. Inclusive civil societies reap the benefits from their diverse citizens. Likewise, organizations, including health institutions, are likely to benefit from a diverse workforce and users by being inclusive in their approaches to diversity.

· ·

Take a moment and think about where tea comes from, even if you do not drink it.
Jot down your responses.

· ·

You may have jotted down, for example, India, China, Sri Lanka, Malaysia, and so on. When we drink tea, we do not think about it as a cultural product with a history not only about culture, but also about diversity. You may have conjured up in your head some exotic places in these countries. Another exotic location is the Cameron Highlands, a hill station in Malaysia where tea is grown and picked. Tea is picked by people who represent diversity, such as Malay, Chinese, Indians,

and Eurasians, and the tea plantations are visited by Europeans, Australians, and backpackers representing various nations. Amongst them are Christians, Hindus, Muslims, Buddhists, atheists, agnostics, young and old people, heterosexuals, lesbians, gays, bisexuals, transgenders, able and non-able people. The same diversity is involved when tea is refined and packaged in another country. We do not necessarily think about the diversity that surrounds tea when drinking it. Yet sometimes, when facing someone who looks different from us, some of us socially construct this person as the 'other' using stereotypes based on assumptions and unfounded information (Narayanasamy and White, 2005). The socially constructed 'other' may get ignored, disrespected, marginalized and excluded. Yet all of us belong to a common humanity as global citizens with a rich diversity. It is a waste of vast human talents when we ignore the diversity that exists, and the richness that this brings to both the workforce and service user experience. As social beings, interdependence on biodiversity and human diversity is necessary for our survival (Barry and Yuill, 2008). Without diversity in social and health care workforces, both services would come to a halt. That is the reality of diversity.

The starting point in responding to diversity is to remember that '*people's differences are an asset rather than a burden to be tolerated*' (Nzira and Williams, 2009: 84). However, an understanding of the meaning of diversity is required before we pursue with further discourses on its many features. Two popular meanings prevail, although various critiques exist about the degree to which equality and inclusivity can be achieved regarding diversity. These are managing diversity and diversity management.

Managing diversity and diversity management

The basic concept of managing diversity concedes that the workforce consists of a diverse population of people. The diversity consists of visible and non-visible differences which include factors such as sex, age, background, race, disability, personality and work style. It is

founded on the premise that harnessing these differences will create a productive environment in which everyone feels valued, where their talents are being fully utilised and in which organisational goals are met.

(Kandola and Fullerton, 1998: 7)

[Diversity management] refers to a strategic organisational approach, organisational culture change, and empowerment of the workforce. It represents a shift away from the activities and assumptions defined by affirmative action to management practices that are inclusive, reflecting the workforce diversity and its potential. Ideally it is a pragmatic approach, in which participants anticipate and plan for change, do not fear human differences or perceive them as a threat, and view the workplace as a forum for individuals' growth and change in skills and performance with direct cost benefits to the organisation. (Arredondo, 1996: 17)

Both definitions emphasize the importance of responding to diversity in organizations and such endeavours will lead to an environment in which people are valued because of their diversity. As with all definitions, these two definitions may not measure up as embracing all aspects of diversity, but they offer a starting point for promoting approaches to diversity in the workplace and service delivery.

The subsequent themes of this chapter are largely based on the social model of care because it focuses on the importance of empowering individuals accessing health care. We now turn to caring to disabled people as the starting point in our approaches to diversity and inclusivity.

Caring for disabled people

To empower disabled people, nurses need to work in partnership with them in determining their needs while caring for them. They should ensure that anti-discriminatory practices are in place for the care of disabled people, because evidence suggests that they

are particularly vulnerable to discrimination. Consistent with social models of disability, it is best to use the term 'disabled people' rather that 'people with disability' since the former emphasizes that people are disabled by a society, since it expects them to adapt rather than the other way around. It is paramount that patronizing languages and stereotypes are avoided. Languages embedded in disabilism have no place in health care or anywhere.

Although nurses are involved in the care of disabled people, there is very little literature on nursing approaches to the care of disabled people, apart from learning disability nursing discourses. The individual model of disability is apparent in medical and health-care (rehabilitative) discourses. This model focused almost exclusively on the individual's incapacity as due to bodily or functional limitation. The functional incapacity is used as a basis for typifying the individual as invalid. This social construction of the person leads to the disability becoming their defining characteristic and their incapacity is generalized (see **Figure 5.1**).

The personal tragedy approach, embedded in contemporary social welfare policies, is attributed to this social construction of disability whereby the individual is pitied as a victim and as someone who requires care and attention, and who is dependent on others (Barnes et al., 1999).

The focus of the medical approach on the personal tragedy of the affected is to put them through a medical regime of cure and rehabilitation involving allied health practitioners, psychologists, and educationalists. The primary concern of the medical profession is to diagnose the bodily or intellectual 'abnormality' and prescribe an appropriate treatment (Barnes et al., 1999). The medical and related professionals exert great power over the impaired person's life by imposing medical and therapeutic action upon the assumed dependent person. In this regard, the individual model is based on the assumption that disabled people are inert: acted upon rather than active. They have no other alternative but to rely on others for care and charity. Their fate and destination is dependent upon policymakers and service providers. They are subjected to a trajectory of compliance and adjustment

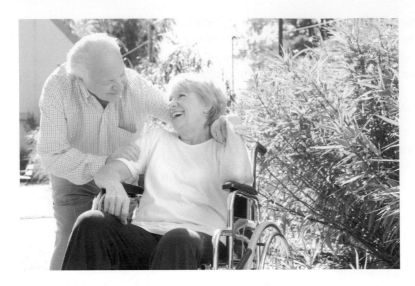

Figure 5.1 Consider how you perceive this lady: is her disability her defining characteristic? © iceteastock–Fotolia.com.

to their disabilities and a future dictated by panels of health experts. The disadvantage faced by the person with disability is perceived as an individual, not a collective, matter. A dichotomous scenario is created in which the disabled person is seen as an uninformed lay client deferring to a professional expert. The unequal power relations and the conflicts between lay and expert values are ignored. The individual model offers the disabled person only a childlike existence with the assumption that they are unable to speak for themselves.

The affected individual is expected to make best use of their situation through individual adjustment and coping strategies. They are required to take on a persona whereby their hopes and aspirations are curtailed to be realistic about life due to their impairment and incapacity to determine things for themselves. Individuals are socialized into a disabled identity whether the impairment was congenital or acquired later in life. The personal tragedy model depicts the person's disability as a pathology in health terms and disability as a social problem in welfare terms (Oliver, 1996). Although the individual model appears to be altruistic and takes moral responsibility for the well-being of people with disabilities, it limits them as persons to be pitied with childlike needs.

Whilst the individual model appears beneficial in the form of state support through Disability Living Allowance (DLA) and related financial support and services, critical disability theorists vehemently reject that the intent of this model is benevolent. Critics argue that the individual model causes the disability and disempowers the affected person. It privileges medical experts in terms of their biomedical knowledge, power in determining treatment plans for powerless patients (Reynolds, 2004). Medical ways of defining and controlling the trajectories of the disabled person's body and mind take prominence over the individual's agency, including experiences, values, and goals concerning their disability as well as treatment, care, and support. However, the individual/medical model is relevant and necessary in case of emergencies and the fixing of reversible bodily impairments and control of diseases, but the respect for patients' agency should be maintained and promoted in medical care in the context of the equal power relations.

While critical disability theorists emphasize the centrality of disabled people's agency, they locate the problems encountered by them in the structure, of which oppression stands out among many other social injustices. Barnes and Mercer (2003: 19) cite evidence of oppression where there is *'highly unequal distribution of material resources and uneven power relations and opportunities to participate in everyday life, compared to those available to non-disabled people'*. Barnes et al.

(1999) deconstruct the individual model of disability and offer the social model as an alternative.

Social model of disability

The social model of disability is advocated as the enabling approach to disability. Such a model offers an analytical framework that critically examines the '*process of marginalization, oppression, discrimination, exclusion, or in other words disablement that affects people with impairment*' (Sapey, 2004: 273). Instead of focusing on the individual's limitation and incapacity, the social model concentrates on a set of causes established externally—that is, obstacles imposed on disabled people—which act as barriers to full participation and citizenship (Finklestein, 1980; Riox and Bach, 1994; Barnes et al., 1999).

The social model of disability offers a progressive approach to disability. It views disability as the disadvantage or restrictions of activity caused by social organizations that take no or little account of the affected person and exclude them from participation in the mainstream of social activities. Disability is associated with social barriers and, in doing so, it does not disregard the reality of impairment. It emphasizes how society renders people with impairment dependent and excludes them in many social and economic activities. Using social theory, Abberley (1997) produces a sophisticated discourse on disability as a form of social oppression. Drawing on comparative social theories of sexism and racism, Abberley identifies and contextualizes experiences of disabled people, locating oppression in hierarchical social relations and divisions. However, Abberley argues that disabled people are more disadvantaged through oppression than those facing racism and sexism (women) due to skin colour and gender, respectively. Physical impairment as a biological element is a reality that limits the disabled person, whereas gender and race are not.

The social model proposes a review of the effects of physical, social, and disabling barriers as lived experiences. In other words, the social exclusion and the impact of anti-discrimination policies need constant review. In developing a critique of the personal tragedy model, the social model of disability is put forward as an effective alternative. Advocates of this model argue for a radical reformulation of our understanding of disability. They attempt to provide radical answers to key questions such as '*What is the nature of disabilities? What causes* [them]*? How* [are they] *experienced?*' (Oliver, 1996: 29–30).

It is clear that the social model of disability demands a more comprehensive examination of the processes and structures connected with social oppression and discrimination at everyday levels, workings of the state, and social policy. It also calls for closer examination of the impact of domination and power over disabled people and the arenas of resistance and challenge posed by disabled people themselves (Barnes et al., 1999). The social model covers a wide range of social and material factors and conditions, including family circumstances, income and financial support, education, employment, housing, transport and the built environment, and many more. Furthermore, the social model treats disabilities and their associated problems not as fixed entities, but as temporal ones, as the disabled persons negotiate and navigate through their life course.

Although the social model of disability is favoured by disabled people, there is contention that the social model should be seen as an analytical model that is open to alternative approaches to disabilities. It should not be used too prescriptively to refer to disability that restricts ideas in its pursuit to enforce conformity or partial adherence (Shakespeare, 1997; Ward, 1997). Instead of being seen as a blueprint, the social model should be used as an analytical framework (Stone, 2001)—a case in point for much of this chapter.

....

Take a moment to reflect on what the following terms mean to you.
Ethnicity
Cultural diversity
Cultural competence
Spirituality and religion
....

Ethnic and cultural diversity

Caring for people from diverse ethnicities and cultures is a characteristic of UK healthcare practices. Therefore, in this section, ethnicity and cultural diversity are addressed within the context of a multicultural UK.

The conceptual and empirical discourses on these dimensions of humanity are developed with further guidance on the promotion of inclusivity regarding ethnicity and cultural diversity. The literature acknowledges the UK as one of the most ethnically diverse countries in Europe (Baxter, 2000; Narayanasamy and White, 2005; Narayanasamy, 2006; Barry and Yuill, 2008). According to the 2001 population census, approximately 9 per cent in England claimed to belong to black and other minority ethnic (BME) groups. Thus it is within this ethnically diverse society that healthcare providers should deliver a service that is culturally sensitive and appropriate to meet specific needs (Narayanasamy, 2006).

Five decades have lapsed since Leininger first recognized the importance of understanding the significance of other ethnicities' cultural 'lifeways' (ways of life) that are based on their value and belief systems. So full of conviction was Leininger regarding the pivotal importance of this fundamental specialist knowledge to the effective practice of nursing that she embarked on a lengthy ethnographic study, resulting in the production of approximately a hundred culture-specific studies. From this work, Leininger developed a body of evidence on cultural awareness and culturally sensitivity care programmes. Although Leininger was criticized for overlooking structural factors such as racial and cultural discrimination, her work was highly influential in the developing the theory of transcultural nursing, which can be defined as:

> **formal areas of study and practice in the cultural beliefs, values and life ways of diverse cultures and in the use of knowledge to provide culture-specific or culture-universal care to individuals, families and groups of particular cultures.**
>
> (Leininger, 2001: 50)

Herberg (1989) believes that nursing care provided '*in a manner that is sensitive to the needs of individuals, families and groups who represent diverse cultural population within a society*' is transcultural nursing.

There is now a body of knowledge that professional nursing can access. Leininger (1997a; 1997b) held the view that care was powerful in healing and that there could be no curing without caring. Thus, she 'gave birth' to the concept of transcultural nursing, the goal of which is to provide culturally congruent care that is tailored to cultural-specific care values and lifeways. Leininger hoped that the research-based evidence from her culture care theory would provide knowledge to support the discipline of transcultural nursing. Leininger's vision was that, by the year 2020, transcultural care would have permeated all aspects of nursing globally (Leininger, 2001). However, critics stress that Leininger's model is a passive statement of good intent based on free will and the assumption that all good nurses want to provide culturally specific care. Her model neglects the real 'heart of the matter': the issues of prejudice and racism (Eisenbruch, 2001; Narayanasamy, 2006).

In the UK, there has been a tradition in the cultural care discourse whereby a transcultural healthcare approach based on research knowledge and competence offered a basis for how to care sensitively for people with cultural needs (McGee, 1992; Rassool, 1995; Gerrish et al., 1996; Narayanasamy, 2002, 2006). Nurse education offers empirically based guidance on cultural care practice. From the perspectives of healthcare users (minority ethnic communities), educators, practitioners and students, Gerrish et al. (1996) propose a model for transcultural healthcare practice that incorporates the development of cultural sensitivity (the practitioner as a tourist), reflexive honesty, a re-examination of ethnicity, intercultural communication and associated stress, measures to eradicate racism (particularly institutional), concerted efforts in improving policies, and procedures related to the recruitment and selection of candidates from ethnic minority communities. In addition to this model, the planning and delivery of transcultural healthcare programmes can be effective if specific learning materials are available (Narayanasamy, 2006).

Much of the literature on cultural care (Parfitt, 1998; Gerrish and Papadopoulos, 1999; Narayanasamy, 2006;

Papadopoulos, 2006; Holland and Hogg, 2009) describes the following as desirable for implementing transcultural health care. An extensive database of healthcare information about culturally determined aspects of health, illness, and care may help to improve transcultural care. This can be enhanced by the provision of culture-specific and culture-sensitive nursing care (Leininger, 1997a), but at the same time placing an emphasis on caring acts as universal, but taking many forms and variations in many cultures (Leininger, 1997b). This approach can be strengthened if healthcare practitioners consider that systems of treatment and care may already prevail in other cultures, and integrate these into current practice (Narayanasamy, 2006). In regard to this, Leininger (1997b) stresses that attention should be paid to the significance of 'folk systems' and that these need to be incorporated into professional approaches to care. However, Gerrish et al. (1996) caution that without opportunities for self-awareness development (subjecting the self to challenges of assumptions), healthcare practitioners are less likely to show sensitivity to other cultural values. Likewise, Baxter (2000) warns that imposing one's own values on others can be offensive and unprofessional; in such circumstances, clients may avoid carers.

Although progress is being made regarding cultural competency in nursing in the UK, a critical discourse on cultural care is emerging. According to Culley (2001), Qureshi (1989) and Rack (1990) have been instrumental in producing distorted notions of cultural cohesive communities in the UK and portraying them with negative stereotypes. Qureshi and Rack use the biomedical discourse in perpetuating the essentialist's view of ethnicity and culture. Such a misguided approach is limiting in homogenizing and perpetuating stereotypical versions of cultural beliefs and practices of the socially constructed 'other'. Cultures framed in rigid and static terms are regarded as British or 'aliens'. People are differentiated as the other or British usually in terms of whiteness or physical and other markers including skin colour, culture, religion, and so on. Diversity and differences are redefined and reproduced by social construction and presented as the 'other'. According to Culley (2001: 111), people are stereotyped using the culturalist's framework:

West Indians, for example, are stereotypically described as resentful of authority, having low educational standards and being involved in drugs and crime. Asian families are seen as close-knit and industrious but very different culturally. In recent years Muslims in particular have been characterised as aliens and intolerant fanatics who pose a threat to the 'British way of life'.

In reality, individuals renegotiate, intersect, transact, compromise, and adapt throughout their life course and trajectories of illness, structural barriers, social divisions, and so on. However, in its defence, the culturalist's approach originating from Leininger's theory highlights the importance of cultural sensitivity in nursing and health care. Despite its colonial legacy and anthropological traditions, transcultural perspectives have an enduring hold on nursing by offering an apparent framework for responding with sensitivity to patients' and clients' cultural, spiritual, and religious needs. Culturalists claim to take an inclusive approach to the cultural needs of patient in a multi-ethnic and multicultural context of health care. However, Gunaratnam (2001) contends that, in doing so, culturalists have created 'fact files' on cultural beliefs and practices that are unhelpful. Such an approach ignores diversity and the individual's agency for negotiating, or simply for being a human requiring holistic understanding rather than a socially constructed person with imagined attributes and categories as the 'other'. Gunaratnam (2001) argues that 'fact files' reinforce a myopic view of culture as one-dimensional, '*frozen in time and context*' (Culley, 2001: 122). The culturalist focus leads to packaging cultural practices with patients' choices and this precedence sidelines or ignores their need for holistic care, including emotional support. The reductionist approach to multicultural practices renders professional interaction highly task-orientated. Until a consensus is reached towards a unitary approach to ethnicity and culture in nursing and healthcare practices, a misguided and untested approach to cultural care will be perpetuated.

As a consequence of the emerging criticism on cultural care, the preferred approach is ethnicity and cultural care in diversity and inclusivity. This may include spiritual care (see Chapter 8), according to the needs of patient/clients. Spiritual care is distinct from religious care, but religion may be part of cultural and spiritual care. It is important not to make assumptions about people's ethnicity, culture, spirituality, and religion. It is always best to be guided by patients or clients, or their next of kin, or their representatives, about their individual preferences regarding the above dimensions of care. In the absence of personal preferences for reasons of incapacity to express wish, if cultural and religious fact files are consulted, these should be used with caution and sensitivity, because none of the cultural and religious lists is fixed.

There is no such thing as a fixed cultural or religious factor. Healthcare practitioners should continue to check with patients and users about the currency of the 'fact files' before imposing interventions based on the cultural/religious list. None of these is a substitute for holistic care, which normally embraces comprehensive care in terms of physical, emotional, psychological, cultural, and spiritual care in partnership with patients. The care plan and interventions should be based on the principles of autonomy and justice. Nursing interventions should embrace the five 'C's (Narayanasamy, 2006):

- **C**are;
- **C**ompassion;
- **C**ommunication skills;
- **C**onnection; and
- **C**ommitment.

Now see **Practice Example 5.1.**

Putting diversity and inclusivity in action

As explored earlier, the social model gets us to reflect critically on the social factors that disable the person and it empowers individuals to take control of their lives. It is empowering because it puts the patients in the centre stage of health care and calls on us to respect individuals' identities and personhood. The three themes—caring by being inclusive, empowering people, and promoting anti-discriminatory practice—are central to actioning care practice that is inclusive of diversity. These are outlined below, after which we will provide the ACCESS model as a framework for an inclusive approach to caring for diverse needs.

Caring by being inclusive

Although most people may have faced some form of discrimination and disrespect in their lives, the groups of people referred to in this chapter are even more vulnerable or become targets of discrimination for being perceived to be different from dominant norms and values. Inclusive practice is characterized as:

- involving caring, compassion, connection, communication, and commitment to patients/clients (the five 'C's);
- promoting equality, empowerment, partnership, working collaboratively, participation, and anti-discriminatory practices;
- promoting individuals' well-being;
- responding with sensitivity to diversity in practice;
- making a difference to people's lives; and
- empowering others.

PRACTICE EXAMPLE 5.1

Ramesh, an Asian young man with autistic spectrum disorder (ASD), is admitted to a medical unit following bouts of diarrhoea and dehydration. Recently, he has been to India to visit his grandparents. Ramesh is partially sighted and has problems getting around the unit because of the unfamiliar environment. Since admission to the unit, he appears withdrawn and uncommunicative. Staff attend to his medical and physical needs, but leave him alone most of the time. They assume that he is non-interactive because of ASD and visual problems.

What might staff do, beyond attending to his medical and physical needs, to make Ramesh's stay in the unit a better one? Remember to take into account in your discussion his diverse needs and to consider a transcultural model of care for Ramesh.

Assessment	Focus on spiritual, religious, and cultural aspects of clients' lifestyles, health beliefs, and health practices
Communication	Be aware of variations in verbal and non-verbal responses
Cultural negotiation and compromise	Become more aware of aspects of other people's spirituality and cultures, as well as understand clients' views and explain their problems
Establishing respect and rapport	A therapeutic relationship that portrays genuine respect for clients' cultural beliefs and values is required
Sensitivity	Deliver diverse culturally sensitive care to culturally diverse groups
Safety	Enable clients to derive a sense of cultural safety

Figure 5.2 The ACCESS model (Narayanasamy, 2006).

Empowering people

Central to anti-discriminatory practices is empowerment. Caring practices should be based on the principles of empowerment because empowerment frees individuals from powerlessness and oppression. Powerlessness generates experiences such as exclusion, rejection, or being treated as inferior, which lead to feelings of inadequacy, helplessness, and dependency (Dalrymple and Burke, 2006), with devastating effects on individuals—especially individuals perceived to be different and constructed as the unworthy 'other'.

Promoting anti-discriminatory practice

One way of ensuring that vulnerable groups are protected is through anti-discriminatory practices. Anti-discriminatory practices can be achieved by personal and professional development, including:

- self-awareness—that is, value clarification;
- critical reflective thinking and positive action;
- challenging assumptions and deconstructing misunderstandings or myths;
- respecting diversity and differences;
- connecting;
- self-empowerment; and
- seeking help if you need to work on value clarification.

To promote anti-discriminatory practice, an awareness of structural factors is necessary—particularly an awareness of legislation related to diversity.

The ACCESS model

The ACCESS model, developed by one of the authors (Narayanasamy, 2006), can be used as a framework for responding to diversity and inclusivity in health care, and for cultural needs assessment and cultural care planning. The rudiments of this model are as illustrated in **Figure 5.2**.

Although the ACCESS model focuses on cultural care, we feel that culture is central to diversity in health care. Our cultural orientations in terms our age, gender, and sexuality, ability or disability, 'race' and ethnicity, and spirituality or religion influence our approaches to life. Culture, in the context of diversity, is the map that enables us to navigate and negotiate our way through the social transactions that we encounter throughout our lives, whether in health or illness. Since diversity covers a range of social and cultural identities, we selectively use these categories to illustrate in the ACCESS model how nurses and healthcare practitioners might respond to the care needs of their patients.

These are now briefly discussed in turn.

Assessment

A comprehensive assessment of (for example, disabled) patients' lifestyles, health beliefs, and health practices will go a long way towards enabling nurses to make decisions and judgements related to care interventions. The disabled person may be young or old, heterosexual or LGBT, religious or secular, black, white, Asian, or of other ethnicity. By paying careful attention to a patient's history, we will be in a better position to understand their biography as well as their journey to health care. A holistic assessment in the context of diversity may enhance the nurse's understanding of the patient's health beliefs and practices, as well as offer insights into the social and cultural dimensions of their lives.

Assessment incorporating answers to the following questions with regard to the patient's beliefs about their illness and its causes, symptoms, and treatment may be thought of as the patient's explanatory model of illness (Kleinman et al., 1978). The term 'explanatory model' is preferable to the term 'folk health beliefs' because this latter has derogatory connotations relating to something primitive and non-scientific. The information obtained from assessment will provide vital understanding of similarities and differences related to the patient's beliefs and attitudes regarding the illness and the nurse's own beliefs and attitudes. The ACCESS model offers opportunities for a conscious and sustained effort on the part of the nurse to focus on the diversity factors such as spiritual and cultural that influence a patient's behaviour and reaction to an illness. Patients' narratives about the progress and difficulties that they experience on a daily basis may provide clues about basic values and attitudes regarding the impact of their illness on activities of daily living (ADLs).

The following questions may be asked as part of the assessment, for example in the context of a patient's culture.

1 Do you know why you receive health care?
2 Do you have specific cultural and/or spiritual/ religious needs?
3 What problems has your illness caused?
4 Some persons forget to take daily medications/ injections. Does this happen to you?
5 What have you done to remind you to take your pills?
6 What worries you about your health?

In the main, cultural assessment should comprise:

- a holistic approach;
- partnership (the patient is the expert);

- a person-centred approach;
- sensitivity to the individual and their identity;
- the preservation of respect and dignity; and
- the avoidance of assumptions and stereotypes.

Care plans and intervention programmes can be developed derived from the above assessment and the subsequent elements of the ACCESS model.

Communication

The crux of transcultural spiritual care is communication (Peberdy, 1997; Narayanasamy, 2001; Johnston Taylor, 2007). It is important for nurses to be aware that groups vary widely in their ideas about appropriate body stances and proximities, gestures, language, listening styles, and eye contact. For example, Narayanasamy (2001) points out that traditional Asians typically consider direct eye contact inappropriate and disrespectful. It is well known that language differences cause prolonged treatment in comparison with that of English-speaking patients (Sherer, 1993). Sometimes, it may seem convenient to use a member of the patient's family as an interpreter to facilitate the communication process, but to save embarrassment in the presence of a family member the patient may fabricate a new problem. Also, the interpreter may interpret rather than translate the patient's problems. The nurse who is unfamiliar with the language may not realize whose views are being expressed. We provide a focus on gender, older people, and ageism to draw attention to the impact that derogatory terms may have in communications pertaining to such groups. The impact of negative references and connotations may have a devastating effect upon vulnerable people categorized in terms of sexism and ageism.

Gender

At the simplest level, we see humans as women and men, and assign physical and other attributes to differentiate gender. Sociologists have challenged the assumptions that gender divisions could be explored merely in terms of biological differences between women and men (Abbott, 2000). Sex is a biological fact, but gender is socially constructed (Barry and Yuill, 2008). Connell (2005) provides useful insights into the theory of gender regarding masculinity and patriarchy. Sex is determined by the anatomical features leading to identification of male and female, whereas gender refers to the social, cultural, and psychological aspects of being a woman or a man. However, both terms are used interchangeably in some discourses with the term gender used synonymously to refer to women. Gender is not as clear-cut, with research showing that the social category of a woman or man is variable. For example, among the Wodaabe tribe in Niger of the African continent, men wear makeup and behave in ways that could be constructed as feminine in some other societies (Barry and Yuill, 2008). As part of their culture, men go through elaborate measures to be attractive to women, but still retain their masculinity; elsewhere these men may be categorized as effeminate or gay.

The language that we use and its discourses about women and men are sometimes sexist. There is the prevailing stereotype that women talk more than men. However, empirical research evidence suggests that men frequently talk more, although not necessarily all of the time, in mixed-sex groups than do women. Furthermore, men will interrupt women more often than women will interrupt men (Tannen, 1993). This is the case in our observations of classroom interactions and management meetings. Feminists' discourses have explained in terms of recurrent observations that men talk more to exploit their power and dominance over women to devalue them. However, others observe that such discourses have overlooked the possibility that women and men are socialized to interact differently because they have different goals of interaction. Consequently, naturally occurring talk targets these goals (James and Drakich, 1993). Other research highlights how girls and boys use language differently, with boys asserting themselves to be dominant by attracting an audience, while girls create and maintain interpersonal relations, criticize others less directly, exercise leadership less directly, and respond to interaction with others differently (Conefrey, 1997). However,

such interactions may not necessarily occur in all situations. A more fluid approach with no clear-cut dominance may prevail in inclusive social discourses.

Take a moment to reflect on interactions between women and men in any settings in health care.
As part of your reflections, consider what you would do to eradicate sexism in workplace practice and user settings.

You may have identified in the reflective activity some of the observations made in this chapter. You may have noted that there is no single discernable behaviour exhibited by women or men in the different health care settings. This may indicate that progress is being made in the right direction regarding equality and inclusivity in terms of sex and gender. However, if differences in the patterns of interactions occur in typically gendered lines, we need to be aware of the potential consequence and impact of such occurrences on recipients. We need to take measures to eradicate individuals exerting dominance over others in interactive situations in health care.

You may have indicated the conscious avoidance of sexist remarks and jokes, patronizing sentiments towards women and men, challenging colleagues and users when respect is infringed through misuse of language. It is important that all healthcare staff set and maintain personal standards in the way in which we use languages that undermine sexual identities. In a civilized society, there is no place for people to use offensive language, or to patronize or exclude anyone. Such gestures sometime make indelible imprints in individuals' minds, severely denting their self-esteem and self-image. As members of healing teams and educators, we have met people with dented self-concepts because of such impact. We had to work hard as carers (us) and cared (dented selves) to restore the selves from damage. There is no place for remarks that compromise people's dignity.

We have explored gender issues regarding diversity and inclusivity, because these potentially occur in our everyday interactions with colleagues and users. Next, we will explore age and ageism regarding older people in the context of lexicons that are used pejoratively, which often damages the self in the older person.

Older people

Although many older people are experiencing fuller lives as citizens, including being prominent socially, culturally, politically, and in many other areas, some are vulnerable due to ageism and prejudices. Some older people are subjected to discrimination for being old and are consequently marginalized in all walks of life, including in health care.

....

Before we proceed to explore ageism and older people, take a moment to reflect on what life will be like for you in fifty years' time.

....

It might be difficult for you to have a sense of what life might be like in fifty years' time, because most of us do not think that far ahead. Depending on our age, some of us may not even be here in fifty years' time. We talk about older people as though they are some 'other', but we are actually talking about us in a few years' time. This exercise will have made you think about yourself in years to come: most of us will have indicated that we would like to be healthy and independent, and continue to live as respected citizens. While most of us treat older people with respect and inclusivity, there are disturbing incidences of disregard for older people's dignity and respect (Patient Association, 2009). This sometimes happens because we construct the older person as the 'other' and use stereotypes that influence our reactions to older people. Needless to say, older people are us—but they have the advantage of having lived for many years and developed great insights into life as a consequence of that lived experience.

Old age confronts all of us in spite of the attempts to find scientific means to avert the ageing process. The body is subjected to ageing and changes from the moment of birth to the time of death. However, the physical, social, spiritual, and psychological trajectories of ageing can be made as bearable as possible with due consideration to fellow humanity through positive attitudes and actions that eradicate ageism.

Ageism can be defined in various ways. Barry and Yuill (2008: 212) offer two definitions:

- a set of beliefs originating from biological variation related to the ageing process; and
- the actions of corporate bodies and their agents, and the resulting views of ordinary people.

Ageism is one of the most resistant forms of discriminatory acts against humanity, although all of us go through ageing process. Ageism occurs at personal and structural levels. At a personal level, individuals may react with ageism towards older people, whilst structural factors may constitute an institutional level, and the context can be widened to a national level at which policies may discriminate against older people. In health care, ageism may occur in direct form whereby older people are denied care and treatment due to discriminatory policies or guidelines. This overt form of ageism can be prevented, but indirect ageism is subtle and prevails because of negative attitudes and assumptions that the health of older people is less significant than that of younger people. These forms of attitude prevail in some of our courses on which intense value clarifications and ethical considerations had to be undertaken to shift negative attitudes among some healthcare students.

....

Consider for a moment the positive and negative images of older people.

....

Apart from physical and emotional abuses, older people are often excluded and subjected to derogatory language. The terms 'old folk' and 'the elderly' are unacceptable terms, while terms such as 'pensioners' and 'senior citizens' may be acceptable to some, but not others. The term 'older people' appears to be acceptable to all. The term 'elders' may be used by some religious groups and minority ethnic communities.

We have explored how language and its discourses may perpetuate stereotypes in terms of gender and age, and we have considered how various aspects of stereotypes and practices might be eradicated.

Cultural negotiation and compromise

A great degree of self-awareness is required on the part of the nurses in order to make cultural negotiation and compromise when using the ACCESS model to respond to the diverse needs in practice. The emancipatory paradigm derived from feminist and postcolonial theoretical perspectives calls us to examine our values in the context of the dominant cultural and heterosexual positions. Values clarification—that is, self examination of our beliefs and values based on dominant culture and practices—may help us to be sensitive to those socially constructed as the 'other'. The other could be persons different from us in terms ethnicity, spirituality, sexuality, age, ability, and many more. For example, as part of cultural negotiation and compromise, the ACCESS model calls us to become more aware of aspects of other people's cultures, although it is recognized that it is almost impossible for all of us to be experts in all cultures, because there are more than 3,000 cultures. Transcultural therapeutic interventions require cultural negotiation and compromise (Goode, 1993). This requires an understanding of how the patient views and explains the problem. It may include, for example, working in partnership with traditional healers and other health practitioners, or herbal therapists along with orthodox medical treatment. It may involve helping patients to arrange culturally orientated ceremonies connected with grieving and loss. In summary, nursing intervention should be aimed at being orientated to patients' value positions, showing sensitivity to the communication process and care expectations.

Establishing respect and rapport

Many of us can recall occasions when we were treated disrespectfully by other people and it may have had a devastating impact upon our self-concept and dignity as a person. Disrespect evokes feelings of being devalued and leading to dents in our self-esteem; being respected produces a more positive effect in us. Nurses can establish respect and rapport as follows. The nurses can portray a genuine respect for the patient as a unique individual with needs that are influenced by cultural beliefs and values (Narayanasamy, 2006). This will enable patients to maintain their self-respect, leading to better self-esteem, which is often at a low ebb during a health crisis. A positive nurse–patient relationship is most likely to establish the rapport between them. This, in turn, will foster an atmosphere of trust in which a therapeutic relationship will be continued. All of these will lead to the development of mutual respect for each other's cultural beliefs and values.

Sensitivity

The primary concern of health care is to understand and deliver diverse culturally sensitive care to diverse cultural groups. The care needs of the patients should be met through culturally adapted approaches. For nursing interventions to be effective, it is paramount that nurses show sensitivity to all aspects of patients' needs, as well as to the communication process involved. As part of this process, nurses require knowledge of expected patient-specific patterns of communication. For example, it is important for nurses to recognize that certain terms, concepts, and distinctions drawn in other languages are not always easily translated into English. In such situations, patients whose first language is not English may sometimes draw from their indigenous vocabulary to make their points. Further understanding of the ways in which style and tone of communication may be used is required.

However, sensitivity needs to be extended to all patients, as explored in the earlier section on 'Communication', and how the use of inappropriate language and derogatory terms pertaining to gender, sexuality, and age may have devastating impact upon individuals. It is therefore needless to stress that sensitivity needs to be in the forefront of our approach to patients in caring practice.

Safety

We now turn to safety, the final element in the ACCESS model. Patients need to derive a sense of cultural safety in the sense of ethnicity, age, sexuality, spirituality, and ability and disability. Conceptualization related to this part of the model is derived from the work of Ramsden (1990; 1993) and Polaschek (1998). Cultural safety as a concept was developed by Maori nurses in an attempt to bring to focus the needs of the indigenous minority in New Zealand. Its strategy is to avert actions that diminish, demean or disempower the cultural identity and well-being of an individual. Therefore, culturally safe nursing practice promotes actions that recognize, respect, and nurture the unique cultural identity of individuals, and *'safely meet their expectations and rights'* (Wood and Schwass, 1993: 5–6; cited in Polaschek, 1998: 254).

It is culturally unsafe if individuals perceive the healthcare environment to be alienating and one that ignores their needs in terms of service, treatment, or attitude. On the other hand, an environment in which cultural adaptation takes place between nurses and patients may promote a sense of cultural safety. Patients who experience a sense of cultural safety are most likely to have trust in nurses and to derive further benefits from the therapeutic relationship, which is vital for interventions designed to meet cultural needs.

....
Consider the following scenario.
Words get around the ward and the hospital that a transgender person has been admitted to the ward, and that some staff are finding it hard to deal with this patient due to a poor understanding of sexuality.
Reflect upon your own understanding of sexuality and the issues this may raise when caring for people who do not fit the convention of heterosexuality.
How would you address the lack of regard for this patient's privacy and preferred identity?
....

There are some people who may not quite fit the mainstream notion of heterosexuality and these include people who regard themselves in terms of 'lesbian', 'gay', 'bisexual', and 'transgender' (LGBT is a collective label for such identities). Some may feel unsafe and resort to concealing their sexual identities to avoid discrimination and reprisals. The caring culture needs to be inclusive and receptive of people who have either disclosed or concealed their identities. While society may have become more tolerant, with 'normalization' due to the assertive work of identity politics involving relentless campaigns by LGBTs, some individuals face exclusion. Our health care, perceived to be feminized, benefits users with a culture of care, compassion, and communication, but the organization may be run as an enterprise with replication of mainstream heterosexual perspectives at the delivery point. Such perspectives may pervade practice in the form of hidden discrimination against people perceived to be deviating from norms of heterosexuality. Caring should not be subjected to practices characterizing exclusions of those not conforming to heterosexuality. Much of the healthcare considerations for LBGTs are covered by the Department of Health (2008). In its document 'Delivering the NHS Plan', the Department offers clear guidance on everything that healthcare professionals need to know about LBGTs (see the end of this chapter for more information and a link to the online publication). It addresses people who are LGBT, illustrating the identities and diversity of such people in various walks of life. In doing so, it proceeds to explore the health needs of LGBT people, including the discrimination, bullying, intimation, and abuses that some people with these identities may face. There then follows an outline of some of the barriers to LGBT health care, and the policies and legislation that relate to the provision of health care for LBGT people are addressed in this document. Finally, this valuable document incorporates the links and resources that are useful for caring for LGBT people.

Further information about the Department of Health's work on sexual orientation and gender identity is available online at the address given in the 'Further reading' at the end of this chapter.

Conclusion

In a chapter of this nature, it has been possible to cover only the essentials for caring ways of working in respect to diversity and inclusivity. Visible and hidden diversity was addressed to highlight that certain groups perceived to be different and socially constructed as the undesirable may become targets of discrimination and stereotypes. Although progress has been made in regard to greater awareness and tolerance of fellow humanity, there is much to be achieved in promoting the social model for more inclusive approaches to diversity and caring. We have used the social model of care as the theoretical framework within which to develop much of the discourse on diversity and inclusivity in caring practice. Various theoretical perspectives underpinned by the social model are explained to develop a practice focus on caring for diverse needs. Rudiments of approaches to promoting anti-discriminatory practices and positive actions have been outlined to guide such measures in caring practice. Various resources and further readings central to diversity and inclusivity are provided at the end of this chapter, and you are strongly advised to visit the resources and undertake further reading, in order that your personal and professional development is responsive to diversity in caring, in which each one of us is a bright colour in the rich tapestry of life.

Further reading

Department of Health on sexual orientation and gender identity **http://www.dh.gov.uk/en/Policyandguidance/Equalityandhumanrights/Sexualorientationandgenderidentity/index.htm**

Equality and Human Rights Commission **http://www.equalityhumanrights.com/**

Ethnicity Online **http://www.ethnicityonline.net/**

References

Abberley, P. (1997) 'The limits of classical social theory in the analysis and transformation of disablement', in L. Barton and M. Oliver (eds) *Disability Studies: Past, Present and Future*, Leeds: The Disability Press, pp. 25–44.

Abbott, P. (2000) 'Gender' in G. Payne (ed) *Social Divisions*, Basingstoke: Palgrave, pp. 55–90.

Arredondo, P. (1996) *Successful Diversity Management Initiatives*, London: Sage.

Barnes, C. and Mercer, G. (2003) *Disability*, Cambridge: Polity.

Barnes, C., Mercer, G., and Shakespeare, T. (1999) *Exploring Disability: A Sociological Introduction*, Cambridge: Polity.

Barry, A-M. and Yuill, C. (2008) *Understanding the Sociology of Health: An Introduction*, 2nd edn, London: Sage.

Baxter, C. (2000) 'Antiracist practice: Achieving competency and maintaining professional standards', in T. Thompson and P. Mathias (eds) *Lyttle's Mental Health and Disorder*, Edinburgh: Bailliere Tindal, pp. 350–8.

Conefrey, T. (1997) 'Gender, culture and authority in a university life science laboratory', *Discourse and Society* 8(3): 313–40.

Connell, R.W (2005) *Masculinities*, Cambridge: Polity.

Culley, L.A. (2001) 'Nursing, culture and competence', in L. Culley and S. Dyson (eds) *Ethnicity and Nursing Practice*, Basingstoke: Palgrave, pp. 109–28.

Dalrymple, J. and Burke, B. (2006) *Anti-Oppressive Practice*, 2nd edn, London: Open University Press.

Department of Health (1998) *Tackling Racial Harassment in the NHS. A Plan for Action*, London: HMSO.

Department of Health (1999) *National Service Framework (NSF) for Mental Health*, London: HMSO.

Department of Health (2001) *National Service Framework (NSF) for Older People: Modern Standards and Service Models*, available online at **http://www.dh.gov.uk/en/Publicationsandstatistics/Publications/PublicationsPolicyAndGuidance/DH_4009449** [accessed 16 June 2011].

Department of Health (2008) 'Delivering the NHS Plan', available online at **http://www.dh.gov.uk/en/Publicationsandstatistics/Publications/AnnualReports/Browsable/DH_5277178** [accessed 16 June 2011].

Department of Health (2009) *Religion or Belief*, London: HMSO.

Eisenbruch, M. (2001) *National Review of Nursing Education: Multicultural Nursing Education*, Canberra: Department of Education, Training and Youth Affairs.

Equality Act 2010 The Equality Act (October 1 2010): need to know for small businesses available online at **http://www.smarta.com/advice/legal/employment-law/the-equality-act-(october-1-2010)-need-to-know-for-small-businesses?gclid=CO6L8eHQuKoCFcMMtAodp3YHmA** [Accessed 5 January 2012].

Finklestein, V (1980) *Attitudes and Disabled People*, New York: World Rehabilitation Fund.

Gerrish, K. and Papadopoulos, I. (1999) 'Transcultural competence: The challenge for nurse education', *British Journal of Nursing* 8(21): 1453–7.

Gerrish, K., Husband, C., and Mackenzie, J. (1996) *Nursing for a Multi-Ethnic Society*, Buckingham: Open University Press.

Goode, E.E. (1993) 'The culture of illness', *US News and World Report* 114(6): 74–6.

Gunaratnam, Y. (2001) 'Ethnicity and palliative care', in S. Dyson and L. Culley (eds) *Ethnicity and Nursing Practice*, Basingstoke: Palgrave, pp. 169–86.

Herberg, P. (1989) 'Theoretical foundations of transcultural nursing', in J.S. Boyle and M.M. Andrews (eds) *Transcultural Concepts in Nursing Care*, Glenview, IL: Scott, Foresman/Little, Brown College Division, pp. 3–53.

Holland, K. and Hogg, C. (2009) *Cultural Awareness in Nursing and Health Care: An Introductory Text*, London: Hodder Education.

James, D. and Drakich, J. (1993) 'Understanding gender differences in amount of talk: Critical review of research', in D. Tannen (ed) *Gender and Conversational Interaction*, Oxford: Oxford University Press, pp. 124–38.

Johnston Talyor, E. (2007) *What Do I Say? Talking with Patients about Spirituality*, West Conshohocken, PA: Templeton Press.

Kandola, R. and Fullerton, J. (1998) *Diversity in Action: Managing the Mosaic*, 2nd edn, London: Chartered Institute of Personnel and Development.

Kleinman, A., Eisenberg, L., and Good, B. (1978) 'Culture, illness and care: Clinical lessons—Anthropologic and cross-cultural research', *Annals of Internal Medicine* 88: 251–8.

Leininger, M. (1997a) 'Transcultural nursing research to nursing education and practice: 40 years', *Image Journal of Nursing Scholarship* 29(4): 341–7.

Leininger, M. (1997b) *Transcultural Nursing: Concepts, Theories and Practice*, New York: John Wiley.

Leininger, M. (2001) 'A mini journey into transcultural nursing with its founder', *Nebraska Nurse* 34(2): 16–17.

McGee, P. (1992) *Issues in Transcultural Nursing: A Guide for Teachers of Nursing and Health*, London: Chapman and Hall.

Murray, R. and Zentner, J.B. (1989) *Nursing Concepts for Health Promotion*, London: Prentice Hall.

Narayanasamy, A. (2001) *Spiritual Care: A Practical Guide for Nurses and Health Care Practitioners*, 2nd edn, London: Quay.

Narayanasamy, A. (2002) 'The ACCESS model: A transcultural nursing practice framework', *British Journal of Nursing* 11(9): 643–50.

Narayanasamy, A. (2004) 'The puzzle of spirituality for nursing: A guide to practice assessment', *British Journal of Nursing* 13(19): 1140–4.

Narayanasamy, A. (2006) *Spiritual Care and Transcultural Care*, London: Quay.

Narayanasamy, A. and White, E. (2005) 'A review of transcultural nursing', *Nurse Education Today* 25: 102–11.

Nzira, V. and Williams, P. (2007) *Anti-oppressive Practice in Health and Social Care*, London: Sage.

Oliver, M. (1996) 'A sociology of disability or a disabled sociology?', in L. Barton (ed) *Disability and Society: Emerging Issues and Insights*, London: Longman, pp. 89–99.

Papadopoulos, I. (2006) (ed) *Transcultural Health and Social Care*, Edinburgh: Churchill Livingstone.

Parfitt, B. (1998) *Working across Culture: A Study of Expatriate Nurses Working in Developing Countries in Primary Health Care*, Aldershot: Ashage.

Patient Association (2009) *Patients … not Numbers, People … not Statistics*, London: Patient Association.

Peberdy, A. (1997) 'Communication across cultural boundaries', in M. Siddle, L. Jones, J. Katz, and A. Peberdy (eds) *Debates and Dilemmas in Promoting Health: A Reader*, Milton Keynes: Open University Press, pp. 99–107.

Polaschek, N.R. (1998) 'Cultural safety: A new concept in nursing people of different ethnicities', *Journal of Advanced Nursing* 27(3):452–7.

Quality Assurance Agency for Higher Education (2001) *Benchmark Statement: Health Care Programmes*, London: HMSO.

Qureshi, B. (1989) *Transcultural Medicine*, The Hague: Kluwer Academic.

Rack, P. (1990) 'Psychological/psychiatric disorders', in B.R. McAvoy and L.J. Donaldson (eds) *Health Care for Asians*, London: Routledge, pp. 290–303.

Ramsden, I. (1990) *Kawa Whakaruruhau: Cultural Safety in Nursing Education in Aotearoa*, Wellington: Ministry of Education.

Ramsden, I. (1993) '*Kawa Whakaarruruhua*: Cultural safety in nursing education in Aotearoa [New Zealand]', *Nursing Praxis* 8(3): 452–7.

Rassool, G.H. (1995) 'The health status and health care of ethno-cultural minorities in the United Kingdom: An agenda for action', *Journal of Nursing* 21: 199–201.

Reynolds, F. (2004) 'The professional context', in J. Swain, J. Clark, K. Parry, S. French, and F. Reynolds (eds) *Enabling Relationships in Health and Social Care*, 2nd edn, Oxford: Butterworth-Heinnemann, pp. 120–34.

Rioux, M.H. and Bach, M. (1994) (eds) *Disability is not Measles*, North York, ON: Roeher Institute.

Sapey, B. (2004) 'Disability and social exclusion in the information society', in J. Swain, S. French, C. Barnes, and C. Thomas (eds) *Disabling Barriers, Enabling Environments*, 2nd edn, London: Sage, pp. 273–8.

Shakespeare, T. (1997) 'Researching disabled sexuality', in C. Barnes and G. Mercer (eds) *Doing Disability Research*, Leeds: The Disability Press, pp. 177–89.

Sherer, L.L. (1993) 'Cross cultures: Hospitals begin breaking down the barriers to care', *Hospitals* 67(10): 29–31.

Stone, E. (2001) 'Complicated struggle: Survival and social change in the majority world', in M. Priestly (ed) *Disability and Life Course: Global Perspectives*, Cambridge: Cambridge University Press, pp. 52–63.

Tannen, D. (1993) *Gender and Conversational Interaction*, Oxford: Oxford University Press.

Ward, L. (1997) 'Funding for change: Translating emancipatory disability research from theory to practice', in C. Barnes and G. Mercer (eds) *Doing Disability Research*, Leeds: The Disability Press, pp. 67–89.

Part 2: Human dimensions of care

6 Caring for communities

SUE THORNTON

Learning outcomes

This chapter will enable you to:

- recognize the social basis for caring and the different social settings in which care can be provided;
- outline ways in which an understanding of key ideas and debates from sociology and social policy can inform caring activities;
- explore the influence of a range of social factors upon the health and well-being of individuals and their communities;
- reflect upon the caring skills and attributes required to respond effectively to the care needs of individuals and their communities; and
- acknowledge and justify the importance of social factors in relation to the holistic and systematic delivery of nursing care.

Introduction

No man is an island, entire of itself; every man is a piece of the continent.

John Donne (1572–1631) Meditation XVII

Providing care for communities might seem to be a self-evident aspect of the nurse's role. However, further examination raises some important questions: what exactly do we mean by 'a community'? Where does this care take place and who does it involve? Does it require any special knowledge, skills, or qualities to ensure that the care that we give effectively meets the holistic care needs of our patients and clients? As a first step in attempting to clarify some of these issues, consider the above quotation.

This popular and much-used phrase by English poet John Donne seems aptly to highlight the interrelatedness and social nature of human relationships. Although people are individuals, they are born, age, and die as members of a wider social community. As nurses, it reminds us of the importance of recognizing the social dimensions of care and the need to try to address this in our caring activities.

This chapter will introduce you to ways in which key ideas, drawn from sociology and social policy, can directly inform nursing. Specific emphasis will be placed upon the potential impact of a wide range of social factors on bio–psycho–social well-being and the implications of these for effective care delivery. A variety of case studies and interactive exercises have been included to enable you to explore, reflect upon, and apply ideas raised within the chapter, and to attempt to relate these to your own clinical experiences.

The need for nurses to appreciate the social aspects of care is reflected in the standards that the Nursing and Midwifery Council (NMC, 2004) have identified that UK students will require both on entry to their branch programme and as registered practitioners. The essential knowledge and skills of care that demand an understanding of the social dimensions of care can be found overleaf.

Professional requirements

Professional frameworks (NMC, 2004; 2008) emphasize the importance of individuality, but also remind us of the collective dimensions of caring. As professionals, we therefore need to address not only the needs of the individual, but also those of the social groups and

Essential knowledge and skills for care

● All nurses must possess a broad knowledge of the structure and function of societies and communities, derived from the behavioural and social sciences as applied to health, illness/disease, disability, ageing, and death.

● You must be aware of the knowledge and skills required to enhance the health and physical and social well-being of patients and clients from diverse care settings.

● You must contribute to the development and completion of comprehensive nursing assessments that include the social needs of patients and clients.

● You will work in partnership with a range of other health and social care professionals, agencies, service users, their carers and families, in all settings, including the community, ensuring that decisions about care are shared.

● You must promote equity in patient and client care by contributing to care in a fair and anti-discriminatory way.

communities to which they belong. For example, the NMC's Code (NMC, 2008: 1) states that you must '*work with others to protect and promote the health and well-being of those in your care, their families and carers and the wider community*'. Because the idea of a community appears to be central to this chapter, then it will be necessary to explore what we mean by this term.

Defining 'communities'

In the first instance, defining a community might seem to be a fairly straightforward exercise. After all, we use the word widely in our everyday conversations and rarely think about its meaning. From a professional perspective, providing care in the community is becoming an increasingly important aspect of a nurse's role (Department of Health, 2006; 2009).

However, as Kelly and Symonds (2003) note, the idea of a community is perhaps more complex than it first appears. The term can be subject to a wide range of different meanings and interpretations, all of which can be seen as particularly significant in how and why we provide care.

What do you understand by the term 'community'?
Write a list of the different ways in which the term can be used.

Many writers on the subject have highlighted the shifting nature of the concept and how our understandings of this can change over time. See, for example, Barry and Yuill (2008: ch. 9) Kelly and Symonds (2003), who have written extensively on the social construction of community nursing.

Box 6.1 highlights some of the popular usages of the term.

In attempting to understand what a community is, you might have noticed that ideas of community seem to be firmly embedded in our views of society. The following section attempts to highlight the significance of the relationship between care, communities, and society, by exploring the settings and basis for care provision.

The social context of health care

All health care takes place in a specific location or social setting. This can range from a person's home to

Box 6.1 Some meanings of 'community' (Cavanagh, 2007)

● Common interests (that is, based upon occupation, education, leisure activities)

● A geographical area (rural, urban, local, national, international, global)

● Networks of social relationships (small-scale family ties, extended family networks

● Shared identity (ethnicity, race, gender, age, religion, sexual orientation)

● Utopian ways of group living (for example, the kibbutz movement)

● Mutual caring (community as an action)

● Cyberspace or virtual environments (online communities)

traditional institutions, such as acute hospitals, and can involve both formal and informal mechanisms of care delivery. Increasingly, with the rising popularity of information technology such as the Internet, the site of healthcare delivery does not necessarily involve a physical location or 'face-to-face' contact with a healthcare professional (Latifi, 2008). With the advent of 'e-medicine', much health-related advice and education occurs within a virtual environment. A good example of this was the strategy for disseminating advice, including diagnostic criteria, during the recent swine flu pandemic (Pratt, 2009).

How many potential care settings can you identify?
Make a list of possible locations of care within your own community.

On reflection, you may have been surprised by the scope of your answer to the above reflective activity. This section attempts to highlight where and why that care takes place—that is, the diverse locations of health care and the social basis for its delivery.

Locations and providers of health care

As you may have noted in earlier chapters, attitudes towards care and ways of providing this appear to be changing. These seem to be moving from a traditional medical model of care to a more socially driven, holistic, and person-centred model (Taylor and Field, 2007).

As a consequence, many aspects of care and caring, traditionally located within acute general hospitals, are now carried out within an individual's home environment or a selection of community-based organizations, which range from health centres, care homes, hospices, walk-in centres, GP surgeries, to private hospitals (Bochel et al., 2005). The range of individuals with a responsibility for caring is equally vast, involving not only qualified health and social care professionals, but also informal carers such as friends, relatives, and the 'third sector' (that is, charities, voluntary agencies, and 'not-for-profit' social enterprises). Some of the key sources of healthcare provision are identified in **Figure 6.1**.

This wide diversity in the providers of health care is sometimes referred to as a 'mixed economy 'of welfare provision (Walsh et al., 2000: 107). In this sense, it reflects the emphasis placed over the last thirty years by successive governments on moving away from dependence on the state for health and other welfare services, towards care provision 'in' and 'by' the community, and the increasing priority that is given to the implementation of primary healthcare services (Department of Health, 2009). These ideas are strongly reflected in the current government's conception of a 'Big Society' in which all individuals are encouraged to make an active contribution to the health and social well-being of their local communities (see **http://www.cabinetoffice.gov.uk**).

Social attitudes to care provision

Social 'shifts' in the location and delivery of health care have been matched by changes in the public's attitudes towards 'who knows best' and the trust that the community places in the judgements and actions of healthcare professionals (Nettleton, 2006). One area that has been subject to particular criticism is the traditional dominance and integrity of the medical profession. This has been highlighted by a number of

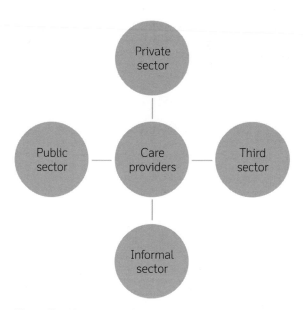

Figure 6.1 Key sources of healthcare provision.

widely publicized scandals and subsequent inquiries, as outlined in **Box 6.2**.

The examples highlighted in **Box 6.2** have undoubtedly tended to reinforce public fears and concerns about the quality of care delivery. According to Anthony Giddens (2009), such changes in attitude reflects a much wider pattern of social change and transformation, whereby traditional values and conventions (such as religion, the family, education, politics, and the legal system) are challenged and replaced by a broader social emphasis upon developing individual choice and identity. People in today's society are much more likely to be aware of their rights and to dispute expert opinion and advice if they feel that it is not in their best interests.

The quality of nursing care has also been exposed to similar public scrutiny. Consider the comments made by the late Claire Rayner, nurse and president of the Patient's Association, highlighted in **Box 6.3**.

The report (Patients Association, 2009) contains several personal accounts that emphasize consistent failings in basic nursing care and infringements on dignity and self determination. In many ways, it reflects increasing public concern that some nurses are not adequately meeting even the most basic care needs of their patients and clients.

· ·

How do you feel about these remarks?
Find the report online at **http://www.patients-association.com** and debate its findings with your colleagues.

· ·

This section has provided an overview of the social nature of care and some of the issues that it raises, including the social setting in which care takes place, who has a responsibility for providing that care, and the influences of changing social attitudes. Ideas drawn from both sociology and social policy can be used to enhance our understanding of the links between society and caring, and the ways in which we can use this knowledge to improve our everyday nursing practice.

The contributions of sociology and social policy

As noted earlier, ideas and insights drawn from the social sciences (particularly sociology and social policy) may be valuable in enhancing nursing practice. There has, however, been dispute about the relevance of sociology in nurse education and exactly how this should be applied, with some commentators suggesting that it has little real application in the everyday world of 'hands-on' nursing (Denny and Earle, 2009).

You might initially agree with this view and regard many of the ideas within sociology as simply 'common sense dressed up in fancy words'. However, understanding the true nature of sociology often involves looking beyond the obvious and 'taken-for-granted' meanings that we use to try and make sense of our

Box 6.2 Relevant reports

- The Kennedy Inquiry (1999)—Excessive death rates for children undergoing heart surgery (Bristol Royal Infirmary)
- The Redfern Report (2001)—The unauthorized removal, retention, and disposal of human tissue, including children's organs (Alderhay Hospital)
- The Shipman Inquiry Final Report (2005)—The prolific activities of serial killer and GP, Harold Shipman
- The Francis Inquiry (2010)—Excessive death rates and poor standards of care (Mid Staffordshire General Hospital) (Department of Health, 2010)

Box 6.3 The Patients Association on poor care standards

For far too long now, the Patients Association has been receiving calls on our Helpline from people wanting to talk about the dreadful, neglectful, demeaning, painful and sometimes downright cruel treatment their elderly relatives had experienced at the hands of NHS nurses. Some found it helpful to talk to us, for they had had scant comfort from trying to make complaints or even seek explanations about what had happened to the people they loved never mind the supportive counselling they should have had.

(The Patients Association, 2009: 3)

social world (Marsh et al., 2009). One famous trad-itional sociologist referred to this as the 'sociological imagination' (Wright-Mills, 1959).

Our ability to become more self-aware and to 'think outside the box' would seem to be very relevant in the increasingly complex world of contemporary nursing, which demands that we maximize our critical thinking and problem-solving capabilities. The need to develop these skills has been emphasized throughout the report of the Prime Minister's Commission on the Future of Nursing and Midwifery in England (2010). This highlights the importance of qualities such as leadership, critical judgement, the capacity for innova-tion, and curious intellect in providing compassionate, high-quality nursing care (ibid: 32)

The next section will introduce you to the nature and interests of sociology and social policy, including some of the key areas of controversy and debate. It will also suggest ways in which you might relate and apply these ideas to your everyday nursing practice. The remaining sections of the chapter intend to provide you with an opportunity to explore in more detail some specific health-related issues that have been of central importance to recent sociological enquiry.

What is sociology?

When attempting to define what sociology is, many authors on the subject comment on the difficulties in providing a clear and simple explanation (Nettleton, 2006; Taylor and Field, 2007; Denny and Earle, 2009). As Barry and Yuill (2008) note, this is largely due to the potential scope and complexity of sociological enquiry, including the competing views of different sociolo-gists. Both of these issues will be further explored. Despite such problems in interpretation, most efforts to define sociology highlight a number of common themes, which tend to characterize the subject. Accord-ingly, sociology, in its most literal sense, can be seen as the 'systematic study of human societies' (Macionis and Plummer, 2008: 2).

Sociology is specifically concerned with how society is organized, the social relations that are involved, and how such factors change over time (Giddens, 2009). 'Society' may be perceived as relating to the system, in

which we live, exerting an external regulatory influence over our beliefs and behaviours (Barry and Yuill, 2008). However, some sociological commentators (for example, Marsh et al., 2009) claim that this rather traditional interpretation tends to portray people in a negative, passive way, with little direct influence over their social surroundings. The debate about the relationship between 'society' and 'individuals', and the specific rel-evance of these ideas to caring, will also be considered in more detail at a later point in the chapter.

Sociology and social policy

How does sociology differ from social policy? In many respects, both of these subjects might seem to share many common interests and areas of concern. Most of the issues having an impact on health and health care that are studied by sociologists also fall into the domain of social policy. Much policy appears to be directed by sociological investigation. However, sociol ogy and social policy are, in fact, regarded as separate disciplines with different origins, aims, and methods. Whereas the prime focus of sociology is its attempts to study and explain the workings of society, social policy focuses upon the formulation, implementation, and delivery of policies that affect the circumstances of individuals, groups, and society, including an emphasis on welfare, well-being, and policy outcomes, and devel-oping social policy concerns (Bochel et al., 2009).

Box 6.4 highlights some of the traditional and con-temporary topics that are of interest to social policy-makers.

Although this chapter will place more focus upon the role of sociology in care and nursing, it will also draw attention to the importance of health and social poli-cies, and ways in which these might influence the care that we deliver. One specific example is the idea of health inequalities and how these might be resolved.

Sociology and social change

Sociology is not only concerned with the individuals, but also focuses upon collective social action—that is, how people behave as members of a group, organization, and

Box 6.4 Traditional and new concerns for social policymakers

Traditional concerns	New concerns
Health	Food
Housing	Environment and sustainability
Education	Transport and travel
Personal social services	ICT
Social security	Work and new forms of money
Employment	Leisure

larger institutions. As already noted, it also has a distinct historical component in that it is interested in the evolution and development of social processes and social relationships. For example, one of the classical sociologists, Max Weber (1904/1930), provided an extensive account of the transformation of traditional agricultural forms of social organization to rational industrialized systems. Anthony Giddens (2009), a more contemporary writer, explores these ideas in greater detail, distinguishing between 'modern' and 'post-modern' societies. This refers to the change of emphasis from views of society as a predictable, logically organized, cohesive structure, to social environments that tend to be characterized by change, diversity, social fragmentation, and uncertainty.

···

How do you think society has changed over the last fifty years?

Try to identify some key differences in each of the following areas.

Attitudes towards men, women, children, ethnic minority groups, people with disabilities, homosexuality, and religious differences

- The role of the family
- Work and recreation
- Travel
- Communication and information technology
- Medical advancements

···

You may have noted that there have been vast and rapid changes to our way of life, including changing social expectations, the emergence of global communities, and the advent of the Internet, leading to a wider and more equitable sharing of knowledge. The social order of communities has also been transformed. According to Giddens (2009), many of the traditional roles and institutions such as the family and religious organizations, which had a strong influence upon how we behave, have been replaced by a much more diverse range of role models, including the media and the rise of celebrity culture. There are numerous examples of the impact of these factors, and how they can 'shape' the attitudes and actions of the general public, ranging from an increased uptake in cervical screening—the so-called 'Jade Goody' effect following the reality TV star's premature death from cervical cancer (Everleigh, 2009)—to a reduction in compliance with national vaccination programmes relating to public mistrust following the much-publicized alleged links between the MMR vaccine and autism (Gardner et al., 2010; Thomas, 2010).

Focus and scope of sociology

As highlighted above, the potential scope of sociological enquiry is broad and varied. Some specific topics that are of particular interest to sociologists include:

- the role and impact of social structures, such as the family, education, health and health care, the church, media, and the legal system;
- social stratification and social divisions, such as gender, ethnicity, socioeconomic status, sexual orientation, and ability;
- social processes, including stereotyping, stigma and labelling, socialization, the life course, and social transitions; and
- social behaviours, such as power relations, crime and deviance, status, roles, and language and communication.

Many of these areas have direct application to health care and, more specifically, to nursing practice. For example, in relation to the idea of social roles, one classical sociologist proposed the idea of a 'sick role' (Parsons, 1951). This refers to a special social status created for people when they become ill and can no longer fulfil their usual social obligations, such as work, parenting, etc. In this context, sickness is viewed as a source of social disruption and requires controlling until the person is well enough to return to their 'normal' social identity.

Other themes of particular relevance include Erving Goffman's classical studies about stigma and social identity (Goffman, 1963). These focused on the means by which certain people are rejected from full social acceptance on the basis of possessing a certain social characteristic that is viewed in a negative way. 'Stigma' may refer to a visible physical characteristic (such as a scar or physical impairment), a 'hidden' personal characteristic (such as substance and alcohol abuse, mental health problems), or social position. Goffman was specifically concerned with how people who were stigmatized responded to and managed their situation, both in their social encounters and their relationships with other individuals.

You may appreciate that the idea of stigma and the way in which this may impact upon the life experiences of people has particular relevance for nursing and caring. It enables us to understand how people may moderate their behaviours to 'fit in' with social expectations of what is considered socially acceptable or 'normal'. The need to conform is a powerful motivator. It is essential that nurses are aware of this when they assess and attempt to meet the care needs of their patients and clients.

The significance of social stratification and social divisions and their potential effect on health may also be seen as central to an understanding of the social needs of communities. As such, it will be explored in more detail in a subsequent section.

Key debates in sociology

Sociology is characterized by a wide range of different views about the nature, organization, and purpose of society. This inevitably gives rise to a number of key areas of debate and disagreement about the explanations for social activity (Giddens, 2009). Some of the traditional areas of controversy can be summarized as follows.

- **Macro versus micro perspectives**

  Should the study of society be concerned with a 'big picture' overview of how this works, or should it focus upon small-scale individual interactions?

- **Conflict versus consensus**

  Is the organization of society determined by the smooth and harmonious functioning of each of its relevant and interconnected parts (social systems such the church, law, education, family, health, and welfare), or is it characterized by conflict between competing social groups (for example, rich and poor, young and old, men and women)?

- **Structure versus social action**

  To what extent is a person's behaviour influenced by broad social factors (that is, poverty and social deprivation, low income, social and welfare policies) or by the individual choice that they make about how to conduct their everyday lives?

- **Science versus interpretation**

  Should sociological investigations apply a scientific approach to explain the nature of society (positivism) or, because of the potential subjectivity of social behaviour, are interpretative methods such as phenomenology and ethnography a more appropriate means of exploring social relations?

- **Biological determinism versus social constructionism**

  Is the way in which we behave in social settings largely influenced by our biology (genetic makeup, hormones, survival instincts) or are our actions largely 'shaped' by cultural and socioeconomic processes? (Note that this line of discussion is similar to the 'nature versus nurture' debate within psychology.)

For ease of interpretation, these arguments have been presented in a rather simplistic way as a clear choice between two clearly defined viewpoints. However, in reality, the questions that they generate and the positions that sociologists adopt in light of these are much more complex. Each of these views reflects the theoretical interests and orientations of many different 'schools of thought' in sociology.

If you are interested in exploring the specific characteristics of competing social theories, then there are a number of informative texts that provide an in-depth account and these are detailed in the 'Further reading' that appears at the end of this chapter.

Application to nursing practice

Several of the issues raised in these debates might be perceived as being of particular relevance to nursing. For example, a large number of nurse researchers have adopted the methods of enquiry that have been utilized within the social sciences to investigate specific aspects of nursing care.

Box 6.5 provides an example of how an interpretative social research approach can serve to provide insight into the experiences and needs of patients with leg ulceration.

The mix of social research methods used to inform this study highlights the potential difference between the patients' perceptions and those of the professionals providing their care. It also suggests ways of overcoming these problems.

Structure and social action

As we have noted, in a sociological sense, 'structure' refers to the broad social forces that shape our behaviour and the social frameworks or institutions in which we operate (Taylor and Field, 2007). Structures provide shared meanings and understandings that guide our experiences and actions. However, we are also autonomous individuals who ascribe meaning to social situations and have the power to actively choose how we want to live our lives. Sociologists such as Giddens (2009) describe this capacity for decision-making as 'agency'.

Ideas of the role of social structure and human agency are particularly relevant when considering the potential social factors that may contribute to health and well-being—for example, what role is played by the 'big picture', where we live, whether we work, how much we earn, our cultural background, whether or not we

Box 6.5 Living with leg ulceration: a synthesis of the literature (Briggs and Flemming, 2007)

The purpose of this study was to attempt to explore the patients' experiences of living with a chronic leg ulcer through a review of the qualitative literature on the subject. Selected articles included phenomenological studies, grounded theory, descriptive interviews, and focus groups. Synthesis of the results revealed that, for patients, physical symptoms and pain tended to dominate the 'leg ulcer journey'. It showed that the priority for these patients was relief from symptoms rather than cure. This appeared to contradict the care priorities of the healthcare professionals and policymakers, who often encouraged healing at the expense of long-term care. It was concluded that healthcare professionals needed to shift the emphasis in care from the acute to chronic events, empowering people to live with the problem rather than attempting a cure. If patients were to learn to manage their condition more effectively, then it was speculated that this would have a positive effect upon wound healing.

own a car or a home? Or, conversely, are our 'health chances' are mostly influenced by the individual choices that we make, such as whether or not to smoke, how much exercise we take, and what we eat?

Practice Example 6.1 is intended to encourage you to think about these ideas and the implications for the way in which we care.

From a nursing perspective, our beliefs about a person's self-efficacy and the extent to which we view them as responsible for their own health problems can profoundly influence how we view their entitlement to care. It can also 'shape' the way in which that care is delivered. For example, many health promotion strategies are aimed at enabling people to make informed active choices about the type of lifestyle that they choose to adopt. These are intended to encourage healthy practices and to reduce health-damaging behaviours. However, there is also a need to recognize and attempt to address the wider structural influences that play a role in determining a person's health status and over which they may have very little direct control. The following

PRACTICE EXAMPLE 6.1

Jamie's 'Lot'

Jamie is 19 years old. She is the single parent of a lively 2-year-old boy, Kyle, and currently living with her mum (also a single parent) on a large housing estate in a busy inner-city area. Jamie, like her mother and the majority of her friends, has never worked in regular full-time employment. Money has always been 'tight', but she gets by on state benefits, earning a 'bit on the side' from casual work. As a young child, Jamie always did well at school and wanted to become a teacher. But in her early teens she fell in with a bad crowd, started smoking and drinking alcohol, and began experimenting with recreational drugs. As a result, she was

excluded from school for disruptive behaviour and non-attendance. She has recently discovered that she is three months pregnant, but is unsure if she wants to continue with the pregnancy. She feels depressed, weepy, and unable to cope

Write a list of the potential social factors that might have contributed to Jamie's current situation. Review these, identifying which are structural in origin and which might be attributed to Jamie's personal choices.

How might our perceptions of the cause of Jamie's circumstances affect our ability to provide her with the best care and advice?

section will enable you to consider these in greater detail, along with ways in which they might be addressed.

Social factors and health

Both social policy and sociology focus attention upon the many social factors that can impact upon the health and well-being of an individual. The World Health Organization (2008) has referred to these different spheres of influence as the 'social determinants of health' (see **Box 6.6**).

The social influences listed in **Box 6.6** illustrate the complex interrelationship between social factors such as material deprivation and social standing and biological, psychological, and environmental variables. Due to the wide scope of these determinants, this section will focus upon one key area that appears to be of particular importance to the idea of 'caring for communities' inequalities in health.

What is 'health inequality'?

The idea of health inequality has assumed a high profile in both sociology and social policy over the last forty years. It is also of specific relevance to the way in

which we organize and deliver care. As such, the concept warrants further exploration.

Health inequality refers to variations in the levels of health experienced between different social groups (Marsh et al., 2009). It has traditionally been viewed as comprising two key dimensions: differences in health status (the amount of health that a person experiences); and differences in their access to and the availability of health care (Townsend et al., 1988; Department of Health, 1998; Bartley, 2004).

Box 6.6 The social determinants of health (adapted from Dahlgren and Whitehead, 1991)

- General socio-economic, cultural, and environmental conditions
- Living and working conditions:
  - agriculture and food production
  - water and sanitation
  - housing
  - education
  - unemployment
  - healthcare services
- Social and community networks
- Individual lifestyle factors (age, sex, constitutional factors)

- **Differences in health status**

  According to Taylor and Field (2007), this is usually defined in terms of:
  - how long a person can expect to live (life expectancy); and
  - the amount of ill health that a person actually experiences.

  When researching health inequalities, these two factors are conventionally measured through rates of death (mortality) and rates of illness (morbidity).

- **Differences in the access to and availability of health services**

  Piachaud et al. (2009) state that this relates to a number of dimensions, including the accessibility, availability, usability, and quality of the health services.

The extent of health inequality has been highlighted by a series of influential reports that have been instrumental in raising public and professional awareness of the existence of social differences in health. These have been concerned with examining the extent, causes, and impacts of health inequality, and have proposed a series of potential solutions to the situation. They include:

- the Black Report (1980) and *The Health Divide* (Townsend et al., 1988);
- the Acheson Report (1998); and
- the Marmot Review (2010).

These reports show that, despite overall improvements in general health and the life expectancy throughout the population, there remains a significant and persistent 'gap' between the richest and poorest members of society both in terms of life expectancy and levels of ill health. As the latest findings have revealed, people living in the poorest neighbourhoods will die on average seven years earlier than those living in the most affluent neighbourhoods. They will also suffer from more debilitating illness and chronic long-term health problems, such as cardiovascular disease, diabetes, stroke and hypertension, and lung cancer. Moreover, risk-taking behaviours, such as obesity, drug use, and violence, also show strong links with social and economic deprivation across all age ranges (Strategic Review of Health Inequalities in England Post-2010, 2010).

These differentials in health continue to exist as we move down the social scale. The wealthier a person is, the better their health. This steep grading in the health experiences of the population according to social circumstance has been referred to as the 'social gradient in health' (Townsend et al., 1988). **Figure 6.2** shows the gap in mortality rate between different social groups based upon their socioeconomic classification.

Figure 6.2 indicates that men in routine jobs (group 7) are 2.8 times more likely to die between the ages of 25 and 64 than men in higher managerial posts (groups 1.1, 1.2, and 2).

What job-related factors might contribute to the health gap between occupational groupings?

In response to this question, you may, in addition to income levels and social status, have considered the impact of occupational characteristics such as job control and security of employment. These are some of the key criteria that are used to define the social National Statistics Socioeconomic Classification (NS-SEC), which is a commonly used tool for the measurement of social variations in health and well-being.

Health inequality is not confined to variations in health and well-being between people of different incomes and occupational groupings. Whereas traditional research into health inequality tended to emphasize the role of social class, more recent studies accentuate the multidimensional nature of this phenomenon (Townshend et al., 1988; Department of Health, 1998). Age, gender, religion, place of residence, ethnicity, sexual orientation, occupation, and ability may interact to compound the experience of social disadvantage (Thompson, 2006). Specific examples include the greater prevalence of anxiety and mental health problems such as depression in women (Wilkins et al., 2008), higher rates of stroke and coronary artery disease amongst people born in the Indian sub-continent (Harding and Maxwell, 1997), and generally poorer health outcomes experienced by people with disabilities (Michael, 2008). Inequality also tends to persist throughout the life

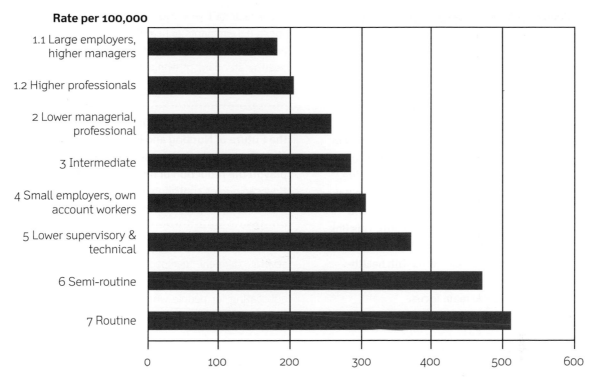

Rate per 100,000

Figure 6.2 The gap in mortality rate between different social groups based upon their socioeconomic classification (Age Standardised mortality rate by NS-SEC: Men aged 25–64 , England and Wales 2001–03). Crown copyright.

cycle, starting at birth and advancing into old age (Department of Health, 2001).

Reports have identified that certain groups of people appear to be particularly vulnerable to poor health outcomes (Piachaud et al., 2009). These comprise individuals who, by virtue of their social circumstances, are unable to participate fully in mainstream society and include the homeless, unemployed, asylum seekers, and members of some ethnic minority groups. Both the processes that exclude these people and the extreme disadvantage that results from this are often perceived as constituting 'social exclusion'.

Inequalities and health care

Social variations in health and well-being are also reflected in the way in which people use the health services. For example, many of the earlier reports suggested that people from the lower socioeconomic groups made less use of the preventative health services and generally received a poorer standard of service in a range of primary and secondary care settings (Townsend et al., 1988; Department of Health, 1998). Gender, age, ethnic background, and sexual orientation may also play a significant role in the ability to access and experience high-quality care.

Indeed, a classical study by a GP (Hart, 1971) identified what he referred to as an 'inverse care law'—that is, a situation in which the level and standard of healthcare provision is far worse in those areas that have the greatest need. For example, areas with the highest levels of poverty and social deprivation often have fewer GP services and other primary care facilities—a situation sometimes referred to as 'service exclusion' (Piachaud et al., 2009).

Causes and responses to health inequality

In the current latest report on health inequalities in Britain, *Fair Society, Healthy Lives*, Professor Sir Michael Marmot, chairman of the review, makes the following opening remark:

> **People with higher socioeconomic position in society have a greater array of life chances and more opportunities to lead a flourishing life. They also have better health. The two are linked: the more favoured people are, socially and economically, the better their health. This link between social conditions and health is not a footnote to the 'real' concerns with health-healthcare and unhealthy behaviours—it should become the main focus.**
>
> (Marmot Review, 2010: 3)

....

Consider Sir Michael's comments.
What is he implying about the causes of health inequality and how these might be addressed?
....

Sir Michael is implying that the health inequality is predominantly linked to the wider structural determinants of health (specifically income and occupation) rather than simply a result of individual lifestyle choices or the quality of healthcare provision. Ways of overcoming the structural basis of these variations in health should take priority over traditional measures, which have focused on changing health behaviours and increasing healthcare provision.

The Marmot Review (Strategic Review of Health Inequalities in England Post-2010, 2010) has also clearly emphasized the way in which health inequality is inextricably linked to other key areas of social inequality, such as educational and occupational opportunities, working conditions, housing, neighbourhood conditions, standards of living, and more generally '*the freedom to participate equally in the benefits of Society*' (ibid: 10–11).

This has resulted in recommendations to address health inequality that extend across a wide range of social factors. These involve measures across all of the social determinants of health, including action on the early years, education, skills and life chances, work, a healthy standard of living, sustainable communities, and ill-health prevention.

....

The report of the Prime Minister's Commission on the Future of Nursing and Midwifery in England (2010) suggests that nurses have a key role to play in the reduction of health inequality.
How can nurses contribute to reducing the types of disadvantage highlighted in the Marmot Review?
....

You might have considered the role of the nurse from several different perspectives, involving providing advice, support, and resources, and empowering and advocating for people who are vulnerable or socially disadvantaged.

Conclusion

Recognizing and responding effectively to the social dimensions of health and well-being seem to be central to the delivery of holistic nursing care. Indeed, as noted in the introduction to this chapter, addressing the social requirements of individuals and their communities might be viewed as an essential prerequisite of professional nursing practice. Consequently, nurses need to develop enhanced insight into the social basis of their caring activities. This includes knowledge of the ways in which a range of socially determined factors can impact upon aspects of healthcare provision.

Ideas drawn from both sociology and social policy can contribute towards a better understanding of the unique social needs of individuals and their communities. This, in turn, can be used to inform nursing practice directly by assisting in the development of skills and qualities, such as increased levels of cultural and social awareness, which will help to ensure that these needs can be met.

....

As a final activity, reflect upon your knowledge of some of the potential social issues that this chapter has identified.

Try to identify specific ways in which a knowledge of these factors might help you to provide better care for your patients and clients.

....

Further reading

The following texts may be useful in offering a more comprehensive understanding of sociology and social policy, and their potential applications in nursing.

Sociology: general texts

Giddens, A. (2009) *Sociology*, 6th edn, Cambridge: Polity Press

Macionis, J.J. and Plummer, K. (2008*) Sociology*, 4th edn, London: Pearson Education

Marsh, I., Keating, M., Punch, S., and Harden, J. (2009) *Sociology: Making Sense of Society*, 4th edn, London: Pearson Education

Sociology: Applied texts

Barry, A. and Yuill, A. (2008) *Understanding the Sociology of Health: An Introduction*, London: Sage

Denny, E. and Earle, S. (2009) *Sociology for Nurses*, 2nd edn, Cambridge: Polity Press

Nettleton, S. (2006) *The Sociology of Health and Illness*, 2nd edn, Cambridge: Polity Press

Taylor, S. and Field, D. (2007) *Sociology of Health and Healthcare*, 4th edn, Oxford: Blackwell Publishing

Social policy: general texts

Bochel, H., Bochel, C., Page, R., and Sykes, R. (2009) *Social Policy: Themes, Issues and Debates,* London: Pearson Education

Walsh, M., Stephens, P., and Moore, S. (2000) *Social Policy and Welfare*, Cheltenham: Stanley Thornes

Some useful websites

http://www.doh.gov.uk The Department of Health's website provides useful information relating to health and social care, and links with other relevant sites

http://www.nhshistory.net/nursing%20commission. pdf The full report and recommendations of the Prime Minister's Commission

http://www.sociologyonline.co.uk Each of these sites provides links with a wide range of sociology and social policy-based resources

http://www.sociology.org.uk

http://socserv.mcmaster.ca/w3virtsoclib/

http://www.patients-association.com Comprehensive information including latest research and reports relating to the healthcare experiences of patients and their carers

http://www.marmotreview.org/AssetLibrary/pdfs/ full%20tg%20reports/social%20inclusion%20 and%20mobility%20t.g.%20full%20report.pdf The full version of the Marmot Review, including the findings of the individual working groups

References

Barry, A. and Yuill, A. (2008) *Understanding the Sociology of Health: An Introduction*, London: Sage.

Bartley, M. (2004) *Health Inequality: An Introduction to Theories, Concepts and Methods*, Cambridge: Polity Press.

Bochel, H., Bochel, C., Page, R., and Sykes, R. (2009) *Social Policy: Themes, Issues and Debates*, London: Pearson Education.

Briggs, M. and Flemming, K. (2007) 'Living with leg ulceration: A synthesis of qualitative literature', *Journal of Advanced Nursing* 59(4): 319–28.

Cavanagh, A. (2007) *Sociology in the Age of the Internet*, Buckingham: Open University Press.

Dahlgren, G. and Whitehead, M. (1991) *Policies and Strategies to Promote Social Equity in Health*, Stockholm: Institute of Fiscal Studies.

Denny, E. and Earle, S. (2009) *Sociology for Nurses*, 2nd edn, Cambridge: Polity Press.

Department of Health (1998) *Independent Inquiry into Inequalities in Health*, London: HMSO.

Department of Health (2001) *The Report of the Public Inquiry into Children's Heart Surgery at the Bristol Royal Infirmary 1984–1995: Learning from Bristol*, Cm 5207, London: HMSO.

Department of Health (2006) *Our Health, Our Care, Our Say: A New Direction for Community Services*, London: HMSO.

Department of Health (2009) *High Quality Care for All: Our Journey So Far*, available online at **http://www. dh.gov.uk/prod_consum_dh/groups/dh_digitalassets/ documents/digitalasset/dh_101674.pdf** [accessed 8 July 2011].

Department of Health (2010) *Robert Francis Inquiry: Report into Mid Staffordshire Foundation Trust*, London: HMSO.

Everleigh, M. (2009) 'Healthcare and the media: The Jade Goody effect', *Nursing in Practice* 47: 1.

Gardner, B., Davies, A., Mc Ateer, J., and Mitchie, S. (2010) 'Beliefs underlying parents' views towards MMR promotion interventions: A qualitative study', *Psychology Health and Medicine* 15(2): 220–30.

Giddens, A. (2009) *Sociology*, 6th edn, Cambridge: Polity Press.

Goffman, I. (1963) *Stigma: Notes on the Management of a Spoiled Identity*, London: Penguin.

Harding, S. and Maxwell, R. (1997) 'Differences in the mortality of migrants', in F. Drever and M. Whitehead (eds) *Health Inequalities*, Decennial Supplement Series DS No.15, London: HMSO.

Hart, J.T. (1971) 'The inverse care law', *The Lancet* 1: 405–12.

Kelly, A. and Symonds, A. (2003) *The Social Construction of Community Nursing*, London: MacMillan.

Latifi, R. (2008) 'The dos and don'ts when you establish telemedicine and e-health (not only) in developing countries', in R. Latifi (ed.) *Current Principles and Practice of Telemedicine and e-Health*, Washington DC: IOS Press, pp. 39–44.

Macionis, J.J. and Plummer, K. (2008) *Sociology*, 4th edn, London: Pearson Education.

Marsh, I., Keating, M., Punch, S., and Harden, J. (2009) *Sociology: Making Sense of Society*, 4th edn, London: Pearson Education.

Michael, J. (2008) *Healthcare for All: Report of the Independent Inquiry into Access to Healthcare for People with Learning Disabilities*, London: Independent Inquiry into Access to Healthcare for People with Learning Disabilities.

Nettleton, S. (2006) *The Sociology of Health and Illness*, 2nd edn, Cambridge: Polity Press.

Nursing and Midwifery Council (2004) *Standards of Proficiency for Pre-registration Nursing Education*, London: NMC.

Nursing and Midwifery Council (2008) *The Code*, London: NMC.

Parsons, T. (1951) *The Social System*, New York: Free Press.

Patients Association, The (2009) *Patients … not Numbers, People … not Statistics,* available online at **http://www. patients-association.com/DBIMGS/file/Patients%20 not%20numbers,%20people%20not%20statistics. pdf** [accessed 16 June 2011].

Piachaud, D., Bennett, F., Nazaroo, J.K., and Popay, J. (2009) *Report of Task Group: Social Inclusion and Mobility*, available online at **http://www.marmotreview.org/ AssetLibrary/pdfs/full%20tg%20reports/social%20 inclusion%20and%20mobility%20t.g.%20full%20 report.pdf** [accessed 16 June 2011].

Pratt, R.J. (2009) 'The global swine flu pandemic 2: Infection control measures and preparedness strategies—Second in a two-part unit', *Nursing Times* 105(35): 16–18.

Prime Minister's Commission on the Future of Nursing and Midwifery in England (2010) *Front Line Care: The Future of Nursing and Midwifery in England—Report of the Prime Minister's Commission on the Future of Nursing and Midwifery in England 2010*, London: HMSO.

Royal Liverpool Children's Inquiry, The (2001) *Report of the Royal Liverpool Children's Inquiry,* London: HMSO, available online at **http://www.rlcinquiry.org.uk/** [accessed 16 June 2011] ('the Redfern Report').

Shipman Inquiry, The (2005) *Shipman: The Final Report, Sixth Report of the Shipman Inquiry,* available online at **http://www.shipman-inquiry.org.uk/finalreport.asp** [accessed 16 June 2011].

Strategic Review of Health Inequalities in England Post-2010 (2010) *Fair Society, Healthy Lives,* **available online at http://www.marmotreview.org/AssetLibrary/pdfs/ Reports/FairSocietyHealthyLives.pdf** [accessed 16 June 2011] ('the Marmot Review').

Taylor, F. and Field, S. (2007) *Sociology of Health and Healthcare,* 4th edn, Oxford: Blackwell Publishing.

Thomas, J. (2010) 'Paranoia strikes deep: MMR vaccine and autism', *Psychiatric Times*. 27(3): 1–8.

Thompson, N. (2006) *Anti-Discriminatory Practice,* London: Palgrave.

Townsend, P., Davidson, N., and Whitehead, M. (1988) *Inequalities in Health: The Black Report and the Health Divide,* Harmondsworth: Penquin.

Walsh, M., Stephens, P., and Moore, S. (2000) *Social Policy and Welfare*, Cheltenham: Stanley Thornes.

Wilkins, D., Payne, S., Granville, G., and Branney, P. (2008) *The Gender and Access to Health Services Study: Final Report,* London: HMSO.

World Health Organization (2008) *Closing the Gap in a Generation: Health Equity through Action on the Social Determinants of Health*, Geneva: WHO.

Wright-Mills, C. (1959) *The Sociological Imagination,* Oxford: Oxford University Press

7 Psychological aspects of caring

GLENN MARLAND AND ANNETTE THOMSON

Learning outcomes

This chapter will enable you to:

- develop your understanding of different approaches in psychology;
- develop your knowledge of theory and research in the areas of 'emotions' and the 'self';
- show how experiences can strengthen individuals' resilience or make them more vulnerable to mental and physical problems; and
- encourage you to reflect on how knowledge of psychological theory and research can inform both self-help and professional helping strategies.

Introduction

One of the most important aspects of caring is understanding emotions. How we feel clearly has a significant effect on our well-being in many ways. Psychology—'*the science of behaviour and mental processes*' (Hewstone et al., 2005: 3)—would seem very well placed to deepen our understanding of the complex emotional facets of caring relationships. How do theories and research in psychology add to the 'toolkit' of knowledge, understanding, and skills that we bring to caring?

Picking up any introductory psychology textbook, you may be struck by the sheer scope of the enterprise. Not only do psychologists have something to say about almost any area of human experience (from memory to

Essential knowledge and skills for care

- You must have a broad understanding of the assumptions that different psychological theories make about the origins of our emotions and how we develop particular views of ourselves and others, which is vital when making sense of caring relationships.

- You must have an in-depth knowledge of common health problems and treatments in your own field of practice, including co-morbidity and physiological and psychological vulnerability. Furthermore, it is also essential to consider what different psychological approaches suggest should be done by the nurse, patient, and family to bring about positive change when things go wrong.

- You must learn and respond to the psychological, as well as physical and social, needs of people, groups, and communities. You will then contribute to the development and completion of a comprehensive nursing assessment that addresses the psychological needs of patients and clients.

- You should plan, deliver, and evaluate safe, competent, person-centred care in partnership with the individual, paying special attention to changing emotional health needs during different life stages, including progressive physical or mental illness, loss, death, and bereavement.

- You must respond appropriately when faced with an emergency or a sudden deterioration in a person's psychological condition (for example, self harm, extremely challenging behaviour, attempted suicide), including seeking help from an appropriate person.

international relations), but they also investigate their area of interest in vastly different ways. One research psychologist might be involved in detailed studies of brain patterns and their relationship to behaviour, using complex apparatus and statistics, while her colleague might be conducting in-depth interviews with only a few individuals on their perceptions of chronic pain, and his aim would be to provide rich descriptions of the experience.

We will not be able to give you a detailed account of *all* that is 'out there' in this huge and fascinating discipline. We are aiming to provide you with an overview of some of the main theories and their historical development, so that you can develop an understanding of how they underpin many of our assumptions about caring. This will hopefully whet your appetite for more. There is no doubt that psychology has the potential to give us important insights about ourselves and others.

Overview of some major psychological approaches

An understanding of the assumptions that different theories make about the origins of our emotions and how we develop particular views of ourselves and others is clearly going to be important in making sense of caring relationships. Furthermore, it is also essential to consider what different approaches suggest should be done to bring about change when things go wrong.

This chapter aims to give you an understanding of some of the key theories in psychology and their applications to health care, and a brief summary can be found in **Table 7.1**.

We will suggest ways in which you can develop such links in your own practice. We also encourage you to look out for how other practitioners from multidisciplinary teams may be drawing on different ideas in their interventions. This will help to develop your understanding of their approaches.

Some of the questions that psychology tries to address have been asked for a very long time—going back to the ancient Greeks. However, as a recognized academic discipline, psychology is relatively young. Its origins can be traced back to the early studies of

researchers such as Wilhelm Wundt (1832–1920), who conducted scientific laboratory experiments into perception. Others regard clinicians such as Sigmund Freud (1856–1939) as key figures in psychology—in particular in relation to developing our understanding of the origins of our emotions (**Figure 7.1**).

In this chapter, we will focus in particular on some of the broad areas in psychology that have had an impact on our assumptions about caring.

As you will see, there are no easy answers for emotional problems. Even within psychology itself, theorists and clinicians may disagree over the causes of difficulties and the remedies that might be helpful. It is therefore particularly important to understand where different approaches are coming from and to reflect on how they might inform practice.

Key theories in psychology

To give you a flavour of these issues, we will introduce you to some of the main strands in the history of psychology.

Sigmund Freud and psychoanalysis

One of the best known figures is Sigmund Freud, founder of *psychoanalysis* (see, for example, Stevens, 2008a). His key contribution was to draw our attention to the importance of the 'unconscious' in guiding, and even determining, our actions. Coming from a medical background, he worked with patients who suffered from neuroses, such as anxiety or obsessional disorders. In his view, these were caused by unconscious emotional conflicts (often assumed to be laid down in childhood). The conflicting demands of societal or parental pressures, on the one hand, and our instincts, or 'drives', on the other, were thought to bring about tension and anxiety. In babies, for example, such tensions might be experienced over feeding and weaning patterns. According to Freud, conflicts over the expression of sexual urges were a major source of anxiety. A popular phrase 'Freudian slip' describes situations in which we say something different from what we meant to say (and what we actually say is assumed to reveal

Table 7.1 Brief summary of some of the major psychological approaches discussed

Approach	Main figure(s)	Key ideas	Application	Legacy
Psychodynamics	Sigmund Freud	Dynamic unconscious Emotional significance of early experiences Defence mechanisms	Psychoanalysis Some counselling approaches	Assumptions about importance of unconscious defence mechanisms
Behaviourism	J.B. Watson B.F. Skinner	Scientific study of behaviour Conditioned reflexes Learning through rewards	Phobia treatments Reward-based behaviour modification	Influence on CBT— see below Behaviour modification techniques in education and health settings
Humanistic psychology	Carl Rogers	Counselling Client-centred therapy Counselling relationship based on empathy, genuineness, and unconditional positive regard	Counselling techniques	Counselling approaches
Cognitive approaches	A. Beck A. Ellis	Cognitive (behavioural) therapy	Specific approach used in therapy based on changing cognitions and behaviour	Cognitive behaviour therapy (CBT)
Biological approaches	Various	Link between brain processes and well-being/behaviour	Medical treatment for depression, for example	Ongoing
Social approaches	Various	Link between individual and social behaviour and experience	Explanations of health behaviours and efficacy of health promotion initiatives	Ongoing

unconscious desires or anxieties, as in the case of the young biologist who meant to talk about 'micro-organisms', but ended up saying 'micro-orgasms'). Other therapists following some of Freud's principles— for example, Erich Fromm (see Thomson, 2009)— assume that a wider range of anxieties about the meaning of life can be the source of our troubles.

Freud thought that we employ 'defence mechanisms' to keep these difficult and uncomfortable emotions at

bay. These include, for example, 'repression', whereby anxieties are pushed into our unconscious. Another such defence mechanism is 'displacement', which describes directing our emotions at a different— perhaps less threatening—target (for example, a frustrated worker might become angry with his family rather than his boss). 'Denial' is another example: we simply deny the reality of what is happening and pretend that things are as we wish them to be. In 'rationalization', we

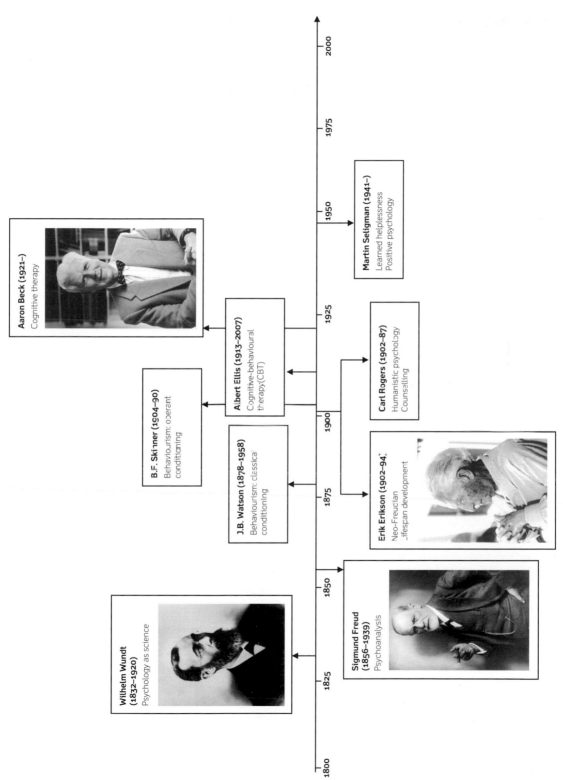

Figure 7.1 Timeline of influential psychologists. Photo of Aaron Beck © Beck Institute for Cognitive Therapy and Research.

William Roberts, a 38-year-old man with a history of schizophrenia, is an insulin-dependent diabetic. On a recent practice placement, your mentor spent a lot of time with William, teaching him how to balance his diet and his insulin, and emphasizing the need for him to reduce his cigarette smoking. You are impressed with your mentor and her knowledge of health promotion.

On your next visit to see William, however, he has increased the number of cigarettes smoked each day and has been surviving on fast food. He says that he needs the cigarettes to 'calm his nerves', 'because all his friends smoke', and 'What is for you won't go past you', and argues that he 'knew a man who smoked 40 cigarettes every day and lived until he was 90'.

Which defence mechanism(s) may help us to understand William's actions?

construct plausible and acceptable explanations to ward off the need to confront tensions that arouse strong and challenging emotions.

Practice Example 7.1 offers a case study that encourages you to think about these mechanisms.

In responding to Practice Example 7.1, we could argue that, in Freudian terms, the main defence mechanism that William uses unconsciously is denial. He resolves the tension between his need for a healthy lifestyle and his difficulties in achieving this by pushing aside any thoughts that he may be harming himself. This allows him to carry on as usual and keeps his anxiety at bay.

It may also be argued that William is leaning on rationalization. He holds on to plausible reasons for smoking, for example 'to fit in with his friends'. Although this may not be the primary reason for his smoking behaviour, it is seen by him to be an acceptable reason that, again, prevents his anxiety. Confronting the dangers to his health head on would cause stress and anxiety, and so this is resolved with the explanations to which he clings.

Freud claimed to be able to access what was troubling his patients through the process of 'psychoanalysis'. This includes methods such as hypnosis, dream analysis, or free association (which basically means getting someone to relax and talk about anything that comes to his or her mind). Healing was thought to come from recognition of the origins of our conflicts. Once we know what past traumatic situations or conflicts may have affected us, we can change that effect and move on.

One technique is the process of 'abreaction'. The patient is encouraged to talk about past situations of psychological trauma that may have been unresolved and repressed from consciousness, but which may be expressed in a physical problem such as paralysis. The trauma experienced by First World War soldiers, for example, was sometimes too terrible to be addressed consciously and so was repressed into the unconscious mind. This became known at the time as 'shell shock'. Doctors at Craiglockhart Hospital in Edinburgh used techniques such as abreaction to bring issues to consciousness so that they could be acknowledged and addressed. Pat Barker (1992) describes this in her book *Regeneration*.

Many psychoanalytically inspired counselling approaches (see, for example, McLeod, 2009) are based on the idea that bringing the origins of our troubles to light will help us to overcome them. Counsellors try to address the questions: why now? What is it about a person's experience that triggers particular emotions at a specific point in time? For example, a relatively minor experience of loss can be amplified by unresolved experiences of a previous event that involved such emotions. Awareness of such links can help people to understand their experiences and, hopefully, to move on. This is illustrated in Becker's (2006) therapeutic approach to a patient experiencing a sense of isolation and fear as part of a 'mid-life crisis'. Aspects of his intervention are based on the ideas of C.G. Jung (1875–1961), another famous psychoanalyst, who wrote about the psychological challenges during adult development. He claimed that, in the second half of life, we need to expand gender aspects of ourselves and integrate masculine and feminine sides into our personalities. For example, women may need to learn to develop their more masculine competitive side (as demands from family life and their roles as mothers change).

More generally, a belief that unconscious issues from our pasts may have a significant effect on us is apparent in many therapeutic encounters. Nelson and Hampson (2008: 1) include a poignant quotation from a victim of childhood sexual abuse:

> **Today I live with a rage and sadness that rules my life. I feel I shall never be a whole human being. My mum used to say you shouldn't live in the past. I don't. The past lives in me.**

However, there were also criticisms of Freud's methods, which many saw as not particularly scientific or open to experimental scrutiny. Discussions continue over exactly what the 'unconscious' might be and how we can investigate this. For example, asking adults about childhood events may not give us a particularly accurate picture of what might have happened to them in their earlier lives. Also, the success of Freudian psychoanalysis is difficult to assess (see, for example, Stevens, 2008a): did Freud's patients get better because of his psychoanalysis sessions or would they have recovered from their difficulties even without any intervention?

Nonetheless, Freud became famous far beyond his own area of work (see Figure 7.1 for a timeline of influential psychologists discussed in this chapter). The idea that we may not be aware of our unconscious desires and conflicts challenged previous views, which assumed that people are rational and self-aware. Furthermore, the suggestion that childhood experiences in particular can lay the emotional foundations for adult personality and relationships has become widely accepted in our common-sense assumptions and in the language that health workers use.

....

Think about your own views on some of the following issues.

Do you think that our childhood experiences determine who we become in adult life? Is it the case—as expressed in Wordsworth's (1802) famous poem 'My heart leaps up when I behold'—that 'the child is the father of the man'?

To what extent do you think we can explain patterns of relationships in terms of previous experiences? For example, might a woman who had a negative relationship with her father be likely to have difficulties in her adult relationships?

Think about situations in your practice in which beliefs around the importance of the unconscious and early experiences have informed people's assessments of others.

....

You might, for example, consider the case of a young woman with anorexia nervosa and explore possible links to parenting patterns during her childhood. Perhaps her attempt to control her food intake is a way of coping with powerlessness in her childhood; her parents may have been overbearing and controlling. Or else her eating disorder may have been connected to her sense of loss and helplessness when her favourite grandmother died. Further factors, such as peer pressure or social ideals on thinness, may also have played a part.

These are complex issues, however, and there will never be easy cause-and-effect answers.

Behaviourism and beyond

Historically, a challenge to the assumptions that psychoanalysis made came from a group of psychologists who are referred to as 'behaviourists'. They believed that the claims made by Freud and his followers were not amenable to controlled experimental study and could hence not be included in academic disciplines. We can only measure what we can see, they suggested, and their focus was firmly on observable behaviour. They believed that our emotional responses are not generated by internal conflicts, but arise from associations with environmental conditions. Freudian references to 'drives' and the 'unconscious' were rejected as spurious and unscientific. Instead, the behaviourists focused on experimental studies of learning in humans and also animals.

Learning associations in our environments

Despite its focus specifically on behaviour, research by behaviourists has also given us insights into emotions and their origins. A controversial experiment (which certainly would not match current ethics standards!) was conducted by J.B. Watson (1878–1958), who was interested in learned fears (see, for example, Gross, 2001). He and his colleague actually taught ('conditioned') a young toddler, 'Little Albert', to fear furry animals. By presenting something of which Albert was afraid (loud bangs behind him) at the same time as something about which he was much more relaxed (a rabbit or rat), Watson conditioned Albert to fear the furry creature because he had learned to *associate* it with a negative stimulus (the loud bang). Watson's plan may have been to remove the fear by breaking this association afterwards—but Albert left the hospital where Watson worked before he was able to progress to this stage.

How have such experiments increased our understanding? One important conclusion is that if fears can be learned, it follows that they can also be 'unlearned'. This then gives us insights into how we can help people to lose their fears. Techniques such as 'systematic desensitization' have been developed as a result. This describes the process by which a therapist encourages a client to relax and then gradually takes him or her through a hierarchy of fear-evoking stimuli. The least fear-arousing ones are tackled first. For example, someone intensely afraid of hospitals might be invited to meet staff and visit a few times prior to an operation, with the hope that familiarity and positive experiences will alleviate some of the anxiety. Hospital-based antenatal classes work on this principle, too.

....

What are your views on the role of environmental factors in learning?

Do you think that our emotions—and in particular fears—are learned through previous negative experiences?

Can you think of an example in your practice in which such associations provide a good explanation of how fears have developed and perhaps also how they have been 'unlearned'?

....

You might, for example, consider a child who, in the past, needed several painful injections, and who now starts to scream and is in obvious distress at the mere sight of a nurse's uniform. Future friendly encounters with nurses should help to eliminate ('extinguish') this response and make the child more relaxed around nurses.

Another example might be a student who has learned to associate exam situations with panic and failure. He finds that just seeing the word 'exam' written on a timetable evokes intense feelings of stress. A series of class tests and relaxation techniques that he is taught by a learning adviser might eventually help him to break this negative association.

And what about emotions other than fear? What associations do we make? For example, some people find that the smell of hospitals makes them feel unwell, or that the sound of the dentist's drill makes them flinch, even though smell and sound on their own should not have such a drastic effect. Studies (for example, Bovbjerg, 2006) have shown how the principles of associative learning can help us to understand why some people experience anticipatory nausea when they embark on a second cycle of chemotherapy. They associate the nausea (the side effects of the first cycle of drugs) with the clinic environment and may feel unwell when they are exposed to (or even just think about) aspects of the situation (for example, the soup served at lunchtime while they were undergoing treatment).

Behaviour and its consequences

Another famous behaviourist was B.F. Skinner (1904–1990), who explored the role of 'reward' and 'punishment' on subsequent behaviour (see Toates, 2009). Skinner's experiments have warned us to consider the consequences of our actions. For example, if a child cries to get sweets at the supermarket checkout and we give in to her demands, we *reinforce* (encourage and strengthen) her behaviour and set ourselves up for further demands on subsequent occasions. Behaviourists suggest that we should reward any steps—however small—towards the desired behaviour. Such reward techniques are still commonly used in the classroom and you may recall reward schemes such as 'gold stars' used by your teachers. Rewards need not

PRACTICE EXAMPLE 7.2

Phil, a mental health nurse, working with Rashid, a young man with a learning disability, praises Rashid's responses when he demonstrates assertive behaviour in role playing and finds that this helps to reinforce the behaviour. If Rashid's newly established assertiveness skills lead to further positive outcomes, for example a successful interview at Jobcentre Plus, the reinforcement will perhaps be even stronger. This helps to promote Rashid's independence and his integration into society.

be specific objects, but can simply be praise for desirable behaviour.

Behaviour modification techniques (successively rewarding small steps towards a target) can also be useful in relation to health behaviours, such as smoking cessation or weight loss. In rehabilitation, too, praising small improvements can be helpful in order to maintain motivation and remind patients that, despite some losses of function, they are making progress. This process of incremental reinforcement is also illustrated in **Practice Example 7.2.**

....

Think about how specific behaviours are seen as useful and desirable, and are reinforced more widely in society.
Reflect on how health professionals can play a role in promoting these.

....

Can you think of any behaviour that you now perform routinely, but which was reinforced initially by rewards from your mother or father?
In what way do you think it is being reinforced in your present environment?

....

Cognitive-behavioural approaches

More recently, behavioural approaches in psychology have been combined with an acknowledgement of the role of 'cognition' to include how we process

information and think about our experiences. Based on the work of Aaron Beck (1976) and Albert Ellis (1975), in combination with the ideas of behaviourism, cognitive-behaviourists emphasize the importance of our interpretations: it is not only our direct experiences that have an effect on our emotions, but also how we make sense of them and what they mean to us. For example, interpreting a pain in one's side as minor and temporary or as a sign of a heart attack will lead to two very different emotional reactions and courses of action. Explanations of panic attacks have made this link (Clark, 1988). If we interpret sensations of feeling unwell as having catastrophic consequences, we are more prone to suffering from panic attacks. We may then benefit from interventions such as 'cognitive behavioural therapy' (CBT) (see, for example, Andersson and Cuijpers, 2008; McLeod, 2009). This is based on the belief that how people feel about a situation and how they act in response to it is influenced by how they perceive and interpret the event to begin with. If we can practise behaviours that are new to us and reflect on their consequences, then we can also begin to interpret situations in a new way, which, in turn, consolidates the new behavioural response. It therefore helps to break the vicious cycle of maladaptive behavioural, emotional, and cognitive responses. We can adapt our thinking patterns to more realistic and positive lines (provided, of course, that our concerns—such as health worries—are unlikely to be related to any significant risk in the first place).

See **Practice Example 7.3** for a case study.

When responding to Practice Example 7.3, you might have suggested that Alison could be helped to *reframe* this event. As a first step, she could be encouraged to consider what she would say to someone else who found themselves in this situation. Rather than dwelling on what is a low risk of infection, she could be led to the conclusion that it would be highly likely that the incident would be without consequence to her health. A clear and concise explanation of how this works is provided by the Royal College of Psychiatrists (2010).

The value of being able to see things differently and 'reframe' a situation can also be seen in **Practice Example 7.4**.

PRACTICE EXAMPLE 7.3

Alison Smith, a student nurse on placement, sustained a needle-stick injury whilst disposing of a needle after giving a subcutaneous injection of fragmen (a medicine used as a blood thinner). She had been supervised by her mentor and was chatting to the patient as she was placing the syringe into the portable sharps box. Holding the box to steady it, she accidentally stabbed her finger through the protective glove with the needle. The patient had been in a residential care facility for seventeen years, had no blood transfusions, and, until admission to the home, had been married to one partner since the age of 18. The student nurse's mentor advised her to follow procedure and go to the accident and emergency (A&E) department. A sample of the student's blood was taken for storage for a three-month period. The student nurse spoke to the charge nurse, who helped her to fill out an accident/incident form and referred her to occupational health. The GP took a sample of the patient's blood to screen for blood-borne viruses. Both the charge nurse and the mentor reassured the student nurse that the patient was very low risk.

That night, Alison started to dwell on the incident and began to panic about all sorts of situations in which the patient could have been involved: for example, her husband could have visited prostitutes when working away from home, or she may have worked at the local hospital and sustained a needle-stick injury herself, but not reported it. Alison then phoned the National Aids Helpline, which also offered reassurance. Later that evening, she spent four hours surfing the Internet reading about blood-borne infections following needle-stick injury. She began to be aware of her heart beating rapidly and that night she was not able to sleep. The next day at work, the only thing that Alison could think of was her fear. The prospect of meeting her friends in the evening held no pleasure.

How might Alison be helped to view this situation differently?

PRACTICE EXAMPLE 7.4

Jim is a mental health branch student on placement in a day hospital. One day, Gordon, a service user, approached Jim's mentor and was visibly upset because, when he said 'good morning' to Rachel, another service user, she 'blanked him' and walked away. Jim's mentor made a cup of tea for Gordon and began to discuss the issue. In a process called 'Socratic questioning', a technique sometimes used in CBT, the mentor sensitively and tactfully began to explore with Gordon possible explanations for Rachel's behaviour. Jim realized that this was beginning to give Gordon a different perspective on the situation: Rachel may not have deliberately blanked Gordon because she disliked him. Realizing that Rachel's behaviour may have had entirely different causes made Gordon feel more positive about the situation.

Humanistic psychology

Both psychoanalysis and behaviourism tend to look at what shapes, or even determines, our behaviour and experience. Such assumptions have been criticized by those theorists who believe that this misses out the importance of choices that we have and the ways in which we are not necessarily passive victims of circumstances. A group of psychologists began to address these issues in the 1950s (see Figure 7.1 for a timeline of influential psychologists discussed in this chapter). The term used for this approach is 'humanistic psychology' and it emphasizes the importance of our ability to grow and develop on a path of our own choosing. One of the key theorists was Carl Rogers (1902–1987), who became well known for his assumptions about 'client-centred therapy' (see, for example, Rogers, 1965). He felt that each client, with his or her hopes, dreams, aspirations, and worries, should be seen and treated as a unique individual and should be in control of his or her own learning and development. Rogers believed that most personal difficulties stem from social pressures on people to be the ideal wife, the perfect boss, or the ever-patient teacher. A counsellor should develop good listening skills along with the qualities of empathy (a deep understanding of another person's world), congruence (relating to the client as a genuine person and not hiding behind the conventions of the role as 'the expert'), and unconditional positive regard (a fundamental acceptance of the client). These ideas can be difficult to pin down and have, at times, been defined in different ways. Their underlying stance goes back to Rogers's '*deep respect for the significance and worth of each person*' (Rogers, 1951; cited in McLeod, 2009: 186). (For more on respect for the individual, see Chapter 4.) This is thought to encourage the development of a caring relationship in which clients feel secure and confident enough in themselves to progress and develop their true selves. Many counselling approaches are based on the importance of good and constructive communication between counsellor and client. However, such qualities underlie other positive caring relationships too and can be seen as essential to building a constructive rapport with people.

···

Be aware of confidentiality and anonymity issues in the following activity.

Listening can be more difficult than we often assume. It is easy to let time pressures, and our own thoughts and assumptions, take over rather than really tune into what someone has to say.

Practise listening with a colleague.

Take turns to talk about a recent placement experience for five minutes. Really *listen* to what your partner is saying.

Discuss how often other thoughts interfered with this process.

Did the 'talker' spot if or when the 'listener's' attention tuned out? Your constructive feedback to each other will be very useful.

···

The psychology of emotions

This brief tour of a few key theories in psychology will have given you an indication of some of the different and varied assumptions that psychologists have made about how to study behaviour and experience, and what can be done when we go through difficult times. In this section, we will focus more directly on specific areas of our experience that affect our emotional well-being.

The area of emotions is particularly useful in showing the complexity of our subject matter and the way in which the many different facets of our lives contribute to our experience. Alder et al. (2009: 25) define emotions thus:

> Emotions are transient, internal experiences involving sensations, feelings and changes in bodily arousal; they connect us to thoughts and images and influence how we react to and communicate with others.

Biological, psychological, and social factors contribute to how we feel. Fundamentally, biological factors are clearly involved. Neurotransmitters in the brain have a major effect on how we feel. For example, low levels of serotonin have been shown to be associated with clinical depression (Nemeroff and Owens, 2009). Medical treatment of depression involves selective serotonin reuptake inhibitors (SSRIs) such as fluoxetine to boost the effects of serotonin. Biological psychology is a burgeoning area of research with exciting new developments, such as brain imaging techniques (see, for example, Toates, 2007).

Then again, our physiological responses are obviously also affected by social situations: you need only to consider your blushing response when someone reveals embarrassing information about you. In this case, a physical reaction—dilation of blood vessels—occurs in response to very specific social meanings. The immediate social context also has an effect on how we interpret the physical symptoms that we might feel. Schachter and Singer's (1962) classic experiments illustrate this. They found that, when their research participants' adrenaline levels were raised without them being aware of this (they were given what they thought were 'vitamin injections'), the social situation affected how they actually felt. In other words, participants interpreted their physical symptoms (increased heart rate and sweating) in line with what was going on in their environment. Those in the company of people who appeared happy reported feeling positive and excited. Those whose companions came across as frustrated interpreted the same physical symptoms as anger.

There is some evidence to suggest that emotions are, at least to some extent, universal (and thus perhaps genetically pre-programmed). For example, Ekman (1994) found that basic emotions—for example, joy, sadness, or surprise—are recognized across many different cultures. He suggests that evolution has predisposed us to be able to communicate these fundamental aspects of experience in a quick and easily recognizable way through our facial expressions.

However, social conventions and culture also clearly play a role in how we express our emotions. 'Display rules' is the term used to describe what is 'encouraged' or 'allowed' in specific situations. At a wedding, for example, happy smiles would be welcomed, while uncontrollable laughter would no doubt attract stares or shaking heads (unless a specific reason for such hilarity was recognized). However, biological and social factors are not the only determinants of emotions. We also have some choice over how and when we convey particular emotions, and how we manage the expression of emotions in interaction with others.

A good illustration of how important it is to appreciate these factors is the management of embarrassment in a nursing context. Lawler (1994; cited in Robb et al., 2004) describes the need for nurses to be aware of social rules (on modesty) and personal meanings (loss of control) involved in carrying out intimate tasks (such as undressing and washing patients), which are normally considered intensely personal and private. Sensitive management of these situations can help to make people feel more comfortable about a potentially distressing situation. This involves nurses reflecting on their own feelings and how to deal with them. It also entails recognizing their patients' emotions and helping them to redefine situations, which may be new and exceptional for them, as 'normal'. Thus the topic of emotions in caring would seem an important one on which to pick up in order to try to make sense of

some of the complexities that our behaviour and experience present to us.

How do you feel? The 'self' and emotions

In Chapter 2, the importance of self was explored. In this section, we will examine three specific areas to show some of the ways in which psychologists have explored:

- how we can make sense of the 'self', and how our perceptions of ourselves and others can have an effect on happiness, well-being, and behaviour;
- how we cope with pain and stress; and
- how our relationships with others can have a significant effect on our emotional and physical well-being (loss, social support) and how we can try to build resilience in ourselves, and also support this in others.

Making sense of the self

Making sense of what we experience as the *self*, or 'I', is clearly a complex task. You will find that there are several terms to describe this, such as 'self', 'identity', or 'ego', all of which reflect different theories with diverse starting points. In further study of psychology, you may want to follow up some of the subtle differences between them. In this section, we will focus on two aspects of this experience: the development of the self; and the way in which a sense of control over our lives can affect the way we feel about ourselves and others.

Developing a sense of self

How do we develop a sense of self? There have been several approaches to shed light on this. We will examine here one example of a theory that tries to show how our personal development is linked to physical maturing, as well as to social issues.

Following in Freud's footsteps, Erik Erikson (1902–1994) developed a theory of life stages, in which he charted our development through a series of eight 'crises', or developmental challenges that we have to resolve. (See Figure 7.1 for a timeline of influential psychologists discussed in this chapter.) During each stage, we have to work on particular qualities, developing our *ego* or *self*. His ideas are still commonly used as a way of exploring how we develop a sense of trust and hope (infancy), autonomy and will (early childhood), initiative and purpose (play age), competence (school age), identity (adolescence), intimacy and love (young adulthood), care for others (maturity), and finally integrity and wisdom (old age). Erikson (1995) thought that if these positive qualities are not developed at the appropriate stage, we then struggle with constructive development at further stages. For example, a baby experiencing erratic and unpredictable care in her first year may develop a sense of mistrust that might stay with her as she grows up.

Erikson used the phrase 'triple bookkeeping' to emphasize the importance of taking into account biological factors, individual ego development, and the social context. For example, at the stage of adolescence, young people have to deal with very specific biological changes during puberty, and particular social contexts are clearly important too. At this stage, Erikson suggests, *identity* issues can be foregrounded (see Erikson, 1968). The way in which teenagers often idolize pop stars or engage in risky behaviours can be easier to understand if we see this as a way of trying to make sense of questions such as 'who am I?' or 'what is my place in society?' Peers and role models—whether teachers, media personalities, or parents—are thought to play a particularly important role at this stage in life.

If peers and role models are particularly important at the adolescent stage, what health messages do you think teenagers are likely to pick up on?

What might this imply for health promotion initiatives?

This suggests that peers and role models will have a powerful influence in consolidating lifestyle choices. If, therefore, the peer group were to be very interested in a particular sport, a teenager may be motivated to join

them. On the other hand, people who find themselves in a group of people who like to smoke cannabis would tend to conform to the rules of this circle. Health promotion initiatives may be more powerful when presented by people seen as positive role models, such as musicians or sports personalities.

Another stage at which social stereotypes and expectations would seem to be particularly important is old age. Erikson suggested that the positive outcome at this stage involves looking back on our lives with a sense of satisfaction despite (or perhaps because of) our awareness that we may not have much time left to live. A negative resolution of this stage would be to become bitter about missed opportunities and remain unable to accept the prospect of death. We may also want to examine to what extent society's messages about staying or looking young at all costs might contribute to some people's negative feelings about their own ageing.

Consider social stereotypes about old age. To what extent and in what ways might these influence health professionals' care?

The idea that older people prefer traditional foods, for example, may lead to them being offered only this kind of food in a nursing home without any regard for individual choice. Similarly, assumptions about music and daytime activities may be based on outdated generational assumptions about what 'they' like.

But Erikson's theory is not without criticisms, for example from those who prefer research methods such as scientific testing to the general observations that Erikson made. He himself called his theory '*a tool to think with, rather than a prescription to abide by*' (Erikson, 1950; cited in Stevens, 2008b: 58) and, in this sense, his suggestions are still useful as a trigger for consideration and reflection.

Developing a sense of control

Erikson highlighted the importance of a sense of trust, will, and competence. These qualities have also been investigated by other researchers who focus less on their development and more on the cognitive aspects of how we make sense of our lives. Whether we feel in control or develop a sense of helplessness and hopelessness has been shown to influence our well-being in several ways.

Rotter (1966) has described this as 'locus of control': do we feel that we have the capacity to change things (an internal locus of control), or do we have a sense of being at the mercy of factors that give us little scope for manoeuvre (an external locus of control)? This can affect health behaviours, for example whether we seek medical help in the first place, or whether we comply with the recommendations given by our doctors or nurses.

In relation to physical health, people may be more likely to take up screening opportunities if they feel that early diagnosis will give them a chance of taking action to avoid more serious problems. Those people who have a sense of personal choice and feel in charge of their lives may be more likely to respond to such schemes. Health belief models (see, for example, Marks et al., 2005) have been developed to provide an illustration of how people make sense of health issues and to predict how they might behave. Health beliefs are developed in interaction with individual aspects, such as personality, and social factors, such as class, gender, and age stereotypes. Commonly cited components of health beliefs are perceived susceptibility to a particular illness and its perceived severity, general health motivation, and perceptions of the benefits of and barriers to treatments. Perceptions of control have also been found to play a significant part. For example, if people believe that their actions will have an effect and that they are able to carry them out, compliance with medical advice is more likely (Alder et al., 2009). Conversely, people who externalize the locus of control may comply totally with medical prescription even if they do not believe themselves to be ill (Marland and Cash, 2005).

In terms of mental health, a thought pattern that emphasizes a person's perceived inability to change negative events has been linked to depression (Sweeney et al., 1986): if we feel that, no matter what we do, bad things will happen anyway, there may seem little incentive to remain positive. Seligman (1975) showed in experimental research that dogs can be conditioned to become apathetic and withdrawn if they

have no opportunities to escape from a negative situation. Even when they are then able to leave their distressing circumstances, they will not do so because of their conditioning. Transferring these findings to people, this pattern has been termed 'learned helplessness', which describes the situation in which '*a person has discovered that efforts at bringing change are futile, and that the outcomes are out of his or her control*' (Kitwood, 1999; cited in Robb et al., 2004: 310). Therapy will then focus on getting us to reframe our thought patterns and our behaviour, and to focus on what *can* be changed (even if this seems very limited).

See **Practice Example 7.5** for a case study.

In response to Practice Example 7.5, Erikson's ideas may suggest that Edward's passive approach was learned in his early childhood, while Rotter's theory would lead us to conclude that he had developed an external locus of control possibly because his adoptive parents did everything for him. Similarly, Seligman's views would point towards Edward's previous inability to avoid negative experiences (his biological parents' neglect and abuse).

You might have suggested an objective such as arranging to have your next visit at a time when the Celtic game is broadcast live on the subscription channel in the local pub. You will go to the pub with Edward. This could be the first step towards encouraging Edward to make a decision (and he may, in the end, still involve his neighbours in the practicalities of subscription if this is what he decides to do).

There is further evidence to indicate that when we perceive a sense of control in our lives, mental and physical health improves. For example, a classic piece of research by Langer and Rodin (1976) suggests that even small changes in how a nursing home was run had an effect. When residents were given more control and choice (for example, over leisure activities), their physical health appeared to be better and they also reported being more content and happy. (For a more recent discussion with Ellen Langer on the significance of her findings, listen to the radio programme available online at **http://www.bbc.co.uk/programmes/b00m0zz3.**)

Similar findings have been made by researchers who look into work satisfaction (Layard, 2006). Opportunities

PRACTICE EXAMPLE 7.5

Whilst on a placement with a voluntary organization providing social support to people with mental and social health needs in the community, your mentor takes you to visit 74-year-old Edward Scott. You have learned that, as a child, Edward was neglected by his mother and physically abused by his alcoholic father, who did not abuse his two siblings. At age 10, a very caring childless couple who doted on him and did everything for him adopted him. Edward continued to live with the couple and gained work as a refuse collector. When his adoptive parents died around ten years ago, Edward inherited their house and all of their savings.

Edward takes little initiative and is reluctant to try anything new. He demonstrates little trust in the workers from the voluntary agency, and depends on his neighbour to fill out forms for him and to help him to make decisions. He says little to the mentor, but does chat about his favourite football team Glasgow Celtic. You are also a Celtic fan and watch games often on a satellite TV channel. You suggest that he also subscribes. Your mentor tells you after the visit that this has been suggested to Edward before, but that he does not carry out any action to follow up his initial interest.

Outline the reasons that Erikson, Rotter, and Seligman may suggest underlie Edwards's passive approach to life.

Give an example of an objective that you might negotiate with Edward. Based on Rotter's and Seligman's ideas, how would you work with him to achieve this objective?

for control and for using our skills appear to play a significant role. A lack of ways in which workers can exercise and develop their competence and have this acknowledged by their employers has been cited as a reason for staff burnout in caring organizations (Kitwood, 1999; cited in Robb et al., 2004).

It is easy to see how positive opportunities might be equally relevant in other spheres of our lives, such as leisure activities. This is perhaps particularly important for people who are unable to work due to ill health or who have been made unemployed.

Coping with pain and stress

Emotions, as we have seen, are extremely complex and cover issues relating to individual and society. This applies to all emotions, even those—such as pain—that, at first glance, appear to be dominated by biological factors such as pain. Melzack and Wall's gate control theory (see Marks et al., 2005: 314) sees pain '*as a multidimensional and perceptual experience, in which … physiological and psychological inputs are equally involved*'. As for the emotions discussed earlier in this chapter, when and how we show that we are in pain is influenced by individual factors and social norms.

Knowing about the different factors that mediate the experience of pain can be extremely useful in helping people to cope when pharmacological pain relief is not appropriate (for example, due to side effects or risks of addiction through prolonged use) or needs to be reduced. Again, a belief in *self-efficacy* (our perceived ability to influence the course of our lives; Bandura, 1977) appears to play a part. A sense that we are able to manage pain or to accept it as part of our identity appears to be a useful way of dealing with chronic pain. It could be suggested that a number of alternative treatments (such as aromatherapy) are reported as being positive because patients feel that they have some control over such treatments (perhaps in contrast to more medically managed interventions). For similar reasons, perhaps, self administered pain relief appears to be more effective (Ballantyne et al., 1993). Giving patients information about what to expect after operations, for example, also seems to increase their ability to cope with pain (Williams et al., 2004).

Can we measure pain accurately? Some physiological signs may be apparent to an observer (for example, facial expressions) or measurable in other ways, such electromyography (EMG), which gives indications of muscle tension and pain (see Upton, 2010). However, none of these measures can replace asking someone what their pain actually feels like to them. Set questionnaires (for example, sliding scales from 'no pain' to 'excruciating pain'), sometimes called 'visual analogue scales', can help with assessment and ultimately the key expert in pain is the person experiencing it.

The challenge for nurses is to assess pain, taking all of these factors into account. This is particularly difficult when patients may not be able to communicate (for example, children or some people with learning disabilities or speech impairments). Many hospitals now have specialized 'pain management teams' to offer specific expertise in this area.

Stress shows a similarly complex pattern. Lazarus (1966) suggests that we come under stress when we feel that we cannot cope with the challenges in our lives. Biological signs can be, for example, biochemical changes (higher blood pressure). People under stress may also report other negative effects on their lives, such as sleep problems and poor concentration. Emotional issues follow on from this: someone going through a particularly stressful time may be irritable or sad.

Different models have been developed in order to give us a better understanding of the causes, consequences, and ways of dealing with stress. Physiologically, stress responses are thought to have evolved to help us to deal with immediate threats, enabling fight or flight responses. Increased amounts of adrenalin in the body can help to add extra energy when needed, for example when running away from an attacker. However, if the threat or stressor continues and fighting or running away are not an option (for example, when work situations are the cause of our stress), such responses are more maladaptive and can result in an increased risk of coronary heart disease (CHD).

Life change models (for example, Holmes and Rahe, 1967) have tried to specify which life events can be seen to score particularly highly in their likelihood to cause stress. Major changes to our lives are at the top of such lists, for example the death of a spouse or partner. Lower down the list would be financial difficulties, for example. However, such models have often been criticized for neglecting the interaction between different personal and interpersonal events. Models that take on board these complexities emphasize the interaction between, for example, someone's personality,

their perception of the stressor, and their coping mechanisms—including relationships.

Research in the 1950s and 1960s suggested that Type A personalities have often been thought to link to an increased risk of CHD. This describes people who come across as very time-pressured and driven (see, for example, Friedman, 1996). Other research, however, has found that high levels of hostility, in particular, appear to be related to higher risks of CHD, while a more relaxed and humorous approach can be beneficial (Williams, 1989). It is important not to oversimplify the role that personality factors play and to avoid stereotyping people. Instead, it may be more helpful to look at ways in which individuals can learn to deal with stress. This includes, for example, relaxation techniques and other lifestyle changes such as exercise (see also Rodham, 2010).

Several mediating factors will contribute to how a particular individual will experience stressful events. These include beliefs and attitudes, perceptions, coping strategies, general health and lifestyle factors, and social support. We may also be reassured when we learn that stress responses to new circumstances can be commonly experienced and are not 'abnormal'.

See **Practice Example 7.6** for a case study.

In response to Practice Example 7.6, you may have noted that Jennifer would have been reassured by Olga's mentor because we tend to judge our own behaviour against our ideas of what is normal in society or in our particular social groupings. The fact that this mother's experience of baby blues was very common meant that she did not feel abnormal. Of course, the health visitor would have remained watchful for signs of post-natal depression and used scales such as the Edinburgh Post-Natal Depression Scale (EPDS) to screen for this. Again, however, the fact that this screening tool is used routinely for all new mothers may in itself be reassuring for each mother.

Dealing with loss

One experience that evokes particularly strong emotions and is commonly encountered in caring situations is loss. Losing a partner, parent, or child can have

PRACTICE EXAMPLE 7.6

Olga, a student nurse on practice placement with a health visitor, observed an interaction in which Jennifer, a new mother with a two-day-old baby, complained of being weepy and irritable and finding it impossible to cheer up. The health visitor explained to Jennifer that this was likely to be 'baby blues', and that it affected most new mothers and therefore was a normal reaction to giving birth.

What might Jennifer have found helpful about the health visitor's response?

a devastating effect on people. However, it is also useful to think of loss as *any* change to our imagined desired future, so that, for example, a diagnosis of infertility is also seen as a 'loss'.

Swiss-born doctor Elisabeth Kübler-Ross (1969) worked closely with terminally ill and bereaved people, and described the process of coming to terms with loss as following a series of phases:

1 **Denial**—The initial reaction is likely to be that a person may refuse to accept a diagnosis with a poor outlook, for example.

2 **Anger**—This is followed by a phase during which people may vent their feelings of frustration about their loss. This may show itself, for example, in unjustified anger towards health professionals or carers (and note that it is extremely important not to confuse this with situations in which people may have cause for complaint).

3 **Bargaining**—The next stage could involve 'bargains' with God, such as 'if I live long enough to see my son get married, I'll go to church every week', or bargains with medical professionals, such as 'if I follow all of the doctor's directions, I'll make it to my next birthday'.

4 **Depression**—A period of depression may follow when, despite all of this, their condition deteriorates and the person realizes the extent of their helplessness to change the situation.

5 **Acceptance**—Kübler-Ross suggests that, with emotional support, we can then come to accept the situation, develop gratitude for what we have had, appreciate the time left to us, and become able to let go of fear and anger.

This model has become widely known in that it was one of the first examples of how health professionals have directly addressed the emotional needs of people going through loss and bereavement.

However, others (for example, Butt, 2008) have highlighted that this model is open to oversimplification. It has sometimes been taken to suggest that there is a 'good' method of dealing with loss. If we imply that other ways may somehow be deficient, we run the risk of putting pressure on patients or clients to 'get it right' and ignore the way in which individuals deal with difficult situations in their own way. Similarly, Corr and Coolican (2010) suggest that recent approaches have moved away from stage- and phase-based theories, to emphasize instead the **tasks** and **processes** that we have to face in grieving and mourning. They point to the importance of avoiding generalizations when dealing with individuals going through experiences of loss. Appreciating the complexity of personal and cultural meanings for each individual is a key factor in providing sensitive and empathetic care.

The important message from Kübler-Ross's work is to recognize that there are emotions that commonly (but not always!) accompany our experience of loss. You may want to reflect on this using an example of a 'light' loss (such as losing your key, book, or mobile phone). Did you experience denial, anger, bargaining, depression, and acceptance? Did you experience any other emotions as well or instead?

Practice Example 7.7 offers another opportunity to consider the ways in which an understanding of the emotions accompanying loss might be useful.

As we have seen earlier, personal meanings and perceptions play an important role in all of these experiences; it is therefore vital for health professionals to be open to different ways of dealing with loss and the personal meanings tied up with it. Finlay's (2003) research illustrates this. Her case study describes how Ann, suffering from multiple sclerosis, regarded a symptom (slight numbness in her hand), seen as 'minor' by

PRACTICE EXAMPLE 7.7

Sarah, a student nurse out on practice placement with a district nurse, was surprised at the reaction of a patient whose daughter is seriously ill in intensive care. The patient said—rather cold-heartedly, Sarah thought— that her daughter would only be in hospital overnight. She did not seem distressed or worried about the situation and went on to discuss everyday matters with no outward show of emotion. In the car, the student's mentor told her that the patient's daughter was being ventilated, was extremely ill, and that her life was hanging in the balance. The student nurse could not understand

why this patient had seemed to be so carefree and found it hard to understand or to empathize with her.

After learning about the reactions to loss, however, Sarah realized that this patient seemed to be detached from the situation of her daughter's life-threatening illness because the reality was too much for her to cope with. The patient seemed to be cold-hearted not because she cared too little, but because she cared so much. The patient was protecting her inner self through the ego defence mechanism called 'denial'.

medical professionals, as a much more significant event because she could no longer feel her baby's skin in the same way and sensed a progressive loss of 'mothering' quality.

PRACTICE TIP

A sensitive, respectful, and non-judgemental approach to those experiencing loss is vital.

Resilience and social support

On what resources can we draw when things go wrong? Research into happiness and *resilience* (our ability to weather the storms of life's challenges) points us to ways of coping with difficult situations. The quality of relationships appears to play a particularly important role. In surveys on happiness, positive relationships with family and friends are frequently near the top of such lists (see, for example, Argyle, 2001).

Supportive relationships (including professional relationships) have been found to contribute significantly to people's ability to cope with challenges. Caring friends can be extremely important when we experience stressful events. For example, one study found that parents whose children go through serious illness were better able to cope with the situation when they had supportive social contact with friends—in

particular, when a partner was perceived as not supportive (Rini et al., 2008).

Social support networks have also been found to play a role in promoting physical health, although the exact relationship between social support and its effects is notoriously difficult to assess (Uchino, 2004). The possibility of such a link does, however, provide some justification for promoting self-help groups, which can offer like-minded individuals opportunities to give as well as take, to share anxieties, and to feel empowered. This also points to the importance of health professionals encouraging and enabling people to maintain and build networks of social support.

······························

List the sources of support for bereaved people that you aware of in your locality.

Do hospitals and other institutions encourage social support? If so, how? If not, what are the barriers?

······························

If you have trouble thinking of all of the sources of support that a bereaved person might access, visit **http://www.patient.co.uk/showdoc/145/**

Further, less-specific sources of support include the person's own unique social support networks. When we are in situations in which we feel vulnerable, this type of support is often particularly important. Consider to what extent hospitals and nursing homes encourage patients to maintain these links, for example through ease of access to the location, visiting times, computer/Internet access, or possibilities of community-based care.

PRACTICE EXAMPLE 7.8

Anton and Susan are both in their 80s and have been married for over fifty years. They have lived in Devon for a long time, and have a good and supportive circle of friends. Several years ago, Susan developed Alzheimer's disease. Initially, Anton was able to care for her in their home, but after Susan had a stroke, residential care was the only realistic option for her. The care home is within easy driving distance of their family home. Anton visits on a daily basis, but also spends some long weekends away with their daughter and family in Edinburgh. After a period of adjustment, Susan has settled well. She visibly enjoys Anton's visits, but appears content on the days when he is not there and takes part in the activities on offer, such as singing.

Anton has joined a carers' group that staff in the residential home have set up. He has made new contacts there and feels that any concerns are listened to and resolved as soon as possible. A long-standing family friend has encouraged Anton to accompany him on fishing trips.

Anton goes through periods of sadness when he misses his old life with Susan, but feels that he has done all he can to cope with the new circumstances and, given the changes he is going through, is as content as the situation allows.

What factors have helped both Anton and Susan to adjust to the changes in their lives?

See **Practice Example 7.8** for a case study.

Some examples of the factors outlined in Practice Example 7.8 are: the social support that Anton gets from friends and the carers' group; Anton's good health; his ability to drive; financial stability (ability to afford trips to Edinburgh); the care home staff making Anton feel welcome; Susan's ability to participate in activities offered by the care home; and Anton's visits. This also illustrates how the care home's concern for residents' carers (and not only for residents themselves) contributes to building resilience in both carers *and* residents.

Why do we care?

Finally, we may want to ask why caring should be seen as so important. At a very basic level, it seems to be a 'natural' reaction for us to want to care when others go through distressing circumstances. Evolutionary psychologists (see, for example, Vine, 1983) suggest that we may have evolved a tendency towards helping behaviours such as altruism due to their potential value in aiding group survival in our prehistoric past. It is perhaps also valuable for us to acknowledge explicitly the creativity of opportunities to use caring skills effectively and sensitively. Arman and Rehnsfeldt (2007) describe how responding to patients with

'human-ness' and compassion can have an immensely positive and transforming effect on patients' experiences. Noticing and acting on even just small aspects of particular patients' preferences can help to make people feel that '*you are a person: not a diagnosis*' (ibid: 377). Different categories of the term 'presence' (physical, psychological, and therapeutic) describe an ability to be centred in ourselves, to develop a sense of empathy and connectedness, and to communicate this to others (Engebretson, 2000; cited in Robb et al., 2004). In this way, even a distressing situation can become 'extraordinarily rewarding' (ibid: 240) in that it gives one person the privilege of sharing another's profound life experiences. Opportunities for using your caring values and skills sensitively and constructively will no doubt also have a positive effect on your job satisfaction (Kitwood, 1999; cited in Robb et al., 2004).

Conclusion

In this chapter, our brief investigation into psychological aspects of caring has shown that our emotional lives involve a rich weave of physiological, psychological, and social factors. A caring relationship can benefit significantly from reflection on these complexities in ourselves and others, and can give us tools 'to think with' (Erikson, 1950; cited in

Stevens, 2008b: 58). Active reflection in relation to research, theories, and experience will help us to understand emotions, develop resilience, and support this in others.

Further reading

There are many psychology textbooks that provide good general introductions to psychology, such as:

Glassman, W.E. and Hadad, M. (2009) *Approaches to Psychology*, 5th edn, Maidenhead: Open University Press/ McGraw-Hill

Gross, R. (2010) *Psychology: The Science of Mind and Behaviour*, 6th edn, London: Hodder and Stoughton

Hayes, N. and Orrell, S. (1998) *Psychology: An Introduction*. Harlow: Longman

Hewstone, M., Fincham, F.F., and Foster. J. (2005) *Psychology*, Chichester: John Wiley & Sons

A number of publications explore the links between nursing and psychology, such as:

Marks, D.F., Murray, M.D., Evans, B., Willig, C., Woodall, C., and. Sykes, M. (2005) *Health Psychology: Theory, Research and Practice*, London: Sage

Rodham, K. (2010) *Health Psychology*, Basingstoke: Palgrave Macmillan

Upton, D. (2010) *Introducing Psychology for Nurses and Healthcare Professionals*, Harlow: Pearson Education

Walker, J. and Payne, S. (1996) *Psychology for Nurses and the Caring Professions* (reprinted 2007 under the title *Social Science for Nurses and the Caring Professions*), Maidenhead: Open University Press

Watkins, D., Edwards, J., and Gastrell, P. (2003) (eds) *Community Health Nursing: Frameworks for Practice*, Eastbourne: Balliere Tindall/Elsevier

For an account of the principles of cognitive-behavioural approaches, see:

Royal College of Psychiatrists (2010) 'Cognitive behaviour therapy', available online at **http://www.rcpsych. ac.uk/mentalhealthinfoforall/treatments/cbt.aspx** [accessed 4 July 2011]

For an introduction to the main concepts of the key theorists mentioned in this chapter, see:

Boeree, G. (2006) 'Personality theories', available online at **http://webspace.ship.edu/cgboer/perscontents. html** [accessed 16 June 2011]

For a more detailed account and contemporary evaluation of some key theorists' ideas, see:

Stevens, R. (2008a) *Sigmund Freud: Shaper of the Unconscious Mind*, Basingstoke: Palgrave Macmillan

Stevens, R. (2008b) *Erik Erikson: Shaper of Identity*, Basingstoke: Palgrave Macmillan

Thomson, A. (2009) *Erich Fromm: Shaper of the Human Condition*, Basingstoke: Palgrave Macmillan

Toates, F. (2009) *Burrhus F. Skinner: Shaper of Behaviour*, Basingstoke: Palgrave Macmillan

References

Alder, B., Abraham, C.S., van Teijlingen, E., and Porter, M. (2009) *Psychology and Sociology Applied to Medicine*, 3rd edn, Edinburgh: Churchill Livingstone Elsevier.

Andersson, G. and Cuijpers, P. (2008) 'Pros and cons of online cognitive-behavioural therapy', *British Journal of Psychiatry* 193(4): 270–1.

Argyle, M. (2001) *The Psychology of Happiness*, 2nd edn, Hove: Routledge.

Arman, M. and Rehnsfeldt, A. (2007) 'The "little extra" that alleviates suffering', *Nursing Ethics* 14(3): 372–84.

Ballantyne, J.C., Carr, D.B., Chalmers, T.C., Dear, K.B., Angelillo, I.F., and Mosteller, F. (1993) 'Postoperative patient-controlled analgesia: Meta-analyses of initial randomized control trials', *Journal of Clinical Anesthesia* 5: 182–93.

Bandura, A. (1977) 'Self-efficacy: Toward a unifying theory of behavioral change', *Psychological Review*, 84: 191–215.

Barker, P. (1992) *Regeneration*. London: Penguin.

Beck, A.T. (1976) *Cognitive Therapy and the Emotional Disorders*, New York: International Universities Press.

Becker, D. (2006) 'Therapy for the middle-aged: The relevance of existential issues', *American Journal of Psychotherapy* 60(1): 87–99.

Bovbjerg, D.H. (2006) 'The continuing problem of post chemotherapy nausea and vomiting: Contributions of classical conditioning', *Autonomic Neuroscience: Basic and Clinical* 29: 92–8.

Butt, T. (2008) *George Kelly: Shaper of Personal Meaning*, Basingstoke: Palgrave Macmillan.

Clark, D.M. (1988) 'A cognitive model of panic attacks' in S. Rachman and J.D. Maser (eds) *Panic: Psychological*

Perspectives. Hillsdale, NJ: Lawrence Erlbaum Associates, pp. 71–89.

Corr, C.A. and Coolican, M.B. (2010) 'Understanding bereavement, grief, and mourning: Implications for donation and transplant professionals', *Progress in Transplantation* 20(2): 169–77.

Ekman, P. (1994) 'Strong evidence for universals in facial expressions: A reply to Russell's mistaken critique', *Psychological Bulletin* 115: 268–87.

Ellis, A. (1975) *A New Guide to Rational Living*, Hollywood, CA: Wilshire Book Company.

Erikson, E. (1968) *Identity, Youth and Crisis*, New York: W.W. Norton.

Erikson, E. (1995) *Childhood and Society*, 2nd edn, London: Vintage.

Finlay, L. (2003) 'The intertwining of body, self and world: A phenomenological study of living with recently diagnosed multiple sclerosis', *Journal of Phenomenological Psychology* 34(6): 157–78.

Friedman, M. (1996) *Type A Behavior: Its Diagnosis and Treatment*, New York: Plenum Press.

Gross, R. (2001) *Psychology: The Science of Mind and Behaviour*, 4th edn, London: Hodder and Stoughton.

Hewstone, M., Fincham, F., and Foster, J. (2005), *Psychology*, Malden: Blackwell.

Holmes, T.H. and Rahe, R.H. (1967) 'The social readjustment rating scale', *Journal of Psychosomatic Research* 11(2): 213–18.

Kübler-Ross, E. (1969) *On Death and Dying*, New York: Macmillan.

Langer, E.J. and Rodin, J. (1976) 'The effects of choice and enhanced personal responsibility for the aged: A field experiment in an institutional setting', *Journal of Personality and Social Psychology* 34: 191–8.

Layard, R. (2006) *Happiness: Lessons from a New Science*, London: Penguin.

Lazarus, R.S. (1966) *Psychological Stress and the Coping Process*, New York: McGraw-Hill.

Marks, D.F., Murray, M.D., Evans, B., Willig, C., Woodall, C., and Sykes, M. (2005) *Health Psychology: Theory, Research and Practice*, London: Sage.

Marland, G. and Cash, K. (2005) 'Medicine-taking decisions: Schizophrenia in comparison to asthma and epilepsy', *Journal of Psychiatric and Mental Health Nursing* 12: 163–72.

McLeod, J. (2009) *An Introduction to Counselling*, 4th edn, Maidenhead: Open University Press/McGraw-Hill.

Nelson, S. and Hampson, S. (2008) *Yes You Can! Working with Survivors of Childhood Sexual Abuse*, 2nd edn, Edinburgh: The Scottish Government.

Nemoroff, C. and Owens, M. (2009) 'The role of serotonin in the pathophysiology of depression: As important as ever', *Clinical Chemistry* 55: 1578–9.

Rini, C., Manne, S., DuHamel, K., Austin, J., Ostroff, J., Boulad, F., Parsons, S.K., Martini, R., Williams, S.E., Mee, L., Sexson, S., and Redd, W.H. (2008) 'Social support from family and friends as a buffer of low spousal support among mothers of critically ill children: A multilevel modelling approach', *Health Psychology* 27(5): 593–603.

Robb, M., Barrett, S., Komaromy, C., and Rogers, A. (2004) *Communication, Relationships and Care: A Reader*, London: Routledge.

Rodham, K. (2010) *Health Psychology*, Basingstoke: Palgrave Macmillan.

Rogers, C. (1965) *Client-Centered Therapy*, Boston, MA: Houghton Mifflin Company.

Rotter, J.C. (1966) *Locus of Control: Current Trends in Theory and Research*, 2nd edn, New York: Wiley Press.

Royal College of Psychiatrists (2010) 'Cognitive behaviour therapy', available online at **http://www.rcpsych.ac.uk/ mentalhealthinfoforall/treatments/cbt.aspx**[accessed 4 July 2011].

Schachter, S. and Singer, J. (1962) 'Cognitive, social and physiological determinants of emotional state', *Psychological Review* 69: 378–99.

Seligman, M.E.P. (1975) *Helplessness: On Depression, Development and Death*, San Francisco, CA: W.H. Freeman.

Stevens, R. (2008a) *Sigmund Freud: Shaper of the Unconscious Mind*, Basingstoke: Palgrave Macmillan.

Stevens, R. (2008b) *Erik Erikson: Shaper of Identity*, Basingstoke: Palgrave Macmillan.

Sweeney, P.D., Anderson, K., and Bailey, S. (1986) 'Attributional style in depression: A meta-analytic review', *Journal of Personality and Social Psychology* 46: 974–91.

Thomson, A. (2009) *Erich Fromm: Shaper of the Human Condition*, Basingstoke: Palgrave Macmillan.

Toates, F. (2007) *Biological Psychology*. 2nd edn, Harlow: Pearson Educational.

Toates, F. (2009) *Burrhus F. Skinner: Shaper of Behaviour*, Basingstoke: Palgrave Macmillan.

Uchino, B.N. (2004) *Social Support and Physical Health: Understanding the Health Consequences of Relationships*, Current Perspectives in Psychology Series, New Haven, CT: Yale University.

Upton, D. (2010) *Introducing Psychology for Nurses and Healthcare Professionals*, Harlow: Pearson Education.

Vine, I. (1983) 'Sociobiology and social psychology: Rivalry or symbiosis? The explanation of altruism', *British Journal of Social Psychology* 22: 1–11.

Williams, D.C., Golding, J., Phillips, K., and Towell, A. (2004) 'Perceived control, locus of control and preparatory information: Effects on the perception of an acute pain stimulus', *Personality and Individual Differences* 36: 1681–91.

Williams, R. (1989) *The Trusting Heart*, New York: The Free Press.

Wordsworth, W. (1802) 'My heart leaps up when I behold', available online at **http://www.pinkmonkey.com/dl/library1/mhluwib.pdf** [accessed 11 July 2011].

8 Spiritual care

WILFRED McSHERRY AND JOANNA SMITH

Learning outcomes

This chapter will enable you to:

- describe the terms 'spirituality' and 'spiritual care';
- reflect on your understanding of these terms;
- identify the drivers advocating spiritual care as a central component of nursing;
- examine the relevance of spirituality and spiritual care within nursing; and
- evaluate the ways in which nurses can meet an individual's spiritual needs.

Introduction

Cultural, religious, and spiritual beliefs are dominant forces that influence how individuals make sense of the world and their experiences. These beliefs can provide comfort, strength, and support in times of stress. Nurses must develop an understanding of these concepts if they are to meet their patients' needs. This chapter is about spirituality and spiritual care. It will provide a definition of these terms and encourage you to reflect on their relevance to contemporary nursing practice. It is anticipated that, by working through the activities in the chapter, you will be able to consider how, as a student, you can meet the spiritual needs of your patients and clients. The Nursing and Midwifery Council expects nurses at all levels to respect the individuals and communities that they serve:

> **Nurses must provide care without prejudice, irrespective of an individual's cultural, ethical or religious orientations. In addition, nurses**

Essential knowledge and skills for care

- You must assume attitudes and behaviours that respect diversity, individuality, and difference irrespective of whether these are different from your own personal beliefs, values, and opinions.

- You must interact with individuals in a manner that upholds and respects their dignity and uniqueness, adopting behaviours and attitudes that safeguard the integrity of the person, and giving consideration to how you, as a nurse, and the caring environment may impact upon care.

- You must appreciate how culture, religion, and spiritual beliefs can have a profound impact on illness and disability.

- You must understand the importance of carrying out a holistic nursing assessment of the individual, giving due attention to spiritual, as well as physical, social, cultural, psychological, genetic, and environmental, dimensions working in partnership with patients, service users, and others through interaction, observation, and measurement.

> **must not convey personal allegiances which may cause anguish or appear to threaten their clients' individual worth.** (NMC, 2004: 16)

The chapter is specifically designed to assist you to meet the competencies that you must achieve to progress through your chosen field of practice, as outlined in the NMC document *Standards of Proficiency for Pre-Registration Nursing Education* (NMC, 2010).

'Spirituality' and 'spiritual care' defined

The way in which 'spirituality' is understood directly influences how it is incorporated in nursing care. Defining 'spirituality' and 'spiritual care' provides a framework through which to understand these concepts and consider their implications across nursing contexts. **Box 8.1** presents definitions of spirituality, spiritual care, and religious care.

In addition to the definition provided, the classical definition of spirituality is that developed by Murray and Zentner (1989: 259):

A quality that goes beyond religious affiliation, that strives for inspirations, reverence, awe, meaning and purpose even in those who do not believe in any good (god). The spiritual dimension tries to be in harmony with the universe, strives for answers about the infinite, and comes into focus when the person faces emotional stress, physical illness or death.

Box 8.1 Spirituality, spiritual care, and religious care defined

Spirituality is universal, deeply personal and individual; it goes beyond formal notions of ritual or religious practice to encompass the unique capacity of each individual. It is at the core and essence of who we are, that spark which permeates the entire fabric of the person and demands that we are all worthy of dignity and respect. It transcends intellectual capability, elevating the status of all of humanity to that of the sacred.

(Developed by Wilf McSherry for use in his inaugural professorial lecture in April 2009)

Spiritual care is usually given in a one-to-one relationship, is completely person-centred and makes no assumptions about personal conviction or life orientation.

Religious care is given in the context of the shared religious beliefs, values, liturgies and lifestyle of a faith community.

(NHS Education for Scotland, 2009: 21)

The word 'god' has been placed in parentheses because numerous citations of the definition have replaced the word 'good' with the word 'god'. Narayanasamy (2001) says that there is no single or authoritative definition of spirituality, implying that a 'perfect' definition may never be constructed. The definition offered by Murray and Zentner (1989) is not without its critics on the grounds that it:

- is not based on or derived from empirical research (Clarke, 2009); and
- implies that spirituality is universal—that is, that everyone has a spiritual dimension or identifies with the concept—which may not necessarily be the case.

Despite some of the criticisms, this definition does seem to legitimize nurses' involvement in the provision of spiritual care because it affirms that nursing is concerned with caring for people facing physical illness, disease, and death. Nevertheless, we cannot make assumptions because not all patients will present with spiritual needs; neither can we assume that all patients will expect support with this aspect of their lives (McSherry, 2004; 2007). This raises some important questions about the nature of spirituality and the provision of holistic care.

What is holistic care?

The Department of Health's *Your Guide to the NHS* states:

NHS staff will respect your privacy and dignity. They will be sensitive to, and respect, your religious, spiritual and cultural needs at all times.
(Department of Health, 2001: 29)

Consider this quotation and ask yourself what this tells you about the concept of holistic care.

The document reflects the government's vision of health care for the general public. *Your Guide to the NHS* has, however, been superseded by the NHS Constitution (Department of Health, 2009a). The Constitution reinforces patients' right to be '*treated* with dignity and respect, in accordance with your human rights' (ibid: 6). Your reflections may have highlighted that people who require nursing care have diverse needs.

In Chapter 4, you were introduced to the concept of holistic care when discussing the importance of respecting the individual. Individuals can be thought of as having four interlinked parts—physical, psychological, social and spiritual—and irrespective of age, gender, sexuality, race, ethnicity, and religious belief, are made up of these same dimensions. Therefore, we would like you to consider and spend a little time reflecting on these four primary dimensions again, as summarized in **Table 8.1**.

....

Think back to a patient/client with whom you have recently worked.

How did the care that you delivered consider the four primary dimensions of being?

....

Your consideration may have concluded that providing 'holistic' nursing care can be complex and not straightforward. Individuals are not only physical beings requiring food, shelter, and warmth, but all are unique, with a distinct personality, having intellectual and emotional needs. Furthermore, individuals are influenced by the environment, society, and culture in which they live and socialize. This means that individuals possess diverse sets of beliefs and values, whether cultural, religious, or spiritual. These beliefs and values can have a profound impact on the way in which people from different regions of the world and within the UK view health and well-being. Hopefully, you are beginning to understand the meaning of holistic care. By ensuring that each individual is supported to meet their specific needs, nurses can help to promote and preserve the dignity of every patient.

Having identified the four primary dimensions, there is now a need to explore why the provision of spiritual care is an essential component of holistic patient care.

Why is the provision of spiritual care an essential component of holistic nursing practice?

Health care has largely followed a medical model of care delivery, with an emphasis on diseases and their treatments, and only to a lesser extent on individual experiences, beliefs, and values. Increasingly, there is greater recognition that individual beliefs, such as faith, hope, and compassion, impact on the healing process (Patients Association, 2009). Nursing is about providing care to help people who are ill, to enable people to manage health issues, and to achieve the best quality of life whatever their disease or disability (Royal College of Nursing, 2003). Nursing is all-inclusive—meeting the needs of communities, families, and individuals of all ages and cultures, with

Table 8.1 Four primary dimensions of an individual (McSherry, 2006: 72)

Dimension	Explanation
Biological	This refers to the physical and biological process or function of an individual that is essential to maintain life.
Psychological	Usually implies the cognitive, intellectual, and emotional aspects of the individual that may shape personality and mental functioning.
Social	The cultural norms, values, and beliefs that influence and classify individuals into different groups or communities.
Spiritual	A vague term used normally to indicate an individual's inner beliefs, commonly related to religious affiliation or belief in the existence of a god or supreme power.

diverse spiritual and religious beliefs. Nursing recognizes the uniqueness of each individual in relation to their experiences of illness and their heath beliefs. Nursing is based on values that '*respect the dignity, autonomy and uniqueness of the individual*' (ibid: 3).

Spiritual care matters because it focuses care delivery on the individual, and recognizes and utilizes patients' own resources, strengths, aspirations, hopes, and experiences (NHS Education for Scotland, 2009). Incorporating spiritual care into nursing practice can enhance recovery, and helps nurses to understand patients' perspectives in relation to health and illness.

Read and reflect on the extracts in **Box 8.2**.

Hopefully, reading about other people's perceptions of spiritual care will broaden your own understanding and knowledge of the concept. The provision of spiritual care is a central component of providing individualized, patient-centred care. Research undertaken by nurses suggests that although nurses value and can identify aspects of individualized care, such as respecting individuality, there is a gap between nurses' knowledge and daily practice (Gerrish, 2000). For example, research undertaken with patients from South Asian backgrounds suggests that the needs of this client group are not always met, and that patients strive to 'fit in' and to cause as little disruption to healthcare staff as possible (Vydelingum, 2000). This finding emphasizes that individualized care is of paramount importance if we are going to provide care that is appropriate and relevant. Caring for individuals is not about expecting individuals to 'fit in'; it is about capturing and celebrating the uniqueness of all people.

Drivers to promoting spiritual care

A range of political and ethical drivers are influencing a renewed focus on ensuring that spiritual care is integral to health care, including the following.

- **Societal changes**
  The National Health Services is an all-inclusive organization and therefore must respond to societal changes, such as an increasingly multicultural society with diverse norms and values.
- **Ethical and moral values**
  It is ethically moral to treat people appropriately, with respect and dignity, whatever their faith, beliefs, gender, age, abilities/disabilities, and sexual orientation.
- **Users' and carers' views**
  The involvement of users and carers in health care includes their contributing to service delivery, being empowered to make care decisions about care delivery, the design of healthcare research, and the training of healthcare professionals, and is central to the modernization of the NHS (Department of Health 2000, 2004, 2009b; The Patients Association, 2009). The overall aim in relation to the involvement of users and carers in health care is based on the need to make health care more responsive to the needs of patients. The NHS Constitution emphasizes that patients can expect to be treated with dignity and respect; this must include their religious, spiritual and cultural needs being respected at all times (Department of Health, 2009a).
- **Legislation**
  Legislation relating to discrimination on the basis of religion or beliefs has been implemented within the UK. Examples include the Equality Act 2010 and the Racial and Religious Hatred Act 2006. Key issues for health services include that it is unlawful to discriminate on grounds of religious beliefs or lack of beliefs, that healthcare professionals' personal beliefs must not have an impact on the care given to patients, and that the NHS should embed issues of diversity

---

Box 8.2 Cases studies: beliefs about spiritual care

Spirituality is part of health, not peripheral but core and central to it. It pervades our every thought and action, each caring moment. Spirituality and health are bonded to each other, inseparable companions in the dance of joy and sadness, health and illness, birth and death.   (Wright, 2005: 15)

Traditional spiritual practices such as the development of empathy and compassion are being shown to be vital active ingredients, even prerequisites, in effective healthcare—in the carer and the cared for they build wellness and happiness. Effective and efficient healthcare must now (re)take into account these core values.   (Reilly, 2005: xi)

into all processes from recruitment and selection of staff, through to the delivery of services.

- **International directives**

  There are a range of international mandates describing the need for holistic care, of which spiritual care is an integral dimension. For example, the World Health Organization has criticized a reductionist view of patients and advocates healthcare professionals valuing the contribution of faith, hope, and compassion in the healing process (WHO, 1998). The International Council of Nurses has stressed that, in providing care, the nurse must promote '*an environment in which the human rights, values, customs and spiritual beliefs of the individual, family and community are respected*' (ICN, 2006: 2).

- **UK health policy**

  A range of policy guides are available to support staff at all levels to meet the individual needs of patients in relation to culture, religion, and spiritual needs, including: *Religion or Belief: A Practical Guide for NHS Staff* (Department of Health, 2009b) and *Spiritual Care Matters. An Introductory Resource for all NHS Scotland Staff* (NHS Education for Scotland, 2009). Key issues include the need for all staff to develop knowledge and skills in relation to meeting individuals' spiritual and religious beliefs, and the need to strengthen the training available to all staff in order that they can gain the skills necessary to deliver competent spiritual care.

- **Professional bodies and codes of practice**

  The 2008 NMC Code for the standards of conduct, performance, and ethics of nurses and midwives clearly states that nurses must '*make the care of people your first concern, treating them as individuals and respecting their dignity*' (NMC, 2008: 1), and must '*not use your professional status to promote causes that are not related to health*' (ibid: 5). Upholding the Code and the reputation of the nursing profession is a requirement of all registered nurses and midwives.

- **Clinical benefits**

  It has been suggested that meeting the holistic needs of patients results in health benefits including increased patient satisfaction and a quicker recovery process.

···

Consider the drivers outlined above.
Do you feel that spiritual care is an integral part of the care that you have observed and to which you have contributed while in practice?
···

For more on how attending to the religious and spiritual needs of individuals may enhance their well-being, see Koenig et al. (2001).

What is spirituality?

We have presented definitions of spirituality and spiritual care that we will now explore in more depth.

···
Before proceeding, take some time out to consider what you understand by the term 'spirituality'.
You may find it useful to jot down your ideas and reflect on them as you progress through the chapter.
···

You may consider spirituality to be universal, in that it applies to all people—those who have a religious belief and those who do not. You may find that your understanding of spirituality may fit into one of three categories:

- a religious belief and faith in God or a deity;
- no religious belief and faith in God or a deity;
- a search for meaning and purpose and fulfilment in life.

However, do not be alarmed if you have never given any conscious thought to spirituality. Research suggests that many patients, and indeed some healthcare professionals, have given no consideration to the meaning of this concept (McSherry, 2004; 2007). Perhaps some of the descriptions in **Figure 8.1** reflect your understanding.

The Department of Health has recognized the different interpretations of the concept of spirituality, reinforcing its uniqueness and deeply personal aspects:

Spirituality is difficult to define, as it can mean different things to different people, and its existence as a discrete phenomenon may be denied by some. In essence it is to do with making important connections which provide

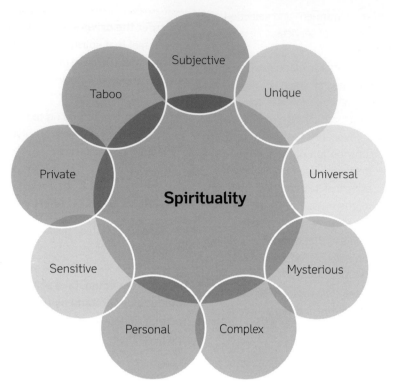

Figure 8.1 Descriptions of spirituality within nursing.

people with hope, purpose and comfort. This may also be confused with religion which relates to a belief system.

(Department of Health, 2009b: 19)

Figure 8.2 illustrates the broad range of interpretations by providing actual descriptions of spirituality provided by healthcare professionals and patients.

The descriptions outlined in Figure 8.2 reveal that spirituality has a broad range of meanings and associations. For some people, spirituality is synonymous with formal religious belief and practice. Yet within nursing, spirituality is concerned with a wide range of meanings, including relationships and connection with the environment. Narayanasamy (2001: 3) provides a useful list of descriptions that people connect with spirituality (**Box 8.3**), some of which may be reflected in your own understanding of the concept.

Box 8.3 Descriptions connected with spirituality (Narayanasamy, 2001)

- Beliefs affecting one's life and how it relates to others
- Something not necessarily religious
- A source of strength
- At peace with oneself
- Inner peace
- A feeling of security
- Love and to be loved
- Self-esteem
- Inner self
- Inner strength
- Searching
- Coping
- Hope and security
- Trusting relationship
- Connectedness

> 'I have not a clue. I really don't know what it means. To me, it is just about religion. I don't know how you describe it, quite honestly. That's why, when you rung up, I thought to myself "I don't know what I am going to say to you", because I don't know what it means.'
> **Female orthopaedic patient**

> 'Never has interested me. Even in illness, it's never interested me has religion. It has done nothing for me.'
> **Male patient, palliative care**

> 'I think it's different to every person. To me, spirituality is what makes me feel—what makes me! The emotional side, the essence of living! It makes somebody feel whole. It's the sparkle. Yeah—it's just je ne sais quoi! I don't know?'
> **Senior nurse, palliative care**

> 'Spirituality... I think it is personal. It depends on what the individual believes. For example, my mother believe spirituality to be psychic, ghosts, and people coming back from the dead. Whereas I think it to be what religion you believe in—your own aspects towards God or however it is that you worship.'
> **Nurse manager, acute care**

> 'My current understanding is that it's threefold! The meaning purpose aspect, which is most often talked about, is only part of spirituality and I would say that equally at least of relationships, and I still struggle to find the right word. A sense of transcendence, awe, wonder, mystery are also important parts of spirituality and spiritual care.'
> **Chaplain, palliative care**

> 'I knew it was about finding meaning in life, whatever that might be—feeling a sense of purpose—and almost like that for me, life is about finding a sense of purpose and meaning, and doing what feels right—what feels your life purpose or path. For me, if I've been doing that, then my life feels more comfortable. If I've been fighting against it, then it's not!'
> **Physiotherapist, palliative care**

Figure 8.2 Healthcare professionals' and patients' understandings of spirituality (adapted from McSherry, 2004; 2007).

This list of items reveals that spirituality is an elastic concept (Paley, 2008) and that it is much broader than a religious belief. Yet, for some people, their spirituality will be inextricably linked with a religious belief and practice. From this section, it should be apparent that spirituality is something fundamental to our human existence—at the core of one's existence—enabling people to discover meaning, purpose, and fulfilment in life. If nursing accepts this premise, then spirituality is central to and crucial to nursing care.

Historical aspects of spirituality

Historical nursing has always had a rich religious and spiritual heritage that seems to have been discarded within contemporary health care in favour of more scientific models of care delivery. Some nursing writers, such as Bradshaw (1994) and Narayanasamy (1999), have described how nursing emerged out of religious traditions. McSherry (2001: 108) underlines this rich religious and spiritual heritage, writing:

> **These communities of priests, monks and brothers sanctified their own souls in works of mercy by sacrificing themselves through caring for the sick, dying and destitute ... The spiritual was not divorced or viewed in isolation, from other dimensions of the person.**

This quotation demonstrates that, historically, nursing, caring, and spirituality were integrated and not separate entities. It also implies that, at some point in the evolution of nursing, there has been an erosion of the spiritual values and principles that were once fundamental to the role of the nurse.

Your reflections may have revealed that nursing is no longer associated or aligned with religious institutions or organizations, and that much of nursing is now carried out in publicly funded and predominantly secular institutions, such as the NHS. Indeed, the National Secular Society argues that publically funded institutions such the NHS should not provide religious and spiritual support (chaplaincy departments) to patients and staff (National Secular Society, 2009). Another argument is that society has changed, and that the role and place of religion has declined, meaning that many people now do not hold or practice a formal religious belief or faith.

Nursing has evolved over the past two decades and it could be argued there has been an adoption of the medical model. The dominance of a medical model of care may have eroded the artistic aspects of nursing, such as caring, compassion, and spiritual dimensions, with greater focus on the scientific and the technical. It is sad when nurses are being accused of not caring. When the Patients Association (2009) published its report *Patients ... not Numbers, People ... not Statistics*, Claire Rayner stated in a Foreword:

> **For too long now, the Patients Association has been receiving calls ... from people wanting to talk about the dreadful, neglectful, demeaning, painful and sometimes downright cruel treatment their elderly relatives had experienced at the hands of NHS nurses.**   (ibid: 3)

The factors that have led to some patients experiencing less-than-dignified nursing care are complex, but perhaps one explanation or contributory factor may be the loss of all of the humanistic elements of care to which spirituality is central.

Providing holistic and spiritual care

Having identified that individuals are composed of different dimensions and that we are all unique, possessing assorted beliefs and values, we now need to explore the practicalities of providing holistic care. The concept of holistic care was first introduced in Chapter 4; this section will develop this further in relation to spirituality. Holistic care is not something new: it has been promoted in nursing for almost two decades to combat the medical model of care. Figure 4.1 in Chapter 4 presented one model of holistic care. If you look again at the pie chart, the four dimensions are equal and of the same value—which raises several key issues:

- can the whole person be divided into four distinct parts?
- do the four parts have equal weighting?
- does this diagram actually represent holistic care?

Nurses are extremely proficient in addressing and meeting the physical, psychological, and social needs of their patients. You may have already discussed the provision of holistic care with your mentors or supervisors. Parts of the dimensions, such as meeting physical needs, are clearly visible—for example, undertaking patient assessments, monitoring clinical signs and symptoms, and the provision of direct care such as assisting with washing and dressing. Nursing theorists such as Roper et al. (1996) describe this as supporting patients to meet their activities of daily living (ADLs). There are some areas of care that are hidden, but again may be observed, such as supporting patients with their social needs and involving families/carers in patient care. However, aspects of holistic care that nurses still feel uncomfortable exploring, such as spiritual needs, sexuality, and death and dying, are often avoided. These have been described as the 'last taboos' of nursing because there is still a great deal of misconception and anxiety surrounding them. If nurses are to provide holistic care in its truest sense, then they must engage with all of these taboo subjects, since they are all important aspects of individualized and person-centred care. 'Person-centred' means that any plan of care developed is done so with the full cooperation, consent, and involvement of the patient. In this way, patients/clients are involved in decisions about their care and can feel empowered. Yet, in some situations, this may not always be possible, for example when dealing with a person with profound learning disability or nursing the unconscious patient. In these situations, the care is usually planned with the involvement of the person's immediate next of kin or primary carer.

....

One of the activities that we use when teaching nurses about holistic care is to ask them to draw a diagram or symbol that sums up their understanding of the concept.
We would now like you to undertake this activity using a blank sheet of paper.

....

In response to the activity above and without exception, students start to gesture with their hands by drawing a circle. They also tell us that they use a circle because this represents the 'whole' person. Using students' diagrams enables a further critique of the common representation of holistic practice outlined in Figure 4.1: dividing the person into four equal parts, or functional units, that can be managed—or even prioritized—does not address the 'whole'. However, this is not to say that this approach is wrong or unnecessary: by focusing on the different parts, we are able to gain an understanding of the different dimensions of a person and what importance each of the dimensions plays in a person's life. Considering the different parts helps us in our understanding of the 'whole'. This is especially important in nursing: for example, when admitting a patient, a thorough nursing assessment is undertaken of their physical, social, psychological, and spiritual needs, which should include whether a person has any specific religious needs. This helps the nurse to gain an understanding of how the patient's illness or condition may impact on their life or to identify what support is required.

Reductionism

By looking only at individual dimensions, we could say that the person has been 'fragmented' or 'broken'—that is, 'reduced' into separate parts. This approach is known as 'reductionism'. The danger with a purely reductionist model is that you do not gain a sense of how all of the parts of a person are interrelated and connected. Furthermore, within nursing, the emphasis in the past has been on the physical and biological parts at the expense of all of the others.

....

We would like you to look again at Figure 4.1 and compare it to Figure 8.3.
Do you think that Figure 8.3 offers a better approach to looking at individuals?

....

The broken lines in Figure 8.3 indicate that all of the different dimensions are interconnected. The fact that spirituality is at the centre reflects some of the definitions of spirituality earlier outlined in Box 8.1, in which health professionals and patients suggest that spirituality is concerned with a broad range of issues. This model of holistic care can accommodate a diverse view of spirituality. The diagram emphasizes that all of the parts are important and related to each other, and that no part is superior to another, because they are all of equal importance.

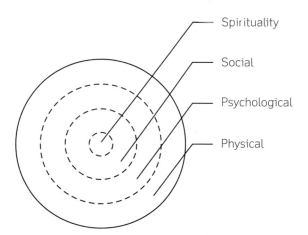

Figure 8.3 An alternative representation of holistic care.

Integrated care

Figure 8.3 can also support the theory of integrated care, which implies that nurses do not only focus on one aspect of care, for example when carrying out personal care with a patient. The nurse, while assisting the patient, enters into a dialogue and, through the qualities displayed and the communication used, is supporting the patient at a number of levels, including physical, psychological, and spiritual.

Spiritual needs

Having explored the meaning of spirituality within the context of holistic or integrated care, there is now a need to explore what is meant by the term 'spiritual needs'. If we subscribe to the belief that there is such a thing as spirituality, then a logical extension of this argument is that we all possess spiritual needs. Think about this as you read **Practice Example 8.1**.

The nursing literature suggests that there are different views regarding what constitutes spiritual needs. Shelly and Fish (1988) suggest that there are three 'basic' spiritual needs: the need to find meaning, purpose, and fulfilment (known as 'existentialism'); the need for love and relatedness; and a need for forgiveness. Narayanasamy (2001: 28) has developed a concept of spiritual needs that includes:

- meaning and purpose in life;
- love and harmonious relationships;
- forgiveness;
- a source of hope and strength;
- trust;
- expression of personal beliefs and values; and
- spiritual practices, expression of a concept of God or a deity, and creativity.

You may want to read Practice Example 8.1 again, reflecting upon the meaning of each of these spiritual needs and identifying which ones are relevant to this situation.

For a more detailed discussion on the concept of spiritual needs, read ch. 3 'Spiritual needs' in Narayanasamy (2001)

John was feeling vulnerable, isolated, and disconnected from his family. He felt alone and may even have felt imprisoned in the unit. The nurse in this interaction treated John as a human being, not only as a young man with a label of 'cancer' or 'leukaemia'. The nurse acknowledged John has a human being, and was trying to alleviate his isolation and need for human contact. Through these acts of caring, a sense of trust developed between John and his carer. The nurse did not do anything extraordinary, but supported John physically, psychologically, spiritually, and socially through the appropriate use of touch. This case study emphasizes the idea of integrated care. The nurse did not say to John: 'Would you like me to support you with your spiritual needs?' The care that she provided was integrated and 'whole', and through fundamental nursing care, and the skills and the qualities that the nurse displayed and used—such as empathy, compassion, kindness, and concern—she supported John both emotionally and spiritually.

PRACTICE EXAMPLE 8.1

Identifying spiritual needs (Anderson and Steen, 1995: 15)

John, a hospitalized 18-year-old, was dying of leukemia. John's family visited infrequently. The first day that John's nurse cared for him, she noticed how depressed and hopeless he seemed. During a quiet moment one afternoon, she asked John if he would like her to rub his back. John readily accepted and stated that she was the first person who had touched him since he had been in the hospital. John had been on the unit for one month and felt totally isolated from people. Through touch, the nurse reached out and comforted John.

What do you think that John's spiritual needs might be?

What are the key lessons that, as healthcare professionals working with vulnerable patients/clients, we can learn from this example?

> **PRACTICE TIP**
>
> Spiritual care may not necessarily be different from fundamental care. A patient, when asked the question, 'Do nurses meet your spiritual needs?' gave the following response: 'Yes—but they don't know that they are doing it' (McSherry, 2004; 2007). This simple illustration indicates that spiritual care may be a hidden and not explicit dimension, because it is often intuitive and integral within the caring relationship.

The danger is that by focusing specifically on spiritual care, nurses may feel that spiritual aspects of care are something separate from and alien to the nursing and caring relationship, rather than a fundamental component of nursing. Nevertheless, if too much emphasis is placed on the term 'spiritual care', nurses may feel that they do not have the skills and knowledge to support individuals with this aspect of nursing care when, in reality, they are probably supporting patients all of the time in this area.

Challenges to promoting spiritual care

Nurses may encounter a range of challenges when attempting to meet individuals' spiritual needs.

Before proceeding, you may want to reflect on the information that you have read so far in this chapter and answer the following question.
What do you believe are the challenges to the delivery of spiritual care?

There are a range of factors that create and present challenges to the delivery of spiritual care. These challenges were identified by nurses as part of a research study exploring nurses' perceptions of spirituality and spiritual care (McSherry, 1997).

- *Physical limitations*—in the sense of a loss of ability to communicate
- *Environmental constraints*—for example, lack of privacy and quiet rooms, and hidden taboos and cultures that operate within professional and health service organizations
- *Psychological*—for example, anxieties, insecurities, and fears of healthcare professionals relating to the concept of spirituality; people suffering from dementia
- *Economic*—perceptions relating to staff not having enough time or money for resources to deliver spiritual care
- *Knowledge and skills*—lack of education about spirituality and spiritual care, and limited focus on developing healthcare professionals' skills in relation to delivering competent spiritual care

These challenges suggest that the barriers to providing spiritual care can often be complex and sometimes are outside the nurse's power or control. However, it must be highlighted that, in order to meet and support patients' spiritual needs, nurses do not need a Master's degree in counselling or need to be experts in this area. On the contrary, the following are all that we feel nurses require to support patients in this area.

- *Self-awareness*—the ability to reflect upon ourselves, identifying our own personal and unique spirituality
- *Interpersonal skills*—the ability to relate confidently to individuals
- *Trust-building skills*—the ability to establish a rapport and therapeutic relationship with patients
- *Non-judgement*—the ability to be accepting and tolerant, acknowledging that we are all unique
- *Prioritization and management of care*—an awareness of own limitations and an ability to identify the need for appropriate referral
- *Education*—we need to develop our knowledge and understanding of the concept of spirituality

This list suggests that providing spiritual care is about self-awareness and knowing what your own personal beliefs, values, and attitudes are with regards spirituality. This level of awareness will enable you to be sensitive to the needs of others, who are perhaps feeling vulnerable. The provision of good nursing care stems from knowing your own personal strengths; where you feel there is a limitation in your knowledge, expertise, or practice, you should make appropriate referral (with the consent of the individual), so that the patient is adequately supported. This may, for example, mean liaising with a patient's own religious or spiritual leader, making a referral to the hospital chaplaincy team, or using other counselling and support services.

Relationship between the personal and professional

In 2008, Caroline Petrie, a community staff nurse, was suspended from duty because it was suspected by her employers that she had breached the nursing code of conduct.

Read the outline of her case presented in **Practice Example 8.2**.

Caroline Petrie's case highlights several important points about the relationship between personal beliefs and values, and how these may impinge on nursing practice. Irrespective of what one thinks of this case, it does raise the important issues of self-awareness and the need not to impose one's own personal beliefs and values on to other people, however well intentioned this may be. The Department of Health practice guidance on religion states:

> **Members of some religions, including Mormons, Jehovah's Witnesses, evangelical Christians and Muslims, are expected to preach and to try to convert other people. In a workplace environment this can cause many problems, as non-religious people and those from other religions or beliefs could feel harassed and intimidated by this behaviour. This is especially the case when particular views on matters such as sexual orientation, gender and single parents are aired in a workplace environment, potentially causing great offence to other workers or indeed patients or visitors who are within hearing.**
>
> (Department of Health, 2009b: 22)

An area of anxiety for nurses relates to praying for or with a patient. We are not saying that it is always 'wrong' to pray with or for a patient—but this is a very sensitive and contentious area. The advice or guidance

---

PRACTICE EXAMPLE 8.2

Personal and professional beliefs: an outline of the Caroline Petrie case

Caroline Petrie, an evangelical Christian, was suspended from duties as a community nurse in December 2008 after asking an elderly patient if she wanted her to pray for her. Although the patient was not offended, she was 'taken aback' by the suggestion and reported the comment to her carer. Caroline Petrie was subsequently suspended on suspicion of failing to *'demonstrate a personal and professional commitment to equality and diversity'*, while the hospital investigated. She was subjected to a disciplinary hearing.

When interviewed, Caroline Petrie stated: *'I'm happy to pray for anybody. I think the issue is* [the patient] *felt possibly there may be somebody who might be* *offended by the question of somebody saying would you like prayer.'*

When asked if she would do it again, Caroline Petrie replied: *'Yes.'* She added: *'I cannot divide my faith from my nursing care; I have to be the person I want to be.'*

Caroline Petrie was reinstated and the trust recognized the fact that Caroline Petrie felt that she was acting in the 'best interests' of her patients.

(Gledhill, 2009)

1 Having reflected on the drivers influencing the need to integrate spiritual care into everyday nursing practice, do you feel that Caroline Petrie should have been suspended?

2 What is your view of the response of the primary care trust?

should always be to take the lead from the patient. The question that must always be asked is: is consent freely given? If consent is freely given by the patient and a nurse feels comfortable in praying with a patient at their request, then there should not be a problem.

Conclusion

Although there is a drive to ensure that spiritual care is an integral part of nursing and health care, there are a range of challenges to ensuring that the spiritual needs of patients are viewed as an ongoing and essential component of care. The idea of providing holistic care and supporting patients with their spiritual needs is clearly presented by the NMC (2004) as a standard of proficiency.

....

Read Box 8.4 and reflect upon this standard of proficiency and consider the following two questions,
Do you feel able to implement and achieve this standard of proficiency in your nursing practice?
If you feel unable to achieve this standard of proficiency, why do you think that is the case?
....

Contemporary nursing is being challenged by several organizations for a perceived lack of care, accusing nurses of cruelty and neglect, and suggesting that nursing has lost its core values and founding principles of care and caring (The Patient Association, 2009). One explanation may be that nurses are now undertak-

ing roles and duties once undertaken by doctors, and that direct nursing care has been undermined and devalued. Whatever the cause, there is a need for nursing to evaluate and redress some of these allegations, so that the patient is once again at the centre of care delivery. A report entitled *Front Line Care recommends that 'Nurses and midwives must renew their pledge to society and service users to tackle unacceptable variations in standards and deliver high quality, compassionate care'* (Prime Minister's Commission on the Future of Nursing and Midwifery in England, 2010: 5). This surely includes attending to the spiritual needs of patients/clients in receipt of nursing care across the full spectrum of sectors and organizations.

To summarize, this chapter describes the terms 'spirituality' and 'spiritual care', examining the relevance of these concepts within nursing. Societies for which nursing and healthcare services provide are increasingly diverse and multi-ethnic. Therefore, nurses must not only recognize and respect the cultures, spiritual, and religious beliefs, and individuality of their patients and families, but also incorporate and address these beliefs within the course of their nursing practice.

Having worked through the activities within this chapter, you should have concluded that there is no authoritative definition of the term 'spirituality' and that the delivery of spiritual care is complex. Part of the complexity of delivering spiritual care relates to its subjectivity, with nurses and the public whom they serve each having their own interpretations and understanding of the term. It should be clear that spirituality is not necessarily associated with institutional religion, although for some individuals spirituality and religion are intrinsically linked. Spirituality consists of many components.

The provision of spiritual care is central to the notion of holistic practice and embedded in government legislation, policy guidance, and professional codes of practice. Nurses must value the uniqueness of their patients and treat them with respect and dignity. Therefore, ensuring that the spiritual needs of patients are met and incorporating spiritual care into everyday practice is not only desirable, but also a requirement. The provision of spiritual care requires healthcare professionals to have the knowledge and

Box 8.4 NMC Standards for Pre-Registration (NMC, 2010)

Domain 3: Nursing practice and decision-making
3 All nurses must carry out comprehensive, systematic nursing assessments that take account of relevant physical, social, cultural, psychological, spiritual, genetic and environmental factors, in partnership with service users and others through interaction, observation and measurement.
(NMC, 2010: 18)

awareness of the issues relating to spirituality, and of the drivers and challenges to implementing spiritual care. Many nurses already possess many of the skills required to take the initiative in dealing with spiritual issues. These skills can be enhanced by additional education relating to spiritual care, which must include providing nurses with the confidence to meet the spiritual needs of their patients and to challenge practices that may be discriminatory and not patient-centred.

Further reading

Narayanasamy, A. (2001) 'Spiritual needs', ch. 3 in *Spiritual Care: A Practical Guide for Nurses and Health Care Practitioners,* 2nd edn, Dinton: Quay Books, pp. 25–35

References

Anderson, B. and Steen, S. (1995) 'Spiritual care reflecting God's love to children', *Journal of Christian Nursing* 12(2): 12–17, 47.

Bradshaw, A. (1994) *Lighting the Lamp: The Spiritual Dimension of Nursing Care*, London: Scutaria Press.

Clarke, J. (2009) 'A critical view of how nursing has defined spirituality', *Journal of Clinical Nursing* 18: 1666–73.

Department of Health (2000) *The NHS Plan: A Plan for Investment, a Plan for Reform*, London: HMSO.

Department of Health (2001) *Patient's Charter: Your Guide to the NHS*, London: HMSO.

Department of Health (2004) *The NHS Improvement Plan: Putting People at the Heart of Public Services*, London: HMSO.

Department of Health (2009a) *The NHS Constitution: The NHS Belongs to Us All*, London: HMSO.

Department of Health (2009b) *Religion or Belief: A Practical Guide for NHS Staff*, London: HMSO.

Gerrish, K. (2000) 'Individualised care: Its conceptualisation and practice within a multiethnic society', *Journal of Advanced Nursing* 32(1): 91–9.

Gledhill, R. (2009) 'Victory for suspended Christian nurse', *The Times*, 7 February, available online at **http://www. timesonline.co.uk/tol/comment/faith/article5675452. ece** [accessed 16 June 2011].

International Council of Nurses (2006) *The ICN Code of Ethics for Nurses*, Geneva: ICN.

Koenig, H.G., McCullough M.E., and Larson D.B. (2001) *Handbook of Religion and Health*, Oxford: Oxford University Press.

McSherry, W. (1997) 'A descriptive survey of nurses' perceptions of spirituality and spiritual care', Unpublished PhD thesis, University of Hull.

McSherry, W. (2001) 'Spiritual crisis? Call a nurse', in H. Orchard (ed) *Spirituality in Health Care Contexts*, London: Jessica Kingsley, pp. 107–17.

McSherry, W. (2004) 'The meaning of spirituality and spiritual care: An investigation of health care professionals', patients' and publics' perceptions', Unpublished PhD thesis, Leeds Metropolitan University.

McSherry, W. (2006) *Making Sense of Spirituality in Nursing and Health Care Practice: An Interactive Approach*, 2nd edn, London: Jessica Kingsley.

McSherry, W. (2007) *The Meaning of Spirituality and Spiritual Care within Nursing and Health Care Practice*, Dinton: Quay Books.

Murray, R.B. and Zentner J.B. (1989) *Nursing Concepts for Health Promotion*, London: Prentice Hall.

Narayanasamy, A. (1999) 'Learning spiritual dimensions of care from a historical perspective', *Nurse Education Today* 19: 386–95.

Narayanasamy, A. (2001) *Spiritual Care: A Practical Guide for Nurses and Health Care Practitioners*, 2nd edn, Dinton: Quay Books.

National Secular Society (2009) *An Investigation into the Cost of the National Health Service's Chaplaincy Provision*, available online at **http://www.secularism.org.uk/uploads/ 3549db17aa47a28474059911.pdf** [accessed 29 June 2011].

NHS Education for Scotland (2009) *Spiritual Care Matters: An Introductory Resource for all NHS Scotland Staff*, Edinburgh: NHS Education for Scotland.

Nursing and Midwifery Council (2004) *Standards of Proficiency for Pre-Registration Nursing Education*, London: NMC.

Nursing and Midwifery Council (2008) *The Code*, London: NMC.

Nursing and Midwifery Council (2010) *Standards for Pre-Registration Nursing Education*. London: NMC.

Paley, J. (2008) 'Spirituality and nursing: A reductionist approach', *Nursing Philosophy* 9: 3–18.

Patients Association, The (2009) *Patients ... not Numbers, People ... not Statistics*, available online at

http://www.patients-association.com/DBIMGS/file/
Patients%20not%20numbers,%20people%20not%20
statistics.pdf [accessed 16 June 2011].

Prime Minister's Commission on the Future of Nursing
in England and Wales (2010) *Front Line Care*, available
online at http://www.nhshistory.net/
nursing%20commission.pdf [accessed 29 June 2011].

Reilly, D. (2005) 'Foreword', in S.G. Wright, *Reflections on
Spirituality and Health*. London: Whurr, pp. ix–xii.

Roper, N., Logan, W., and Tierney, A. (1996) *The Elements
of Nursing: A Model for Nursing Based on a Model of Living*,
4th edn, Edinburgh: Churchill Livingstone.

Royal College of Nursing (2003) *Defining Nursing*,
London: RCN.

Shelly, J.A. and Fish, S. (1988) *Spiritual Care: The Nurse's
Role*, 3rd edn, Westmont, IL: Inter Varsity Press.

Vydelingum, V. (2000) 'South Asian patients' lived
experience of acute care in an English hospital: A phenomenological study', *Journal of Advanced Nursing* 32(1): 100–7.

World Health Organization (1998) *WHOQoL and Spirituality, Religiousness and Personal Beliefs: Report on WHO
Consultation*, Geneva: WHO.

Wright, S.G. (2005) *Reflections on Spirituality and Health*.
London: Whurr.

Part 3: Contexts of care

9 Communicating care

CATHERINE McCABE AND FIONA TIMMINS

Learning outcomes

This chapter will enable you to:

- understand what is meant by 'communication' and 'communicating care';
- reflect on the key dimensions of communication in the context of care;
- explore models of communication; and
- appreciate the importance of communication in nursing.

Introduction

It is clear from the preceding chapters that caring in the healthcare context is a complex concept with many facets to consider in terms of recognizing what constitutes good care. In nursing, we deliver care using innate and/or learned communication behaviours. The communication skills or behaviours that a nurse chooses to use and the way in which they are used when providing care will dictate whether or not the patient perceives that they are being cared for. This chapter aims to enable you to reflect on approaches to communicating care delivery, explaining how these may help or hinder us in providing personalized care that respects the dignity of each individual. Communication is the foundation stone of all human expression, interaction, and relationships. It is the medium through which we experience our lives and express our values and beliefs about the world to others. This chapter explores how nurses use personal and professional communication skills to communicate care to patients.

We encourage you to reflect on clinical situations and, in turn, help you to reflect positively and constructively on your *own* nursing practice. These reflections will enable you to build up a comprehensive picture of how nursing care can meet the holistic needs of individuals and their families within a diverse society. This chapter builds upon concepts and values discussed in other chapters such as respecting the individual (Chapter 4), diversity in care (Chapter 5), spiritual care (Chapter 8), and partnerships in care (Chapter 11).

The chapter is designed to enable you to feel more confident in communicating care to patients. The content of the chapter will also help you to develop

Essential knowledge and skills for care

- You must recognize that communication is an essential and fundamental component of nursing caring, demonstrating an awareness that all communication in nursing should be focused on the needs of the individual (patient-focused), supporting them with their specific needs.

- You must have a thorough understanding of the wide range of strategies and interventions, including the use of communication technologies, which enable nurses to communicate effectively in diverse situations.

- You must use excellent communication and interpersonal skills in all of your interactions with people, ensuring that your own communications are always safe, effective, compassionate, and respectful.

- When people have a disability, you must be able to work with them and others to obtain the information needed to make reasonable adjustments that promote optimum health and enable equal access to services.

communication skills that support the five caring attributes that are further discussed in Chapter 4—that is, self-awareness, respecting differences in individuals, listening and attending, and recognizing one's own limitations and acknowledging the need for referrals.

Theorists and the nature of care and caring

Many theorists explore the nature of care and caring, (Warelow, 1996; Boykin and Schoenhofer, 2001; Watson, 2005; Warelow and Edward, 2007) and concur that it is human nature to care for others. Furthermore, in a profession such as nursing, caring is grounded in a human endeavour that uses specific knowledge and skills, based on an appreciation of individuality, to care for people. Warelow et al. (2008) conclude that caring is the fundamental, identifying component of the nursing profession and should be encouraged, supported, and facilitated in and through communication actions and behaviours at all levels of nursing. However, theories and conceptual models of nursing that incorporate caring as a key component, such as that outlined by Watson (2005), are not in widespread use in clinical practice. Furthermore, there is ongoing debate and discussion as to the overall usefulness of using conceptual models of nursing, particularly in light of new ways of planning and delivering care such as care pathways. Therefore it would be wrong to assume that all nursing practice is based on caring theory; rather, it is accepted, from both theoretical and historical perspectives, that caring is a core component of what nurses do.

Thus, having accepted caring as a core competency in nursing, this chapter aims to unpack one key component of all caring behaviours: communication. Communication is an essential and fundamental component of caring. Communication in nursing is said to be either focused on the *tasks* of nursing (nursing-focused) or concerned with the centrality of the patient within all elements of healthcare delivery (patient-focused) (Morse et al., 1992). Ultimately, *patient-focused* communication is that which is most likely to yield positive results in terms of achieving an outcome of communication and improving the patient experience (McCabe and Timmins, 2006). It is also the most likely communication to be considered as caring by the patient.

Consider **Practice Example 9.1**.

Practice Example 9.1 gives you an example of nurse-focused communication. All communications related only to the tasks at hand, and did not really consider you as a person. You may have noted that you felt very depersonalized and unimportant in the busy hospital schedule. Or you may not have been too concerned about this, instead feeling pleased that all of the necessary tasks were completed efficiently: after all, correct surgical intervention with no complications was your main aim.

....

Think for a moment whether there could be any negative effects of this type of communication.
....

You may have said that this type of communication does not show caring and this is a correct assumption.

PRACTICE EXAMPLE 9.1

A patient in hospital

You are a patient in hospital. You are admitted as a day case for surgical removal of two of your wisdom teeth and you are about to undergo a general anesthetic for the procedure. You become aware, during your admission, that while all relevant practical elements of your treatment seem to be delivered with efficiency, no one has really taken the time to call you by your name, introduced themselves, or addressed you in any personal way. You feel very much like a 'patient'. All relevant checks, observations, and preparations are carried out, but when you arrive in theatre with the attendant and the nurse the theatre staff asks your accompanying nurse, rather than you: 'Is this the wisdom tooth?'

Take a moment to consider how you might feel in this situation.

Although patients will desire optimal treatment within healthcare settings, they also find that positive nurse–patient interaction enhances their journeys. They feel less anxious and also are less likely to take on the powerless patient persona. This powerlessness, although not always obvious, can lead to lack of confidence about personal health care and health promotion, or even about decisions in health care.

Of course, we are focusing our discussion in this chapter primarily on the patient, to demonstrate and explain core elements of communicating care. Our suggestions and advice about communication relate equally to patients' families who engage with the health service. The level and extent of family involvement in nursing varies according to the specific facility and the healthcare needs of the patient. Within children's nursing, for example, parents and guardians may be active participants in all elements of the child's care and thus, in this situation, the term patient-focused communication may be replaced with *family-focused* communication. A patient's family may be less involved in other services, for example when a young adult is admitted to day surgery, except perhaps to deliver and collect.

It might be useful to look again at Practice Example 9.1 and for you to reflect as if you were a nurse caring for a patient admitted for the same procedure. You are probably familiar within your educational programme with using a framework for reflection on practice. To facilitate your reflection on this scenario, you are invited to use Gibbs's (1988) model of reflection to support your analysis (see **Table 9.1**).

From this scenario, you will have learnt that patient-focused communication is important, but that this type of communication applies equally to key carers and that the same principles apply. Thus, by starting out with a premise that your communication must be patient-centred, you are already beginning to demonstrate care.

Defining caring and communication

Caring

Care is the ultimate goal of nursing (Gamez, 2009). Caring in the context of communication in nursing is concerned with being an authentic human within the

Table 9.1 Suggested stages of Gibbs's model of reflection (Gibbs, 1988)

Stage	Action
1	Describe what happened (in the above scenario).
2	How does it make you feel (as a nurse)?
3	Evaluate this situation. (What sense can you make of it? Why do you think it happened or could happen?)
4	Analyse the situation. (For example, what key components of communicating care are missing? Why did it turn out as it did?)
5	Conclude this situation. (Summarize what happened and why. Identify the key elements within the interaction.)
6	Action plan. (What would you do differently in this situation or in your future practice to prevent this situation occurring?)

nurse–patient relationship. Milton (2008: 20) describes this as '*human becoming: a special way of being in the nurse–patient relationship*'. This involves being with the patient, listening, and also being oneself. Caring means retaining the centrality and importance of communication in an increasingly technological healthcare environment (Loscin, 2006). Being with the patient and interacting with them becomes increasingly important as technologies and interventions become increasingly 'dehumanizing' (Parse, 2007: 310).

In nursing, communicating care requires that the individual nurse understands and values human connection as the basis of caring. This connection can only occur in forming and nurturing positive relationships with patients (Warelow et al., 2008) and will be evident in whether the patient perceives the nurse as 'genuine'. This is supported in a qualitative study by Kagan (2008) that explored the structure of the lived experience of being listened to. Participants in this study describe feeling listened to as reassuring because 'somebody is paying attention', that person is non-judgemental, and it provides validation for their feelings. Others described the perception of being listened to as a connection with someone and linked this with eye contact.

According to Warelow et al. (2008: 147), '*Caring enables connection within the nurse–patient relationship*'; they suggest that it is this connection that allows a nurse to intuitively discern problems and to jointly find solutions and implement care that is patient-centred. The converse of Warelow et al.'s suggestion is also true: that this connection enables caring and it is perhaps the connection that communicates the caring—in other words, gives the patient the perception that they are being 'cared for'.

Communication

Gamez (2009: 126) suggests that all care in nursing practice recognizes two basic principles: that communication is the 'basic pillar' of relationships, and includes listening, empathy respect, and understandable use of language; and that professional codes of ethics must apply to nurse–patient relationships.

Further to this, communication is a fundamental skill that underpins all nursing practice; indeed, McCamant (2006: 335) suggests that nursing, by its very nature, is a 'lived dialogue' between the nurse and patient. During interviews with nurses who were describing their understandings of caring relationships with patients (Berg et al., 2006: 47), an underlying theme (competence) revealed that the nurse constantly '*observes, creates, and provides opportunities for conversations with … patients*' and that these conversations 'lay the foundation' for the work of the nurse.

Patient-focused communication

Patient-centred communication is defined as '*communication that invites and encourages the patient to participate and negotiate in decision-making regarding their own care*' (Langwitz et al., 1998: 230). Stein-Parbury (2009: 39) describes a '*connected relationship as one in which the nurse and patient become involved to the degree that they perceive each other as people first, and their roles as patient and nurse become secondary*'. The relationship stays within the boundaries of the healthcare and professional context, but it is still personal. Authenticity and integrity are essential characteristics for both the nurse and the patient in order for a positive, connected relationship to develop. This means that if a nurse does not truly regard the patient as an individual who is equal and important, then it is highly likely that the patient will pick this up from how the nurse communicates. Although principally concerned with patients receiving care, these principles of other-centredness and the necessity of identifying the other's needs apply also to patient's families.

The nurse–patient relationship

The nurse–patient relationship is crucial in nursing (Peplau, 1991). Indeed, the very essence of nursing is thought to occur in the interpersonal relationship between the nurses and the patient (Pearson et al., 2000). The interpersonal relationship fosters patient recovery and rehabilitation, but also allows the '*individuals to understand their health problems and to learn from their experience*' (Pearson et al., 2000: 170). This one-to-one approach helps to improve communication, information-giving, and emotional support given by nurses. Although there is a concern that over-involvement at a personal level may occur, there is an emphasis on professional closeness (Stein-Parbury, 2009).

Self-awareness

Self-awareness is as '*a continuous and evolving process of getting to know who you are*' (Burnard, 1997: 25). While humans (as opposed to animals) usually possess awareness of self, this awareness can be explored and developed to improve communication skills (Burnard, 1997). Self-awareness is essential for successful implementation of the nurse–patient relationship (Arnold and Underman-Boggs, 2006).

While authenticity and 'human-ness' are essential elements of modern nursing, these must be acted out within ethical principles (Gamez, 2009). Self-awareness allows you to become aware of elements of your own behaviours that may not be suitable and their effects on others, to uncover your own prejudices, and so on. Without this, there can be communication difficulties (Betts, 2003). For example, your past experiences, attitudes, and responses to specific client populations or circumstances can affect your behaviour and adversely affect the patient.

Respecting differences in individuals

Respecting patients as individuals is very important in nursing practice, and patients often report being treated according to their condition rather than as an individual, with individual needs (McCabe and Timmins, 2006). In contrast to this, public health policy in the UK clearly emphasizes a person-centred approach to patient care, and many health promotion and educational interventions are now espoused to be based upon individual preferences and needs (Department of Health, 2004; 2007). While the scope of this discussion is too broad for this chapter, it is the context of communication using an approach that is patient-centred and focused on individuals that will ensure that individual differences are respected.

Listening and attending

Listening involves both hearing and internalizing what has been said by another. Effective listening involves '*the active process of taking in, absorbing and eventually understanding what is being expressed*' (Stein-Parbury, 2009: 111); it requires both energy and concentration (ibid). Attending, on the other hand, is the '*outward, physical manifestation of a nurse's readiness to listen*' (ibid: 119). Attending behaviours let the patient know that the nurse is really paying attention and attaching significance to the conversation.

The importance of listening to patients is highlighted in Kagan's (2008) study whereby one participant described the feeling of being listened to as '*an uplifting exploration escalating like a spiralling energy. It is healing and gives a sense of well-being and completeness*'. They also provide a very apt definition of being listened to:

> **[It] is just being with interested people in the quietness of nonjudgmental acceptance. It is a gratifying connection of understanding and intimate sharing during the back and forth exchange between people. It is freedom to express oneself that flows when barriers do not occur.** **(Kagan, 2008: 61)**

Knowing one's own limitations

Knowing one's own limitations transcends many areas of nursing practice and is one of the five caring attributes discussed in relation to other elements of care in other chapters. In relation to communication and communicating care, knowing one's own limitations is linked to self-awareness. As a nurse, building up self-awareness helps you to question your own assumptions. If you find, through this awareness, that you do not have sufficient communication skills to carry on with a patient interaction, you will have to acknowledge your own limitations. This is particularly important when you are still a nursing student, because, in learning situations, you will not always have the answers.

Knowing your limitations also refers to remaining professional in the nurse–patient relationship. This does not mean maintaining a distant aloof stance, but rather not burdening patients with superfluous personal information (Stein-Parbury, 2009). While, at the same time, selective disclosure (perhaps to empathize with a patient) may be relevant and professional discretion is required, you may need to recognize your own limitations if, for example, you have had recent personal experience of an event, similar to that of a patient, and you feel unable to maintain focus on the patient's experiences rather than your own.

Acknowledging the need for referrals

Acknowledging the need for referrals is also linked to self-awareness. Awareness of one's own knowledge and skills and scope of practice, relative to the grade in which you are working, will enable you to refer patients to other colleagues should it be warranted. This happens ordinarily, for example, when requesting advice from the multidisciplinary team. However, even within communication interactions, it is important to realize that you may seek advice from or refer a patient directly to a nurse colleague (for example, you may find dealing with the patient difficult, be too close emotionally to the issue, or simply lack the particular knowledge or skills required to deal with the situation).

Theory, rationale, and evidence base

There are many models that illustrate the components of communication and the factors that influence how we communicate. These include Berlo's (1960) very simple model, which suggests that communication consists of a sender, a message, and a recipient. Nurses often use this linear model of one-way communication when caring for patients. While it does, to some extent, explain elements of communication, it is very restricting.

Nurses confined to this simplistic level of communication may profess to be too busy to deal with the unexpected and possibly difficult concerns that patients may have, or they may also feel that they just do not have the time actually to listen. One-way communication allows nurses to control the interaction and when nurses feel that they have a lot of work to do or tasks to complete, this is a useful way of communicating. This results in nurse-centred communication, and may occur not only due to the use of this linear model of communication, but also due to professional distancing—that is, deliberate detachment from the human interactions required in nursing (Kirkham et al., 2002).

The consequence of this type of communication is that the patient is not recognized as the centre of care, but rather the nurses' need to complete the task takes precedence over the needs of the patient. Interestingly, a change towards patient-centred communication does not necessarily take up more of the nurses' time; rather, it is simply portrayed by nurses in the words and body language that they choose to use when approaching patients. This notion and its relationship to the concept of patient-centred communication forms the basis of Morse et al.'s (1997) model and will be discussed in greater detail.

Comforting interaction–relationship model

The 'comforting interaction–relationship model' (Morse et al., 1997) comprises three components, which include nursing actions, patient actions, and the evolving relationship. Nursing actions refers to comfort strategies, styles of care, and nursing patterns of relating. These three aspects are presented separately in the model, but Morse et al. clearly indicate that the aspects are interrelated. Comfort strategies include communication skills, such as touch and listening, to provide comforting talk for patients. Styles of care refers to the unique patterns of communication or styles of care that a nurse develops when caring for particular types of patient, for example they may speak differently to a person in their 20s compared to an older person.

The third component of nursing actions when caring for patients suggests that these patterns of relating become normative and standardized as a nurse gains experience. Morse et al. (1997) say that these patterns of communication are distinctive nursing behaviours and distinguish nurses from other healthcare professions. This implies that because nursing is a 'caring' profession, patterns of relating are positive and patient-focused; however, this is not always the case, with some patients commenting on feeling 'uncared for' by nurses (McCabe, 2004).

Morse et al. (1997) are somewhat contradictory, although quite correct, in indicating that the development of these patterns of behaviour is influenced by how nurses are socialized, and that this is primarily driven by the culture and environment of the organization and profession. In an economic climate in which health services are cost-driven by the need for increased efficiency with fewer resources, the completion of nursing tasks may be seen as more valuable than patient-centred care.

Warelow et al. (2008) propose that healthcare systems that are grounded in corporate ideology stem from a society that is organized around economics rather than improved quality of life and health outcomes for patients, and suggest that this is at odds with the aim of nursing to provide quality care. This does not bode well for nurses in modern healthcare systems in which the culture and environment clearly reflect just that. Parse (2007) expresses concern that future healthcare planning based on such ideologies will not be concerned with human dignity and quality of life.

It is clear that working in such cultures will increase pressure on nursing to retain and continue to provide quality care. There is, however, another factor that is equally influential in the provision of quality nursing care and that is the individual nurse. Morse et al. (1997), in their comforting interaction–relationship model, suggest that patients also exhibit patterns of relating and that the nature of these depend on how nurses respond to their distress, discomfort, and patterns of relating, and whether, on the basis of this, they perceive the nurse as a caring person and trustworthy.

Fosbinder (1994) and Morse et al. (1992; 1997) both provide somewhat dated, but nonetheless pertinent, accounts of behaviours that can communicate care. Fosbinder's (1994) study identified information-giving, explaining, being friendly, humour, trust, and 'going the extra mile' as being key communication behaviours that patients described when they perceived that a nurse was caring. The last point about 'going the extra mile'

relates to patients perceiving that the nurse did more for them than their role required and did those things in an informal way. This suggests that boundaries were crossed—but perhaps it is just the way a nurse communicates that can make a patient perceive this.

To explain fully why patients perceived that nurses went the 'extra mile', it would be necessary to interview the nurses involved in these interactions. It is possible that patients' perceptions that nurses went 'the extra mile' stemmed from the way in which they communicated and the subsequent trusting relationship that they developed with the nurses rather than the nurse 'doing' anything beyond their role. McCabe's (2004) study on patients' perceptions of nurse–patient communication supports this suggestion by concluding that the quality of the interpersonal interaction is the key to whether the relationship is positive or negative and that the nurse, rather than the patient, is the primary influence on this.

Self-awareness

Self-awareness is also crucial to the nurse–patient relationship and is an essential component to communicating care (Kantcheva and Eckroth-Bucher, 2002). A lack of self-awareness, or self-understanding, can interfere with the nurse–client relationship, because if we do not understand ourselves, then we will find it more difficult to understand others (ibid). Therefore, negative reactions, biases, prejudices, and stereotyping must be recognized and explored through self-awareness.

For suggested reasons for the development of self-awareness in nurses, see **Box 9.1**.

Burnard (1997) proposes a simplistic model of self, suggesting that the self is made up of several

Box 9.1 Reasons for developing self-awareness

- To improve self-understanding
- To facilitate acceptance of self by others
- To develop skills that enable us to deal with difficult situations
- To foster self-regulation and personal autonomy

interrelated aspects of self that come together to form a whole (**Box 9.2**).

Self-awareness requires exploring and becoming acquainted with these various aspects of self. To develop self-awareness, texts such as Burnard (1997) provide a useful resource, with a range of excercises aimed at improving this awareness. Other methods to promote self-awareness include those suggested by the American Society for Training and Development (ASTD, **http://www.astd.org/**). ASTD suggests building personal strength from acknowledging weakness. This can be done by asking others for feedback, and asking someone (with the relevant experience) to be your 'reputable coach' (perhaps your mentor), who would talk you through your strengths and weaknesses. There are also a range of personality tests (such as those found on **http://www.queendom.com/tests**) that can help you to identify your strengths and weaknesses. You might also keep a diary, listing situations that you find challenging or that spark emotional reactions, or simply to journal your thoughts, feelings, and daily events in a way that will help you to get to know yourself more.

Developing self-awareness has many benefits for both your personal and professional life, as outlined in **Box 9.3**. Skills of self-awareness also help you to sustain your energy and resilience, to deal with difficult situations, and to learn from your mistakes (NHS Modernisation Agency Leadership Centre, 2009).

In the National Health Service in the UK, levels of self-awareness have been identified in the context of leadership (NHS Modernisation Agency Leadership Centre, 2005; cited in McCabe and Timmins, 2006).

Box 9.2 Interrelated aspects of self (Burnard, 1997)

- The real self
- The ideal self
- The self-for-others
- The social self
- The spiritual self
- The darker aspect of self
- The physical aspect of self
- The sexual self

Box 9.3 Benefits of developing self-awareness (Burnard, 1997)

Self-awareness helps you to:
- identify your personal strengths and weaknesses;
- identify your learning needs;
- ensure that people feel cared for;
- understand other people's needs;
- learn to help others;
- learn to work with children;
- learn the skills of nursing;
- develop a better understanding of your colleagues;
- get on better with your friends and family; and
- plan your day and your life better.

This provides a useful measure to consider one's own level.

0 Level 0 is the point at which you fail to consider your own emotions: you are not aware of them, do not consider them, and are at times surprised by people's reactions to them.
1 At level 1, you have an awareness of the presence of emotions and when they are present.
2 At level 2, you begin to understand your range of emotions and possible triggers.
3 At level 3, the highest level, you are able to understand the consequences of emotions and are alert to your own limitations.

Peplau's (1952) work was central to the consideration and reconfiguration of the importance of nurses developing a therapeutic relationship with patients. In the past, there has been a tendency towards professional distancing, but this has been replaced by a more patient-centred, humanistic, friendly approach to care (Stein-Parbury, 2009). The aim of nurses using therapeutic communication skills is not to treat or cure a disease or disorder, but to provide a sense of well-being for patients by making them feel relaxed and secure. This helps to establish rapport and trust between the nurse and the patient, and enables the nurse to develop a relationship that is focused and beneficial to both in terms of the achievement of mutually agreed outcomes of care.

Patient-centred communication

If therapeutic communication is about making a patient feel relaxed and secure, then another essential ingredient in establishing a therapeutic relationship is patient-centred communication. McCabe and Timmins (2006) describe this as communication based on an equal partnership between the nurse and patient in terms of identifying patient needs and appropriate care. As discussed earlier, this makes patients feel that they are respected as individuals, that nurses have a genuine concern for their well-being, and that they have control over the care that they receive. The absence of a patient-centred approach to communication will inhibit the development of a therapeutic nurse–patient relationship. The key characteristics of therapeutic nurse–patient communication include a perception of caring, openness, warmth, genuineness, empathy, and purpose on the part of the nurse. For undergraduate nursing students and newly qualified nurses, therapeutic communication may be perceived as a complex and time-consuming process, but it is about communicating understanding and respect to others.

Patient-focused communication behaviours include expressions of pity, sympathy, consolation, commiseration, compassion, and reflexive reassurance. An example of this is where a nurse would put an arm around a patient who has received bad news or is just having a bad day in the way that he or she would with a friend. Other more professional, or learned, patient-focused behaviours refer to humour, reassurance, confronting, comforting, and therapeutic empathy. This includes providing information to reassure a patient, but in a way that demonstrates awareness of their individual needs. Nurse-focused communication behaviours include guarding, shielding, dehumanizing, withdrawing, distancing, labelling, and denying: for example, if a patient seeks information about bad test results and a nurse appears distant and withdrawn, responding that she will get the doctor without engaging on a personal level with the patient's concerns. Interestingly, Morse et al. (1992) also include pity as a nurse-focused communication, along with professional rote behaviours and false reassurance in both categories.

This work has been criticized (Alavi, 2006) because of its implication that nurses control the level of engagement in nurse–patient interactions. Pity as both a patient-focused and nurse-focused communication response appears contradictory, but can be explained by considering the manner in which nurses use this response: for example, a nurse may communicate pity in a way that makes the patient feel that their feelings and emotions are justified, and this can be reassuring. However, if the nurse does not take the time to understand the patient, pity can be patronizing and unhelpful.

Reynolds (2006) also criticizes this work by Morse et al. (1992) because, although he agrees that emotional empathy (sympathy) is valued by patients, he disagrees with their contention that empathy is a concept more suited to clinical psychology than nursing. He devised the 'Reynolds Empathy Scale' for the purpose of measuring what patients want from the nurse–patient relationship (Reynolds, 2000). Two studies that used this scale reported that patients valued active listening, sensitivity, and information (ibid; Forchuk and Reynolds 2001). This may be the case, but it is important for nurses to understand that the way in which they use communication skills and behaviours when caring for patients is not only a professional issue; it is also actually primarily a personal act that is heavily influenced by individual life experiences, values, and beliefs, and is guided by professional boundaries and roles. McCabe and Timmins (2006) integrated elements of these explanatory theories and models, and developed a framework for understanding the communication process within nursing (see **Figure 9.1**).

Communicating care with patients

This section of the chapter will help you understand how you play a key role in communicating care with patients. This will be done through discussion, exercises, and scenarios related to self-awareness, genuineness, respect, and positive regard for others. You will begin to realize that, although you may be

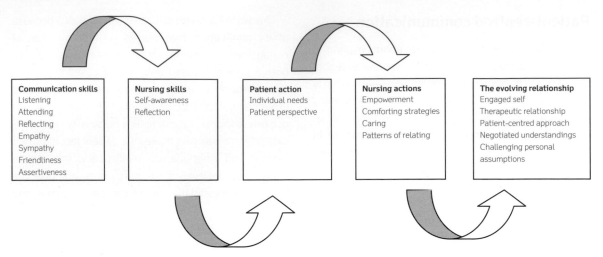

Figure 9.1 Explanatory model of communication in nursing practice. Adapted from McCabe and Timmins 2006 *Communication Skills for Nursing Practice* London: Palgrave Macmillan with permission.

efficient and have an excellent knowledge and ability related to the technical aspects of nursing, without a patient-centred approach to their communication and practice, it will be impossible for you to communicate care to others.

··

Ask yourself the following questions.
Why did I choose to become a nurse?
Do I always value patients as equal and important?
How do I communicate this every day when I am caring for them?

··

Basic communication skills that most people have to a greater or lesser degree include listening, touch, questioning, developing rapport, and non-verbal communication. In nursing, these skills form the basis of how we care for patients. We use these skills to provide reassurance and comfort in such a way that patients perceive that they are equal, respected, and the focus of nurse communication and actions. Listening, which is one of the most important communication skills, is an active process that requires that we give our time, commitment, and complete attention to others. It is physically and emotionally demanding: for example, if you have a friend who is having trouble with her boss at work and is very upset, you will support him or her by giving time and listening, over a glass of wine or a cup of coffee, to him or her telling you all of the details about what happened and when, and how he or she feels. You may do this for several hours, days, or even months, and although it may become tiresome, you do it because you like your friend and you want to make him or her feel better.

McCabe and Timmins (2006) highlight how easy it is for patients to feel that nursing tasks are more important than expecting nurses to talk to patients because nurses are so 'busy'. However, they suggest that it does not have to be a choice for the nurse as to whether they should listen to the patient or complete the task. Both can happen without the nurse spending long periods of time if they simply focuses on the patient while they talk rather than think about the next task. Thinking ahead and prioritizing your work is important, but it must not prevent making a commitment to the patient and giving them your absolute attention for however long is required.

Attending

Showing commitment in an interpersonal interaction is also known as 'attending', or 'being present'. It is reflected in our behaviours and physical actions: for example, when you listening to your friend recount various difficulties that he or she has with a boss, your friend would not feel convinced that you are really interested if you were to keep one eye on the television or interrupt to talk about similar situations that you have had.

The same applies in nursing: when attending to a patient, the nurse needs to assume what Stein-Parbury (2009) refers to as the 'attending posture'. This is an open, relaxed posture with some eye contact and an even tone of voice, but most importantly, the nurse should not focus on other activities, for example continuing to document something in the patient's notes or monitoring equipment while also perhaps even giving an inappropriate verbal response to the patient's queries. This sends the message to the patient that the nurse is not genuine or is very busy and that the patient must not be a nuisance, or they may feel that the nurse is just not interested, which can make the patient feel lonely and/or anxious.

This negative emotional response means that the patient will not trust the nurse and will respond to them accordingly, with the result that this relationship will be detached and functional:

> **What you sound like is what you are. The way you speak more than the words you use marks you down as someone who should be listened to. Tone of voice, clarity, accent, the whole package of paralanguage defines you more than any other single factor in your entire make-up.**
>
> (Shea, 1998: 91)

Shea also suggests that it is our body language that forms the visual impression that is our 'presence' and that humans focus more on this non-verbal communication than the actual words we speak.

....

How do you communicate non-verbally?
In your next communication with someone, be aware of your posture.
Are you arms folded, or outstretched?
Have you adopted an open, relaxed stance, or are you tense?
Reflect on how you communicate with patients when you feel that you are very busy.
Do you think that it influences your interactions with patients?
If so, how does it influence your communication?

....

Respecting others

Attending, or 'being present', reflects both a 'professional' and a personal communication skill that stems from what Tschudin (1999: 30) says is more than just respect: it is an individual's central belief that '*People matter, completely and utterly and simply "respecting persons" is perhaps no longer an adequate enough concept*'. Perhaps this explains why some nurses are not viewed as good communicators, and also helps us to understand the concept of unconditional regard and non-judgemental communication that patients valued in Kagan's (2008) study.

If a nurse perceives and accepts a person as unique and valuable, then this will be reflected in how they carry out nursing actions and procedures (see also Chapter 4). There is no doubt that nursing takes place in a very transient environment in which patients and nurses experience each other for very short periods of time, with discharge often occurring on the same day and often after complex surgical procedures.

Nurse–patient interactions are short, so they need to be focused. However, this does not mean that a nurse does not have the opportunity to attend to patients. Of course, not every nurse–patient interaction requires 'attending'; some interactions are superficial by their nature—for example, confirming details for discharge or even having a quick chat in passing about how the patient is recovering—and it can be a challenge for inexperienced nurses to recognize when they need to move from one type of communication to another.

Stein-Parbury (2009) acknowledges the physical difficulties in adopting an 'attending' posture, but stopping other nursing activities or tasks, having some eye contact with an open posture, and adopting an even tone of voice or silence is often sufficient to indicate to patients that the nurse is paying complete attention.

It is important that nursing students realize that the ever-increasing transient nature of contemporary healthcare services, for example those provided in day surgery or five-day units, does not mean that patients need less reassurance. McCabe (2009) identifies

PRACTICE EXAMPLE 9.2

What is your experience?

A nurse working on a five-day surgical ward, on which most of the patients undergo laparoscopic surgery and are discharged within 24 or 48 hours, is telling his friend over lunch how much he likes this new job. When the friend asks why he likes working on this ward, he says that it is because patients are up and about and independent very quickly. The friend seems surprised by this and says that it was not his experience of working on this ward. He comments that

patients often had procedures related to life-threatening or chronic conditions, and required not only regular analgesia and advice on discharge, but also time for reassurance, and were often quite scared about going home so soon after surgery. The work was physically demanding and ensuring that the patients received the care that they needed was also sometimes emotionally draining.

Think about which of these nurses' experience you identify with most.

---

that simple communication behaviours such as smiling, eye contact, and even minimal interpersonal engagement can reassure a patient as long as that behaviour is patient-centred.

Although care is provided in the context of care pathways, nurses need to plan and implement care through direct engagement with the patient and not only through following a standardized care document. In other words, a nurse can probably assume correctly that a patient is pain-free post-operatively because analgesia has been administered, but patient-centred communication requires that the nurse engages with the patient in confirming the assumption. This is communicating care based on the nurse's belief that patients 'matter', and that their fundamental professional role and responsibility is to help patients feel better physically, emotionally, and psychologically when required (please read **Practice Example 9.2**).

Whether we believe or not that nurses control the level and type of engagement with patients, it is essential that nurses are aware of the type of engagement that they have with patients because it is this that will determine if a patient perceives that they have been cared for. In developing nursing behaviours that communicate caring or even beginning to understand and recognize how they currently communicate, individual nurses need to become self-aware. This requires taking responsibility for how they communicate and the influence that this has on whether patients perceive or feel 'cared for'.

PRACTICE TIP

A very simple exercise that McCabe and Timmins (2006) propose as a method of learning about how you communicate is consciously to make eye contact and smile at the shop assistant the next time you are at a checkout. If this seems alien to you, then it may not be something that you do very often. Observe the difference in the nature of the interaction from previous encounters with the shop assistant: it will feel more positive for you even if the shop assistant does not respond to your open friendly communication! Try smiling and using eye contact more in your workplace, and take note of the difference in how people respond to you.

Questioning is also a very useful tool for finding out about patients, but when communicating care, nurses need to be careful of how some types of question can communicate judgement or lack of understanding. For example, a patient might say that she had noticed a breast lump a few months earlier, but did not see a doctor straight away. An immediate reaction might be to ask: 'Why not?' This can make the patient feel judged and that it was her own fault that she now needs surgery. Communicating care in this case requires sensitivity to the guilt that the patient may be feeling.

Taking it further

Once you have begun to understand the fundamentals of communicating care, it can be useful to give consideration to the barriers that exist to this in the healthcare setting. While nursing has become synonymous in popular culture with feminine attributes such as caring and kindness, this is not to say that all communications within the healthcare setting are optimal. There are many barriers within either the nurse or the patient (or both), or within the environment.

Inadequate listening skills of nurses, for example, have been found to deter communication and nurse–patient relationship development (Keating et al., 2002). There are also a range of mechanisms within individuals that can distort the receipt of the communication message. These are known as 'filters' (Hindle, 2003). These can arise from defence mechanisms, attitudes, beliefs and values, prejudices, and perceptual disturbances. These can adversely affect communication in the healthcare setting. The presence of these 'filters' hampers the open, honest communication that patients desire (McCabe, 2004) and which is essential to good communication and the therapeutic relationship. While an acceptance and understanding of these defence mechanisms in patients is required by nurses, their presence in nurses needs to be explored through self-awareness and personal development in order for the nurse to function effectively in the healthcare setting.

Conclusion

Care is the ultimate goal of nursing (Gamez, 2009). Caring means making a human connection between the nurse and the patient regardless of the context or environment. Caring, in the context of communication within nursing, is concerned with using an authentic, genuine approach within the nurse–patient relationship and exhibiting a range of facilitative communication behaviours.

In nursing, we deliver care using innate and/or learned communication behaviours. This chapter aimed to explore how nurses use personal and professional communication skills to communicate care to patients. In contrast, nurse-focused communication is also witnessed in the healthcare setting. An implicit element of nurse–patient communication is the development of (and disengagement from, if relevant) the nurse–patient relationship. Patient-focused communication involves giving of oneself as a nurse in the act of care. Nurse-focused communication cannot fully communicate caring.

Nurses often use a linear model of one-way communication when caring for patients. However, Morse et al.'s (1997) 'comforting interaction–relationship model' provides a more holistic caring approach that guides nursing actions, patient actions, and the evolving relationship. Central to communicating care is the nurse–patient relationship. Indeed, the very essence of nursing is thought to occur in the interpersonal relationship between the nurses and the patient. Self-awareness is essential for successful implementation of the nurse–patient relationship. Knowing your limitations also refers to remaining professional in the nurse–patient relationship.

It is easy for patients to feel that nursing tasks are more important than expecting nurses to talk to patients because nurses are so 'busy'. The absence of a patient-centred approach to communication will inhibit the development of a therapeutic nurse–patient relationship. The key characteristics of therapeutic nurse–patient communication include a perception of caring, openness, warmth, genuineness, empathy, and purpose on the part of the nurse. In nursing, these skills form the basis of how we communicate care for patients.

Further reading

American Society for Training and Development (ASTD)
http://www.astd.org/
Watson's Caring Science Institute
http://www.watsoncaringscience.org/

References

Alavi, C. (2006) 'Expanding our body of knowledge', *Journal of Advanced Nursing* 30th Anniversary Issue: 89–90.

Arnold, E. and Underman-Boggs, K. (2006) *Interpersonal Relationships: Professional Communication Skills for Nurses*, 5th edn, Philadelphia, PA: Saunders Co.

Berg, L., Skott, C., and Danielson, E. (2006) 'An interpretive phenomenological method for illuminating the meaning of the caring relationship', *Scandinavian Journal of Caring Science* 20: 42–50.

Berlo, D. (1960) *The Process of Communication: An Introduction to the Theory and Practice*, New York: Holt, Rinehart & Winston.

Betts, A. (2003) 'Improving communication', in R.B. Ellis, B. Gates, and N. Kenworthy (eds) *Interpersonal Communication in Nursing Theory and Practice*, 2nd edn, London: Churchill Livingstone, pp. 73–85.

Boykin, A. and Schoenhofer, S. (2001) 'The role of nursing leadership in creating caring environments in health care delivery systems', *Nursing Administration Quarterly* 25(3): 1–7.

Burnard, P. (1997) *Effective Communication Skills for Health Professionals*, 2nd edn, Cheltenham: Nelson Thornes.

Department of Health (2004) *Winning the War on Heart Disease*, London: HMSO.

Department of Health (2007) *National Service Framework for Older People*, London: HMSO.

Forchuk, C. and Reynolds, W. (2001) 'Clients' reflections on relationships with nurses: Comparisons from Canada and Scotland', *Journal of Psychiatric and Mental Health Nursing* 8(1): 45–51.

Fosbinder, D. (1994) 'Patient perceptions of nursing care: An emerging theory of interpersonal competence', *Journal of Advanced Nursing* 20: 1085–93.

Gamez, G.G. (2009) 'The nurse–patient relationship as a caring relationship', *Nursing Science Quarterly* 22(2): 126–7.

Gibbs, G. (1988) *Learning by Doing: A Guide to Teaching Learning Methods*, Oxford: Oxford Brookes University.

Hindle, S.A. (2003) 'Psychological factors affecting communication', in: R.B. Ellis, B. Gates, and N. Kenworthy (eds) *Interpersonal Communication in Nursing Theory and Practice*, 2nd edn, London: Churchill Livingstone, pp. 53–71.

Kagan, P.N. (2008) 'Feeling listened to: A lived experience of humanbecoming', *Nursing Science Quarterly* 21(1): 59–67.

Kantcheva, D.A. and Eckroth-Bucher, M. (2002) 'Self-awareness in psychiatric nursing: Philosophical basis and practice of self-awareness in psychiatric nursing', *Journal of Psychosocial Nursing and Mental Health Services* 39(2): 32–9.

Keating, D., Bellchambers, H., Bujack, E., Cholowski, K., Conway, J., and Neal, P. (2002) 'Communication: Principal barrier to nurse–consumer partnerships', *International Journal of Nursing Practice* 8: 16–22.

Kirkham, M., Stapleton, H., Curtis, P., and Thomas, G. (2002) 'Stereotyping as a professional defence mechanism', *British Journal of Midwifery* 10(9): 549–52.

Langwitz, W.A., Eich, P., Kiss, A., and Wossmer, B. (1998) 'Improving communication skills: A randomized controlled behaviorally oriented intervention study for residents in internal medicine', *Psychosomatic Medicine* 60: 268–76.

Loscin, R.C. (2006) 'Machine technologies and caring in nursing', in L.C. Andrist, P.K. Nicholas, and K.A. Wolf (eds) *A History of Nursing Ideas*, Sudbury, MA: Jones and Bartlett, pp. 121–6.

McCabe, C. (2004) 'Nurse–patient communication: An exploration of patients' experiences', *Journal of Clinical Nursing* 13: 41–9.

McCabe, C. (2009) 'Communication issues in day surgery', in F. Timmins and C. McCabe (eds) *Day Surgery: Contemporary Approaches to Nursing Care*, Chichester: Wiley-Blackwell, pp. 122–36.

McCabe, C. and Timmins, F. (2006) *Communication Skills for Nursing Practice*, London: Palgrave Maccmillan.

McCamant, K.L. (2006) 'Humanistic nursing, interpersonal relations theory, and the empathy-altruism hypothesis', *Nursing Science Quarterly* 19(4): 334–8.

Milton, C.L. (2008) 'Boundaries: Ethical implications for what it means to be therapeutic in the nurse–person relationship', *Nursing Science Quarterly* 21(1): 18–21.

Morse, J.M., Bottorff, J., Anderson, G., O'Brien, B., and Solberg, S. (1992) 'Beyond empathy: Expanding expressions of caring', *Journal of Advanced Nursing* 17: 809–21.

Morse, J.M., De Luca Havens, G.A., and Wilson, S. (1997) 'The comforting interaction: Developing a model of nurse–patient relationship', *Scholarly Inquiry for Nursing Practice* 11(4): 321–43.

Parse, R.R. (2007) 'The humanbecoming school of thought in 2050', *Nursing Science Quarterly* 20: 308–11.

Pearson, A., Vaughan, B., and Fitzgerald, M. (2000) *Nursing Models for Practice*, 2nd edn, London: Butterworth Heinemann.

Peplau, H.E. (1952; 1991) *Interpersonal Relations in Nursing A Conceptual Frame of Reference for Psychodynamic Nursing*, New York: Springer.

Reynolds, W. (2000) *The Measurement and Development of Empathy in Nursing*, Aldershot: Ashgate.

Reynolds, W (2006) 'Barriers to empathy do not mean that empathy is not needed', *Journal of Advanced Nursing* 30th Anniversary Issue: 88–9.

Roach, S. (1992) *The Human Act of Caring*, Ottowa, ON: The Canadian Hospital Association.

Shea, M. (1998) *The Primacy Effect: The Ultimate Guide to Effective Personal Communications*, London: Orion.

Stein-Parbury, J. (2009) *Patient and Person*, 4th edn, London: Churchill Livingstone.

Tschudin, V. (1999) *Nurses Matter: Reclaiming Our Professional Identity*, London: Macmillan Press Ltd.

Warelow, P. (1996) 'Is caring the ethical ideal?', *Journal of Advanced Nursing* 24: 655–61.

Warelow, P. and Edward, K. (2007) 'Caring as a resilient practice in mental health nursing', *International Journal of Mental Health Nursing* 16(2): 132–5.

Warelow, P., Edward, K., and Vinek, J. (2008) 'Care: What nurses say and what nurses do', *Holistic Nursing Practice* 22(3): 146–53.

Watson, J. (2005) *Caring Science as Sacred Science*, Philedelphia, PA: FA Davis.

10 Pathways of care

SHARON D. BATEMAN AND JANE A. GIBSON

Learning outcomes

This chapter will enable you to:

- define the term 'pathways of care';
- outline how pathways of care may influence the provision of nursing practice and patient care;
- understand the purpose, process, and value of implementing pathways of care;
- appreciate the evidence-based foundations of pathways of care;
- identify the individual patient journey across the pathway of care;
- recognize and take the appropriate action of variance in the implementation of pathways of care; and
- identify the benefits of pathways of care.

Introduction

The chapter introduces you to the concept of pathways of care, focusing upon their contribution and value in relation to patient care provision. The chapter also explores the development of pathways of care in relation to clinical practice and the nursing process of assessing, implementation, and evaluation of care. Through increasing your awareness and knowledge of pathways of care, you will be able to provide a consistent care approach that works across multidisciplinary boundaries, enhancing healthcare delivery and the robust maintenance of patient safety.

'Care pathways' defined

'Care pathways', 'integrated pathways of care', 'the patient journey', and/or 'the patient pathway' could all arguably be described as referring to the same thing

> **Essential knowledge and skills for care**
>
> - You must recognize the importance of care pathways within nursing, their role in nursing assessment, and when care planning for the person, their carers, and their families.
>
> - In partnership with the person, their carers and their families, you will make a holistic, person-centred, and systematic assessment of physical, emotional, psychological, social, cultural, and spiritual needs, including risk, and together develop a comprehensive personalized plan of nursing care.
>
> - You will be able to distinguish between information that is relevant to care planning and information that is not.
>
> - You will recognize the significance of information and act in relation to who does or does not need to know.
>
> - You will take appropriate action in the sharing of information to enable and enhance the care pathway.
>
> - You will encourage integrated team working within the care pathway, through involving the patient, carers, multidisciplinary teams (MDTs), and agencies.
>
> - You must monitor and record progress against the care pathway, reporting any variations.

(Nursing and Midwifery Council, 2011). The ultimate purpose of a care pathway within this chapter, as defined by Walsh (1998), is to offer a plan of care for patients with the same clinical problem, setting out stages that they should reach with the passage of time, and defining outcomes that can be measured to assess clinical progress. Furthermore, the NMC (2011) recognizes the importance of care pathways within nursing by stating a care pathway is:

a system of care delivery that organises a service user's care from their first contact with health services to the end of their episode. Care pathways aim to improve continuity and coordination across different professions and sectors.

Care pathways can be undertaken as a multidisciplinary exercise and there is allowance for individual variation within the pathway. Poirrier and Oberleitner (1999) stipulate that certain complex healthcare needs require deviations from the core clinical pathway format to ensure that care outcomes are reached. Variances within care pathways are usually documented on a variance form, which is attached within the core care pathway document. The basic criteria of any given care pathway should include the following:

- *planned intervention*—such as taking a patient's blood pressure;
- *the time and date of the planned intervention*— such as the pre-administration of hypertensive medication;
- *expected outcomes*—such as the acquisition of a blood pressure reading to aid decision-making; and
- *variances*—such as a bariatric patient requiring an extra-large cuff to enable the intervention to take place.

The core elements of care pathways consist of pre-established structured clinical interventions, milestones, and desired care outcomes, which, when required, are flexible to accommodate the potential variance in individual patient's healthcare needs. Coffey et al. (1992) stipulate that care pathways can provide a structural means of developing and implementing local protocols and guidelines related to evidence-based care packages. Grimshaw et al. (1995) have demonstrated that the use of evidence-based care pathways has a positive clinical effect upon improved patient care and clinical outcomes, aided by a consistent approach to care and effective communication at the front line. From a patient safety perspective, care pathways also provide an 'alert' and thus highlight areas of clinical care that are insubstantial through the provision of daily recorded data within the pathway documentation, alongside those outcomes of provisional care that have not been pre-empted (Campbell et al., 1998).

To demonstrate the use of a generic pathway process, the everyday practice of making a cup of tea will be used as an analogy, alongside a daily clinical practical task, to aid understanding of the care pathway concept. Both of these practices are common, and are therefore familiar to us in our daily home environments and in our nursing roles (**Tables 10.1 and 10.2**).

Table 10.1 Explaining the generic pathway process by focusing on making a cup of tea (Cooper, 2010)

Problem	Goal	Intervention
Unable to make a cup of tea	To make a cup of tea	Boil the water Add tea to container Add water to tea Add other ingredients Stir
A sloughy, macerated leg ulcer requires bacterial diagnosis to optimize treatment	To identify bacteria to enable correct therapy to be prescribed	Inform patient and gain consent Clean and prepare the wound bed Moisten wound swab tip Move the swab across the wound bed surface Return swab to the swab container Complete relevant documentation Transfer immediately to the laboratory for processing

Table 10.2 Incorporating variance within the generic pathway process by focusing on making a cup of tea

Problem	Goal	Intervention with variance
Unable to make a cup of tea	To make a cup of tea	
A sloughy, macerated leg ulcer requires bacterial diagnosis to optimize treatment	To identify bacteria to enable correct therapy to be prescribed	

Now reflect upon the common practice of making a cup of tea and taking a wound swab.

Provide a list of variances that you feel may occur within both processes that may alter expected outcomes.

Add your pre-empted variances to the generic pathway in Table 10.2.

The origins of care pathways

Ford and Walsh (1994) suggest that, historically, the nursing profession previously lacked a scholarly and academic foundation when compared which other healthcare disciplines, which often left nursing vulnerable to ritualistic practice and 'big new ideas' in regards to patient care provision. Traditionally, nursing decision-making within clinical practice was, and continues to be, founded upon fundamental ways of knowing, summarized by Carper (1978) as:

● personal knowledge and experience;
● aesthetics and the art of nursing;
● empirical elements of the science of nursing; and
● ethics and the principles of caring.

The expansion and development of nursing training and educational research-based programmes have enabled the nursing profession to gain momentum and equality compared with other more traditionally led professions, producing new ways of working within the clinical field (Walsh, 1998). Within the last three decades, some of these new ideas have evolved into key methods of promoting organized nursing practice and patient outcomes, such as primary and secondary care sectors (Poirrier and Oberleitner, 1999), nursing models (McGee, 1998), managed care packages (Middleton and Roberts, 1998), and more recently care pathways (Middleton et al., 2010) focusing upon a collaborative approach to patient care provision and healthcare outcomes. Keegan (1987) argues that the need for organized and consistent care frameworks and models has evolved from the nursing profession demanding a drastic move forward from traditional and ritualistic practice towards a rational process in which the nursing profession can justify its actions and implement change that benefits patients, carers, and the organization holistically.

Care pathways, according to Poirrier and Oberleitner (1999), originated in part from project management techniques utilized within non-healthcare sectors, such as manufacture, industry, and construction. Within today's healthcare remit, care pathways are variably referred to as 'clinical paths', 'critical paths/pathways', 'care maps', 'care paths', 'collaborative plans of care', 'multidisciplinary action plans', and 'anticipated recovery paths' (ibid). Middleton and Roberts (1998) argue that pathways of care are constructed to overcome common problems such as ineffective communication, inconsistent monitoring and evaluation processes, and timing of completion of care delivery.

··

Review a basic care pathway document in a chosen clinical area.

What skills and knowledge might you require to implement the core elements of the care pathway with your patient group?

··

To implement the core elements of a pathway of care with your patient group, it is important to act on the following. Vanhaecht et al. (2007a) suggest that pathways of care follow alongside the nursing process of assessment, planning, implementation, and evaluation, allowing for variances that are expected within some individuals' care journeys. Ineffective communication and information given associated with the design and implementation of care pathways tend to arise when teams are working in different departments or locations, and are not involved in the initial design, development, and implementation of a care pathway. Effective care pathways, according to Vanhaecht et al. (2007b), are developed by encouraging and engaging members of the MDT in establishing the key elements of the care package required within the pathway and the anticipated patient expected outcomes of care.

> **PRACTICE TIP**
>
> Acquire the relevant knowledge and skills prior to designing and implementing the pathway. Establish the type of pathway and justify why it is required, highlighting the potential impact of the pathway on the patient experience of care.

··

Reflect on the benefits and challenges of using a care pathway within your clinical area, giving consideration to clinical practice, education, research, and patient teaching.

··

The benefits of care pathways

The increase in health demand within the UK and across the world is rising (Ham, 2004). With an ageing and growing population, this upward trend is predicted to continue in all aspects of health and social care (Department of Health, 2009). Health interventions are, in the main, increasingly more technical and costly. Not surprisingly, this increase in demand and expenditure has an unprecedented demand on financial resources and on health service employees (ibid). With the majority of the population having high expectations of the National Health Services, care pathways soothe these competing demands. Since their evolution, care pathways have proven to enhance patient care, ensuring that practitioners' time is used appropriately while reducing financial cost (Middleton et al., 2010).

There needs to be enough demand for an intervention before a care pathway should be considered. This could be a local demand, a national one, or a clinical need of a significant cost. Care pathways can translate national guidance into local practice or evolve local need into a structured pathway. Either way, the construction of any pathway should inform patient-centred care, be evidence-based, and enhance professional accountability (Campbell et al., 1998).

Patient-centred care

Because pathways run the entire length of the patient journey, all of those who have involvement in care provision along this pathway should be included in the construction, including the patient.

There is a realization that patients can do more for themselves to reduce the financial burden and lessen the demand on health services (Department of Health, 2010). In addition to this theory, they can also inform health, and indeed social provision, that is charged to care for us (Department of Health, 2007). Furthermore, organizations will not escape liability if their pathways fail to reach an acceptable standard of care. In the same way, a customer is more likely to receive a meal that they will find enjoyable if a waiter asks what they want rather than simply bringing the customer a meal of the waiter's choice.

Evidence-based care

A plethora of knowledge has evolved since the birth of evidence-based care. It is time-consuming to search and interpret this data accurately. Nonetheless, it is vital that care pathways are based on the most up-to-date evidence (Poirrier and Oberleitner, 1999). To a great extent, these pathways are requested by the Department of Health from arm's-lengths bodies, such as the National Institute for Health and Clinical Excellence (NICE), individual royal colleges, and research projects that feed into systematic review bodies such as the Cochrane Database Review. However, many locally developed care pathways are still evident and robust. A crucial element post-development is implementation to ensure that the pathway achieves optimum effect. Undoubtedly, the successful implementation of a pathway relies heavily on local ability (De Luc, 2001).

A significant advantage of a clinical pathway (see **Practice Example 10.1**) is that it can 'travel' with the patient across organizational and disciplinary boundaries. Therefore there is less duplication of questioning, it is more time-efficient for staff and less frustrating for the patient, and it enables care to be provided in a timely manner. It doubles as the patient record; it collects real-time data that can be used to inform performance. It demonstrates the meeting of set standards of care; it can also be used in the evaluation of care, due to the amount of variances documented, which can inform a need for change.

Professional accountability

To be charged with the duty of care of another human is a privileged position—one that should be taken with due understanding and respect. The Nursing and Midwifery Council's Code (NMC, 2008) clearly states the expected level of professional practice and accountability of a registered nurse. A nurse contributing to the creation of a care pathway will have equal responsibility over its validity to that of any other colleague—that is, all professional colleagues who contribute to the creation of a pathway carry tangible responsibility for the content.

All guidance and evidence used within a pathway should be referenced: if a case goes to court against the pathway, this evidence will be required. However, good quality care pathways will demonstrate that the organization has examined the clinical care that it provides, has sought expert clinical advice, has clearly defined the standard of care to be delivered, and has a built-in system to monitor the care provided (De Luc, 2001). Panella and Vanhaecht (2010) reinforce the basis of the care pathway being embedded into the heart of quality care and patient safety, and that this must be the priority of all healthcare organizations that implement such tools.

Pathways are not prescriptive and should not be followed blindly; those applying the pathway of care could face liability if there were to be a failure to adhere to professional duty of care—for example, if the pathway advocates substandard care, if a practitioner deviates from the pathway and fails to document when and why, or if a practitioner misapplies the pathway in any way. Furthermore, individual organizations hold their own liability for housing substandard pathways (Dykes and Wheeler, 1997).

According to Staunton and Chiarella (2008), the '*Bolam* test' is applicable, in which the defendant's actions will be judged on whether they are considered 'reasonable' by his or her peers; with the modern-day focus on evidence-based practice, however, what is reasonable may drift nearer to what is considered 'best

PRACTICE EXAMPLE 10.1

Elsie is a 72-year-old lady who has successfully recovered from a fractured neck of femur following a fall at home. She was transferred to a care of the elderly rehabilitation ward and discharged within a week of admission. The successful outcome of Elsie's stay in hospital could be attributed to the fact that the journey of care was mapped out from admission to discharge within the fractured neck of femur pathway of care. The pathway identified key stages and roles of professional colleagues within the care processes that only served to enhance the quality of care, along with the professional accountability of the health and social care providers.

practice'. Furthermore, organizations will not escape liability if their pathways fail to reach an acceptable standard of care.

With the progressive nature of today's evidence, care pathways can easily become dated and some criticism can be levelled that, due to the speed at which evidence is created, they play catch up. Conversely, they offer a net through which no one should fall, while allowing clinical flexibility to combine the most current areas of research alongside national guidance. Health care requires those who practice, sometimes at the limits of science, to constantly move care forward.

....

Think about the following questions.
Can you import a care pathway from elsewhere?
Do care pathways stifle clinical autonomy?
Are care pathways implemented as a cost-effective measure within healthcare provision?

....

Care pathways can be used in a variety of situations; we will now focus on a wound care scenario in **Practice Example 10.2** and then on its development in **Practice Example 10.3**.

Evaluation

Evaluation has been described as a form of a feedback loop (Reece and Walker, 1992), and has emerged in clinical practice from integration of professional autonomy and accountability within healthcare processes. Within care pathways, evaluation is vital to ensure that clinically, on a day-to-day basis, clinicians are made aware of whether care end points have been achieved or not, as set out within the document. Clinical evaluation will provide key information that will highlight whether the patient remains upon the pathway, whether the document requires amendment due

PRACTICE EXAMPLE 10.2

You have admitted a patient under your care who you deem is at risk of developing a pressure ulcer. Your care pathway is illustrated in **Table 10.3**.

Table 10.3 Preventing a pressure ulcer

Problem	Goal	Intervention
Patient is at risk of developing pressure ulcer due to immobility	Skin will be intact with no red broken areas	1–2 hour position changes
		Appropriate mattress in situ
		Explain importance of skin hygiene
		Ensure skin hygiene needs are met
		Explain the importance of diet and fluid intake
		Ensure dietary and hydration needs are met
		Ensure risk assessment chart is completed

The aetiology of pressure ulcers has been recognized for many years, and both local and national initiatives have been available to educate professionals in pressure ulcer prevention and management. Yet pressure ulcers and associated problems continue to persist, and costs from both a financial and humanistic perspective keep rising (Butcher, 2001).

The cost of pressure ulcers to the NHS has been estimated by Bennett et al. (2004), with average figures for treating a grade 1 at £1,064 and a grade 4 at £10,551. Collier (1999) suggests that a clinical audit demonstrated that the true cost of managing a grade 4 pressure ulcer amounts to a figure of £40,000 per patient. The cost of pressure ulcers to the NHS annually has been highlighted to be in the region of between £1.4 billion and £2.1 billion—that is, 4 per cent of the total NHS budget (Bennett et al., 2004). Some wound care experts suggest that this figure is, in reality, only the tip of the iceberg due to an ageing population and associated co-morbidity (European Pressure Ulcer Advisory Panel, 2010). And these figures represent only the financial cost to the organization with regards to managing pressure ulcers and do not bring into the equation the holistic effects that this particular wound has on the patient, carer, and healthcare professional.

PRACTICE EXAMPLE 10.3

A patient has been admitted under your care with a grade 4 (EUPAP) pressure ulcer to their sacrum, which has been present for four months whilst being cared for at home following a stroke (cerebral vascular accident).

Complete the following care pathway to ensure that your patient's needs are met and outcomes are achieved, highlighting any variances that you feel may be applicable. The first intervention has been given as your first point of care provision.

1 Do you feel that the care pathway represents the true clinical nursing practice provided?
2 Do you feel that the care pathway meets all of the needs of your patient group?
3 Do you feel that any clinician can follow the care pathway, consistently achieving set outcomes?
4 Do you feel that the care pathway allows individual needs to be met through the variance route?

Table 10.4 Treating a pressure ulcer

Problem	Goal	Intervention	Variances
Patient has a grade 4 pressure ulcer to the sacrum	Provide a healing environment and prevent deterioration Reduce risk of infection	1–2 hourly position changes	

to variances, or whether the patient should be removed from the pathway as a result of journey completion. Periodic care pathway evaluation, as an operational process, is also essential if clinicians are to measure the impact upon factors such as length of stay, care provision, and patient experience of the care journey (Walsh, 1998).

Conclusion

A care pathway is an evidence-based, multidisciplinary outline of anticipated care within a set time frame to allow a patient with a particular condition to travel through health services in different settings at different times, whilst seamlessly achieving positive outcomes of care.

Care pathways allow variances to be acknowledged and addressed, with the ultimate aim of meeting all of the individual needs of the patient within the disease process. Care pathways can also reduce unnecessary

variations in patients who receive care and resulting outcomes, by enabling clinicians to practise and deliver care in a safe, coordinated, consistent, and robust manner. These tools can be used to enable organizations to embed local and national guidelines and policy, to promote patient safety, clinical risk, and governance agendas into everyday clinical practice and patient care outcomes.

When designing and implementing care pathways, a multidisciplinary approach to production must be employed at the outset if relevant and appropriate care pathways are to be utilized in the delivery of efficient and effective care.

Further reading

Nursing organizations

Nursing and Midwifery Council (NMC)
http://www.nmc-uk.org
Royal College of Nursing (RCN)
http://www.rcn.org.uk

Patient organizations

NHS Choices
http://www.nhs.uk/Pages/HomePage.aspx
Patient.co.uk
http://www.patient.co.uk/about.asp
The Patients Association
http://www.patients-association.com

Sources of information

Map of Medicine Health Guides
http://healthguides.mapofmedicine.com/choices/
map/index.html
NHS Evidence
http://www.library.nhs.uk
NHS Institute for Innovation and Improvement
http://www.institute.nhs.uk/

Podcast

National Mental Health Development Unit
http://www.nmhdu.org.uk/our-work/improving-men-
tal-health-care-pathways/

References

Bennett, G., Dealey, C., and Posnett, J. (2004) 'The cost of pressure ulcers in the UK', *Age and Ageing* 33(3): 230–5.

Butcher, M. (2001) 'NICE Clinical Guidelines Pressure Ulcer Risk Assessment and Prevention: A review', *World Wide Wounds*, 26 July, available online at **http://www.worldwidewounds.com/2001/july/Butcher/NICE-pressure-ulcer-review.html** [accessed 16 June 2011].

Campbell. H., Hotchkiss, R., Bradshaw, N., and Porteous, M. (1998) 'Education and debate: Integrated care pathways', *British Medical Journal* 316(7125): 133.

Carper, B. (1978) 'Fundamental patterns of knowing in nursing', *Advances in Nursing Science* 1(1): 13–23.

Coffey, R., Richards, J., Remment, C., and Leroy, S. (1992) 'An introduction to critical paths', *Quality Management in Health Care* 75: 45–54.

Collier, M. (1999) 'Pressure ulcer development and principles for prevention', in M. Miller and D. Glover (eds) *Wound Management, Theory and Practice*, London: NT Books EMap, pp. 88–94.

Cooper, R. (2010) 'How to: Ten top tips for taking a wound swab', *Wounds International* 1(3), available online at **http://www.woundsinternational.com/article.php?issueid=303&contentid=122&articleid=8914&page=1** [accessed 11 July 2011].

De Luc, K. (2001) *Developing Care Pathways*, Oxford: Radcliffe Medical Press.

Department of Health (2007) *World Class Commissioning 3: Engage with Public and Patients*, London: HMSO.

Department of Health (2009) *Tackling Demand Together: A Tool Kit for Improving Urgent and Emergency Care Pathways by Understanding 999 Demand*, London: HMSO.

Department of Health (2010) *The NHS Constitution: The NHS Belongs to All of Us*, London: HMSO.

Dykes, P.C. and Wheeler, K. (1997) *Planning, Implementing and Evaluating Critical Pathways: A Guide for Health Care Survival into the 21st Century*, Springhouse, PA: Springhouse Corporation.

European Pressure Ulcer Advisory Panel (2010) 'Pressure ulcer treatment', available online at **http://www.npuap.org/Final_Quick_Treatment_for_web_2010.pdf** [accessed 16 June 2011].

Ford, P. and Walsh, M. (1994) *New Rituals for Old*, London: Butterworth Heinemann.

Grimshaw, J., Freemantle, N., Wallace, S., Russell, I., and Hurwitz, B. (1995) 'Developing and implementing clinical practice guidelines', *Quality in Health Care* 4: 190–3.

Ham. C. (2004) *Health Policy in Britain*, 5th edn, Basingstoke: Palgrave Macmillan.

Keegan, l. (1987) 'Holistic nursing', *American Operating Room Nurses Journal* 46: 499–506.

McGee, P. (1998) *Models of Nursing in Practice: A Pattern for Practical Care*, Cheltenham: Stanley Thorne Books.

Middleton, S. and Roberts, A. (1998) *Clinical Pathways Workbook*, Wrexham: VFM Unit.

Middleton, S., Barnett, J., and Reeves, D. (2010) *What is an Integrated Care Pathway?*, What is ..? Series, available online at **http://www.evidence-based-medicine.co.uk** [accessed 16 June 2011].

Nursing and Midwifery Council (2008) *The Code*, available online at **http://www.nmc-uk.org/Nurses-and-midwives/The-code/** [accessed 16 June 2011].

Nursing and Midwifery Council (2011) 'Standing orders', available online at **http://www.nmc-uk.org/About-us/ The-council/NMC-standing-orders-2011/** [accessed 16 June 2011].

Panella, M. and Vanhaecht, K. (2010) 'Is there still need for confusion about pathways?', *International Journal of Care Pathways* 14(1): 1–3.

Poirrier, G.P. and Oberleitner, M.G. (1999) *Clinical Pathways in Nursing: A Guide to Managing Care from Hospital to Home*, Springhouse, PA: Springhouse Corporation.

Reece, I. and Walker, S. (1992) *Teaching and Learning*, 4th edn, London: Business Education Publishers Limited.

Staunton, P. and Chiarella, M. (2008) *Nursing and the Law*, 6th edn, Sydney: Churchill Livingstone.

Vanhaecht, K., De Witte, K., and Sermeus, W. (2007a) *The Impact of Clinical Pathways on the Organisation of Care Processes*, Leuven: ACCO.

Vanhaecht, K., De Witte, K., and Sermeus, W. (2007b) 'The care process organisation triangle: A framework to better understand how clinical pathways work', *Journal of Integrated Care Pathways* 11: 1–8.

Walsh, M. (1998) *Models and Critical Pathways in Clinical Nursing, Conceptual Frameworks for Care Planning*, 2nd edn, London: Baillière Tindall.

11 Partnerships of care

ELEANOR BRADLEY AND TIM LEWINGTON

Learning outcomes

This chapter will enable you to:

- describe the term 'partnerships of care';
- reflect upon your understanding of this term;
- identify some of the key drivers advocating partnerships of care;
- examine the relevance of partnerships of care for nursing practice; and
- evaluate the implications and benefits for developing partnerships of care.

Introduction

This chapter will explain care in the context of partnership working in health care. The chapter focuses on the principles and best practice of partnership work, and will address working with patients and carers to meet their needs. The chapter also examines how nurses work with other professions and agencies to deliver care.

· ·

Before proceeding with this chapter, reflect on what you understand by the term 'partnerships of care'.

· ·

Essential knowledge and skills for care

- You must be able to work autonomously, confidently, and in partnership with the person, families, and carers, to ensure that needs are met through contextually relevant care planning and delivery, including strategies for self-management, care, and peer support.

- In partnership with the person, their carers, families, and multi-organizational staff, you will make a holistic, person-centred and systematic assessment of physical, emotional, psychological, social, cultural, and spiritual needs, including risk, and together develop a comprehensive personalized plan of nursing care.

- You will provide safe and effective care in partnership with people and their carers, within the context of people's ages, conditions, and developmental stages, evaluating against the care plan.

- You will work collaboratively with people, carers, and families to respond to feedback and other sources to develop and improve personalized care.

- In partnership with the person, their carers, and families, you will work as part of a team to offer holistic care and a range of treatment options in order to develop person-centred approaches to care and achieve concordance.

Partnerships: between the public and the private

Following the Second World War, the UK had a 'mixed economy': a private sector, the principal purpose of which was the generation of profit through the production of goods and services; and a public sector, the role of which was the provision of public services based primarily on need. Although interconnected, these sectors were both conceptually and operationally distinct. The particular division between the two sectors was historically determined by several factors, including the perceived national interest (for example, the need for basic industries, such as steel, coal, gas, electricity production, and distribution), the failure of the markets to provide certain goods in sufficient quantities (for example, decent quality social housing, and water and sewerage utilities), and the special status of some commodities as 'public goods' (transport infrastructure, national defence).

The post-war period in the West was marked by relative stability, during which markets were regulated and the economy was managed. Education had long been recognized as a prerogative of the state and the post-war settlement also included social welfare provision (child support, unemployment and disability benefits, social care for older people) as a right of citizenship. A geographic division of public service provision emerged in the UK whereby local councils were responsible for development controls, with some local services paid for by local taxes, and others provided and administered by the state. David Harvey (2007: 11) provides a useful overview:

> **This form of political-economic organisation is now usually referred to as 'embedded liberalism' to signal how market processes and entrepreneurial and corporate activities were surrounded by a web of social and political constraints and a regulatory environment that sometimes restrained but in other instances led the way in economic and industrial strategy.**

The benefits included extended life expectancy for everyone, not only the privileged few, and a better educated and healthier population. In the UK, this organization of public/private sector provision began to change in 1979 with the election of Margaret Thatcher as Conservative Prime Minister, and her steady separation of the private and public sectors in the name of efficiency, productivity, and choice. This opening was taken further with the introduction of 'New Labour' in 1997, with the drive to modernize the UK government and a high number of policies designed to facilitate this explicit modernization agenda. Nevertheless, 'for-profit' provision in health care was constrained and kept to the margins, with the overall direction and momentum directed to public provision and the public planning of healthcare services.

In May 2010, in Britain, the Conservatives and Liberal Democrats joined forces to form a coalition government. Shortly afterwards, a new NHS White Paper (Department

of Health, 2010a) was published, outlining plans to abolish current systems for commissioning, removing primary care trusts (PCTs), and placing the responsibility for commissioning with GP consortia. There is a continued emphasis on patient choice and the delivery of flexible, accessible services for service users.

⋯⋯⋯⋯⋯⋯⋯⋯⋯⋯⋯⋯⋯⋯⋯⋯⋯⋯⋯⋯⋯

At this point, we would like you to think about the proposed changes to the National Health Service. What impact might they have upon partnerships of care?

⋯⋯⋯⋯⋯⋯⋯⋯⋯⋯⋯⋯⋯⋯⋯⋯⋯⋯⋯⋯⋯

Partnership working: a 'third way'?

The introduction of the White Paper represents the latest of a series of policy imperatives aimed at healthcare services in England over the past decade (see Department of Health, 1997; 1999; 2000; 2001). These were prompted by the explicit 'modernization' agenda introduced by New Labour in 1997, and have promoted partnership working with the voluntary and private sectors, and explicated a 'third way' in the delivery of welfare and health care (Giddens, 1998). Partnership working has been an increasing presence within policy documentation, and the evidence of partnership working across health and social care has become a key part of commissioning and service provision.

It is important to note at this point the role that informal carers also play in the care of those with health and social care needs. Whereas formal carers act in an agency–client relationship, are paid, and are trained to be carers, informal carers are commonly family members who take on an informal caring role often without training or support provided to them. There are benefits to be derived from the receipt of informal care—most notably an enhanced provision of emotional and general tasks support. However, the burden of informal care can impact on carers as well as those in receipt of care. In April 2001, there were 5.9 million informal carers in the UK (ONS, 2001). The same census demonstrated that 114,000 of these were children aged between 5–15 and more than 1 million people were aged 65 or over (Doran et al., 2003). The support received by informal carers and their links with other providers of care is variable. With respect to financial support, in 2011, the UK government announced proposals to replace Disability Living Allowance (DLA) with a new personal independence payment and the future of the Carer's Allowance remains unclear. Under the current system, direct payments for carers are local council payments available for anyone assessed as needing help by social services. The payments can be used to pay for services from an organization (not including public sector services) or to employ somebody to provide assistance. However, many informal carers are not in contact with social services and so remain unpaid for their efforts, with potential impact not only on their financial, but also emotional, well-being.

Despite this, the White Paper *Our Health, Our Care, Our Say* (Department of Health, 2006) describes an ambition for community-based care and enhanced well-being in communities, as well as plans to support people to look after their own health and well-being, and the further promotion of engagement.

This has shifted the debate around the ways in which services should be delivered explicitly towards partnership working and integrated care (England and Lester, 2005), and is set to be extended yet further with the introduction of ideals such as the 'Big Society' implemented by the coalition government including incentives for those introducing social enterprises that will compete with the public sector for commissioned services.

Defining 'partnerships of care'

Partnerships of care occur in numerous forms, vary in depth of involvement, number, and diversity of members, and are established through negotiation. As a consequence, definitions of 'care partnerships' vary. The term is used in a variety of ways across different sectors (health, social care, private and third-sector organizations) and can refer to a range of variable practices within these contexts (**see Figure 11.1**). There have been few aims or objectives outlined that either specify how to measure the outcomes of care partnerships, or discuss the delineation of key factors associated with successful/unsuccessful partnerships either within health or social care organizations (between staff and service users/carers, within and/or between teams), between health or social care organizations, or across different sectors (including the private or voluntary sectors).

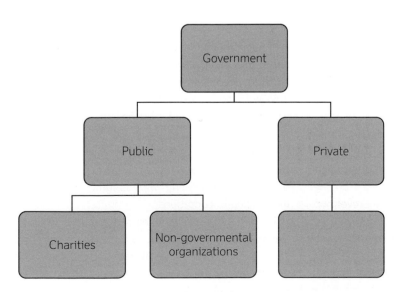

Figure 11.1 Diverse partnerships of care.

As well as the political drivers for partnership working, this increasing emphasis has been attributed by some to an explosion in chronic disease prevalence, anticipated to place an increasing demand on service provision across sectors in the UK, and indeed worldwide, in the coming decades. Partnership working has been one response to address the increasing demands of a population with chronic, often complex, healthcare needs (Butt et al., 2008). The multiple and complex needs of this population commonly extend beyond the remit and capacity of single organizations, and require multi-organizational and agency partnerships in order to meet needs.

Governance of partnerships of care

Within the UK, partnership is vital to provide the wide range of health and social care required, and there are several agencies and charities in place to support, promote, and regulate health and social care services. The Social Care Institute for Excellence (SCIE) is an independent charity, funded by the Department of Health and devolved administration in Wales and Northern Ireland, which aims to identify and spread knowledge about good practice in all aspects of social care throughout the UK. Within healthcare treatment, procedure and care is increasingly governed by guidance issued to the NHS from the National Institute for Health and Clinical Excellence (NICE). NICE is an independent organization responsible for providing national guidance on the promotion of good health, as well as the prevention and treatment of ill health. NICE guidance, along with local commissioning, plays an ever-increasing role in decision-making about care and treatment within the NHS, and the role of multidisciplinary

working, particularly around the promotion of good health and prevention of ill health, is emphasized within the guidance. The Care Quality Commission (CQC) is the independent regulator of health and social care in England, regulating care provided by the NHS, local authorities, private companies, and voluntary organizations. With respect to partnership working, it is one of the key priorities for the CQC to look at how well health or social care services are working together in order to improve services. Another key player in the area of health and social care improvement, established in 2008, is the local involvement network (LINk)—networks of local people and groups who have joined forces to improve health and social care services.

Internationally, the treatment of chronic conditions such as diabetes are also subject to nationally defined guidelines (for example, those of the American and Canadian Diabetes Association and the International Diabetes Federation), which emphasize multidisciplinary approaches in order to achieve specific targets (De Civita and Dasgupta, 2007). In the USA, there is a longer history of multi-agency collaboration than there is in the UK. This is due to the nature of health and social care provision in the USA, which relies more heavily on a market-oriented, private/voluntary sector provision, compared with welfare state-reliant or state-provided (or state funded) services, or state-mandated involvement of the third sector (Rummery, 2009). As discussed, the landscape within the UK is constantly evolving, with an increasing influence of private/voluntary sector provision. Indeed, with respect to commissioning, NHS services are increasingly competing with the private/voluntary sector to provide services that have been historically provided by the NHS. Where services are recommissioned to the private/voluntary sector, this further necessitates inter-agency working between the NHS and these sectors—in particular for those services dealing with chronic physical and mental health conditions.

There may be much to learn from the USA about the management of formal care partnerships of this type, as they are necessitated on a larger scale across the UK, although few studies to date have been conducted to evaluate the outcomes of these partnerships (discussed further in the section below). Traditional patterns of service delivery within the UK have been criticized as inefficient, insufficiently responsive to user demand, and delivered in organizational 'silos' (Papdopoulos, 2003; cited in Rummery, 2009). Integrating public health and mental health programmes will be essential to maintain and prevent ill health across physical, mental, and social well-being. Requirements of the current health system are to foster innovation, to promote prevention and self-care, and to develop team-based approaches to improve the delivery of care (Freeman et al., 2010). Within public health, there is an increasing need to look at ways in which to integrate mental health and physical health, so that policies, programmes, care, and training are all more holistic and 'person-centred', for example promoting depression screening and management as standard practice (ibid). Integration on this scale requires NHS and local organizations to share information and resources in order to provide 'joined-up' care. However, practice around partnership working varies widely around the country (Cook et al., 2007) and formal partnerships frequently fail due to the complexity in administering partnerships, the time-consuming nature of partnership working, the investment required, and the potential to lose decision-making control (Butt et al., 2008).

Cook et al. (2007) highlighted four main areas of concern in respect of effective and sustainable partnerships:

- delivering outcomes for service users and carers, including through whole-system working;
- building better partnerships with service users and carers;
- mainstreaming partnership working; and
- developing the evidence base for partnership working.

This chapter will focus on these four issues, looking at specific roles in place within the NHS designed to deliver outcomes for service users and carers, through close partnership working between service users, carers, and NHS staff.

Do care partnerships work for service users and carers?

As described above, partnership working can be diffuse, including partnering between individuals, roles, teams, and organizations. Concerns about what constitutes a partnership have hindered attempts to evaluate successful partnerships, leading to questions about the efficacy of partnership working in relation to service user outcomes (Rummery, 2009). Dowling et al. (2004) reviewed health and social care partnerships, and found very few studies (11 per cent) that had addressed outcome factors and little systematic evidence base for the UK government policy objective to support health and social care partnerships. One of the key challenges in the evaluation of outcomes for partnerships is the difficulty of attributing process to outcomes (Cook et al., 2007). As with the evaluation of many health and social care initiatives in the 'real world', the sheer number of variables, factors, and influences represents a key challenge in establishing any cause and effect, with most initiatives evaluated on a case-study basis, with few generalizable outcomes outlined as part of the evaluative process (see Pawson and Tilley, 1997, for further discussion of this issue). Of those studies that have been conducted to evaluate the outcomes of partnerships in practice, the majority have focused on specific policy issues, mostly aimed at those groups of people whose needs fall between the interface of 'traditional' health and social care services, including older people, mental health service users, and children (Rummery, 2009).

In order to consider the possible outcomes of care partnerships for service users and carers, we can focus as an example on the implementation of a relatively new role for nursing within the NHS: the role of the non-medical prescriber.

The nurse prescribing role

The non-medical prescribing (NMP) role was introduced in the UK in the early 1980s, but was restricted to community nurses—particularly district nurses and health visitors. NMP was extended across nursing in 2003 and suitably qualified nurses from all disciplines were able to practise as non-medical prescribers (NMPs). The role was specifically developed to support the care of those people with long-term, chronic conditions, and relies heavily on the formation of a strong partnership between service user and prescriber.

Personalized models of care

The central focus of chronic care models is on self-regulatory theory and recognizes that there must be an effective partnership between clinicians and patients if outcomes (relevant to patients) are to be maximized (Von Korff et al., 1997). Personalized models of care were felt to offer a range of opportunities for partnership without the need for inter-agency working (Cook et al., 2007). Nursing practice has long emphasized patient education and collaborative decision-making and the value of a collaborative patient-centred approach has been documented. Nurses are commonly charged with liaising between professionals across multidisciplinary teams (MDTs), and between primary and secondary care, in order to establish streamlined consistency of care for service users. There were a number of drivers behind the development of the NMP role, and the increasing number of people with chronic conditions and reducing number of medical prescribers were just two of these. There were some initial doubts about the introduction of the role across all disciplines, but patients reported feeling positive about the introduction of NMPs (Berry et al., 2006; Williams and Jones, 2006) and happy to be prescribed medication by a nurse with whom they had an existing relationship (Bradley and Nolan, 2007).

Benefits of partnerships of care

There are particular areas in health care in which nurse prescribing has been found to derive benefits to care. Within mental health care, service users experience particular difficulties with adherence to medication, as well as poor satisfaction with prescribing decisions. A mean non-adherence rate of 41.2 per cent has been reported amongst patients diagnosed with schizophrenia (Lacro et al., 2002), with 75 per cent reportedly

discontinuing their prescribed medication within 18 months (Lieberman et al., 2005). There are serious effects to this non-adherence, which include:

- reduced treatment efficacy (Gray et al., 2002; Haynes et al., 2008); and
- an increased risk of relapse (Gray et al., 2002).

Several interventions have been developed to increase adherence, but few have been consistently successful (Zygmunt et al., 2002; Haynes et al., 2008). This is likely due to the fact that many patients across health care, and in particular within mental health care, have concerns about their medication, feel that they are not fully included with prescribing decision-making (Gray et al., 2005), and have described feeling disempowered when meeting with doctors (Hemingway and Ely, 2009).

....

Reflect on your experiences of forming partnerships.
Have these partnerships informed your knowledge of those in receipt of care, their carers, and their families? How have you utilized this knowledge to inform care planning or decisions about treatments?
What communication skills were necessary to engage in this way?
How might outcomes have differed?

....

Qualitative research has suggested that the relationship between professional and patient could be key to improved adherence (Vermeire et al., 2001; Gray et al., 2002). Indeed, Norman et al. (2007) found that patients reported better relationships with their NMP mental health nurse than with their psychiatrist. Some studies have been conducted to examine the outcomes of nurse prescribing in practice (Luker et al., 1998; Latter et al., 2004; Bradley and Nolan, 2007; Courtenay et al., 2009; Norman et al., 2010). Studies have found nurse prescribing to be safe and the independent prescribing role to be steadily increasing in areas in which it has previously been slow to develop (for example, mental health nurse prescribing). With respect to service user experiences of nurse prescribing, a number of studies have found patients to be satisfied with the care delivered by NMP. Courtenay et al. (2009) found that nurses spend longer with patients discussing medicines and feel more able to tailor prescribing decisions to needs of patients.

McEvoy (2004) found that patients particularly appreciated the practical support that they were offered during prescribing consultations with nurses, and felt that they had been offered more advice about their medication in a consultation with a nurse than they were in consultations with a doctor (ibid; cited in Courtenay et al., 2009). It has been suggested that this satisfaction stems from the different consultation style that nurses adopt when compared with doctors (ibid), with nurses being perceived as more approachable, better at listening, and more likely to offer support. Stenner and Courtenay (2008) suggest that the complete episode of care delivered by nurse prescribers enhances relationships with patients, enabling more effective communication and improved concordance. Government policy within the UK continues to increase the emphasis on treatment within the community rather than hospital settings for those with chronic health conditions (Department of Health, 2009b). This emphasis places responsibility on patients to self-manage their medication, and demands that patients are educated and informed about their medical regimens, as well as happy with the prescribing decisions being made in relation to their treatment.

Nurses have been found to adopt a holistic, individualized approach to prescribing (Stenner and Courtenay, 2008), and the value base of nurse prescribing could enhance patient choice and concordance (Jones and Jones, 2008). The ability of nurses to engage with patients, to make accurate assessments of need, and to form prescribing partnerships has been demonstrated in a number of studies, but largely undertaken from the perspective of nurses themselves rather than that of the patients (Brooks et al., 2001; Fisher and Vaughan-Cole, 2003; Bradley and Nolan, 2007; Jones et al., 2008; Courtenay et al., 2009). A critique of this new role in practice demonstrates that key elements underpinning the success of the role depend on the formation of a strong partnership with service users

(and carers), the ability of a prescribing professional to communicate well with the service user, and trust between the professional and patient (leading to better concordance, and potentially adherence, with medication). Communication style, the ability to form a 'prescribing partnership' with service users, and the ability to use this partnership to inform prescribing decision-making that fits with service user experience, social context, and health beliefs all demonstrate the importance of forming an effective partnership between healthcare professional and patient.

The ability to impart information in a way that is meaningful, and to be able to interpret responses from service users and carers and utilize these to inform care planning and prescribing decisions, is a skill that goes beyond prescribing knowledge and the attainment of prescribing competencies. There are many nursing roles that resemble the nurse prescribing role in that they require service users and carers to be fully engaged with care, and to have formed a partnership of care with the nurse and healthcare teams. However, the nurse prescribing role provides a good example of the specific impact that some of these partnership skills can have on service user satisfaction and, potentially, medication management.

Other examples of care partnerships in practice

Box 11.1 details another example of partnership working in relation to dementia care.

In **Practice Example 11.1**, we see an example of how partnerships of care are important at the individual level.

Building better partnerships with service users and carers

Service user involvement is increasingly promoted within health and social care practice and policy. **Figure 11.2** demonstrates that service users and carers should be at the centre of partnerships of care. This diagram implies that service users and their carers have a powerful influence, shaping both health and social care.

Box 11.1 Dementia care

There are estimated to be over 750,000 people with dementia in the UK and numbers are expected to double in the next thirty years in line with an increasingly ageing population. The government's *National Dementia Strategy* (Department of Health, 2009a) makes it clear that raising the quality of care for people with dementia and their carers is a major government priority. Partnerships of care are at the heart of the strategy, with the role of the Department of Health becoming that of an enabler of care, assuming less of a directive role in care provision. Indeed, the strategy, and accompanying quality outcomes document (Department of Health, 2010b), is directed specifically at health, social care, and delivery partners. Community personal support services—provided by a range of formal agencies, but also those providing informal care within the community—are integral to the strategy and essential to meet the four main priorities for care delivery (ibid):

- good quality early diagnosis and intervention for all;
- improved quality of care in general hospitals;
- living well with dementia in care homes; and
- reduced use of antipsychotic medication.

Partnership working, and the formation of effective care partnerships between those in receipt of care, informal carers, health care organizations, and social care organizations, as well as those providing services and care in the third sectors (voluntary and private sectors), is necessary to ensure effective information transfer as well as the delivery of optimal, personalized care.

PRACTICE EXAMPLE 11.1

Importance of good partnerships to individual patients

Jean is 58 years old and has worked for fifteen years as a health care assistant in a local residential home for young disabled adults. Jean has been married to James for thirty years, and they have three adult children and two grandchildren. All of their children live nearby in the town. Until last year, Jean had been fit and well, with no serious health problems.

Over the last year, her husband and colleagues at work have noticed that Jean is becoming increasingly forgetful, irritable, and increasingly withdrawn. At home, Jean is restless, arguing with her husband and children for no apparent reason. They have noticed that she keeps talking about the past, fixating on her mother who died over fifteen years ago.

Initially, Jean's GP treats her for depression, but after several months of medication, there are no improvements in her mood, memory, or behaviour. In fact, if anything, there is deterioration: Jean is no longer attending work and has lost interest in herself. Once a very self-conscious person, taking pride in her appearance and meticulous with her make-up and dress, these now seem to be neglected and of little significance. Together with her husband, Jean goes back to speak with her GP, who is worried about the rapid deterioration in her memory and behaviour. He carries out a mini mental state examination (MMSE). The GP is concerned with the score of 26, indicating that there may be some underlying memory loss.

He makes urgent referrals to the local memory clinic and a consultant psychiatrist for a more in-depth assessment.

1 Which partnerships of care are important for Jean and her family?
2 Which colleagues are central to Jean's care?
3 How would you facilitate good communication with Jean, her family, and with colleagues across the whole care pathway?

There is evidence that services developed in collaboration with service users and carers provide more effective, holistic services, better service outcomes, and improved skills of professionals, as well as promote better communication between professionals (Rummery, 2009).

PRACTICE TIP

When in practice, always remember that meeting the needs of the patient or service user and their primary carer(s) should be the priority determining care delivery.

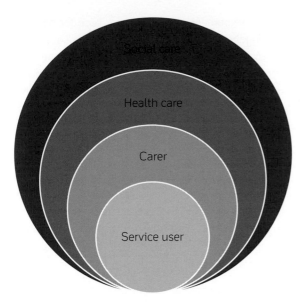

Figure 11.2 Service user involvement.

Furthermore, user involvement has been found to improve the skills and education of healthcare professionals. Some of the benefits seen from service user and carer involvement in service development work include (Cook et al., 2007):

- raising issues otherwise not seen as important;
- access to honest feedback from service users;
- sending messages to other service users and carers that their views are being considered;
- demonstrating what users and carers can contribute, thereby challenging stereotypes;
- fresh perspectives and skills; and
- a challenge to medical and illness models by bringing a vision of recovery and independent living.

Despite this, user involvement is undeveloped within the UK, particularly in those services dominated by health providers. This may be in part due to the relatively weak position of service users and carers in the service commissioning process (Repper and Breeze, 2007; Wendhausen, 2006, cited in Rummery, 2009), and is reflected in services not always reflecting the needs or priorities of service users and carers. Specific tensions seen from service user and carer involvement in service development work include (Cook et al., 2007):

- fear of losing identity as a user or carer;
- difficulties balancing corporate responsibilities with advocacy;
- feelings of not being respected as an equal by professional colleagues; and
- being the sole voice for users and carers, and a lack of support with practical issues such as admin and expenses.

Making partnerships of care work

Key individuals have a central role in making existing partnerships work (Hudson, 2007a; cited in Cook et al., 2007). However, as Chesterman et al. (2001; cited in Rummery, 2009) point out, it is difficult to link user satisfaction and outcomes generally to specific service inputs—and this can be problematic when encouraging, then sustaining, partnership working. It is important that users are increasingly seen as partners in the production and delivery of welfare (particularly health and social care services), but evidence suggests that the development of user involvement towards this requires significant investment (Truman, 2005; cited in Rummery, 2009). It has been suggested that the move towards increased service user involvement in feedback about services, but also service improvements and planning, has arisen from pressure on managers responsible for the delivery of care to provide 'evidence' about impact. Much of this evidence to date has been gathered directly from service users and carers, in the form of narrative about patient journeys and experiences of care. Although consultation of this kind represents a 'partnership' of sorts with service users and carers, there has been criticism from within the academic literature that this can also place pressure on service users and carers to be the providers of 'evidence', rather than exploring wider opportunities for service user and carer partnerships, as well as wider opportunities for the generation of appropriate evidence about service success (see Glasby and Beresford, 2007; cited in Rummery, 2009).

A number of steps can be followed in order to form partnerships with service users and carers and bring about change (Freeman et al., 2010):

1 Make the case for the need for change and gain support at an early stage.
2 Recruit a 'champion' at every level.
3 Form a team by identifying and assembling change agents into a working group.
4 Develop local projects with time-specific, measurable objectives related to a specific population, and select where positive outcomes and early wins can be achieved.
5 Track and evaluate change.

Examples of a range of social care partnerships in place across England are given in the Green Paper *Independent Well-Being and Choice: Our Vision for the Future of Social Care for Adults in England* (Department of Health, 2005), which also suggests a number of ways, encompassing strategic and supportive mechanisms, in which the government could support local working and voluntary and community engagement in social care provision.

Partnership working must be a means to an end, not an end in itself (Cook et al., 2007). Banks (2002) noted concerns that the narrow focus on partnerships to reduce pressure on the acute sector has limited the development of partnerships.

Developing the evidence base for partnership working

Rummery (2009) highlights the importance of including a wide range of outcome measures that reflect user priorities rather than simply measuring the effectiveness of input and output from commissioner or provider perspectives. The impact of the full involvement of service users and carers in research and evaluation work has yet to be assessed. Certainly, service users and carers derive satisfaction from involvement activities, but, as described earlier, the full impact of this involvement on the commissioning process and subsequent service development and delivery has been minimal. Theoretical approaches to developing the evidence, as derived from Pawson and Tilley (1997), are useful in considering

future development of the evidence base for partnership working, which could be considered a social programme of sorts. The efficacy and effectiveness of partnership working are difficult to answer within the experimentalist paradigm, which conceives of programmes as unified entities through which recipients are processed and contextual factors are conceptualized as confounding variables that should be controlled (Blamey and Mackenzie, 2007). With much partnership working, the contextual elements are key to the success of programmes, and context should be considered as part of any evaluation and be key to uncovering circumstances in which partnership working is successful (or unsuccessful). A realistic evaluation approach considers the adoption of four steps (ibid), including:

● understanding the aim of the programme in question;
● mapping out potential mini theories that relate the various contexts of a programme to the multiple mechanisms by which it might operate to produce different outcomes;
● building up a quantitative and qualitative picture of the programme in action; and
● exploring context, mechanism, and outcome, and developing tentative theories of what works for whom and in what circumstances.

In December 2009, the Department of Health published an update on work under way to develop new performance indicators for adult social care and health and social care partnerships. Proposed person-centred outcome themes for adult social care included 'quality of life', 'choice and control', 'health and well-being', 'inclusion and contribution', and 'dignity and safety', and the contextual difficulties involved in measuring outcomes from care partnerships were highlighted (Department of Health, 2009b). Further work was proposed for 2010 onwards.

Conclusion

This chapter has explored the importance of partnerships in care. It has highlighted that partnerships are fundamental to providing high-quality care across diverse care settings. The chapter demonstrates that partnerships of care exist across diverse sectors, whether public, private, or charitable. The chapter affirms that partnerships working involves all health-care professionals working collaboratively, communicating effectively with all involved in care delivery. Above all, the chapter underlines the need for the patient/client and their carers to be at the centre of all partnerships. They need to feel that they are equal partners, and their contribution to enhancing partnership working needs to be valued and accepted.

References

Banks, P. (2002) *Partnerships under Pressure: A Commentary on Progress in Partnership Working between the NHS and Local Government*, London: Kings Fund.

Berry, D., Courtenay, M., and Bersellini, E. (2006) 'Attitudes towards, and information needs in relation to, supplementary nurse prescribing in the UK', *Journal of Clinical Nursing* 15(1): 22–8.

Blamey, A. and Mackenzie, M. (2007) 'Theories of change and realistic evaluation: Peas in a pod or apples and oranges?', *Evaluation* 13: 439–55.

Bradley, E.J. and Nolan, P. (2007) 'A qualitative study to investigate the impact of nurse prescribing in the UK', *Journal of Advanced Nursing* 59(2): 120–7.

Brooks, N., Otway, C., Rashid, C., Kilty, E., and Maggs, C. (2001) 'The patients' view: The benefits and limitations of nurse prescribing', *British Journal of Community Nursing* 6(7): 892–909.

Butt, G., Markle-Reid, M., and Browne, G. (2008) 'Interprofessional partnerships in chronic illness care: A conceptual model for measuring partnership effectiveness', *International Journal of Integrated Care* 8: 1–14.

Cook, A., Petch, A., Glendinning, C., and Glasby, J. (2007) 'Building capacity in health and social care partnerships: Key messages from a multi-stakeholder network', *Journal of Integrated Care* 15(4): 3–10.

Courtenay, M., Carey, N., and Stenner, K. (2009) 'Nurse prescriber–patient consultations', *Journal of Advanced Nursing* 65(5): 1207–17.

De Civita, M. and Dasgupta, K. (2007) 'Using diffusion of innovations theory to guide diabetes management program development: An illustrative example', *Journal of Public Health* 29(3): 263–8.

Department of Health (1997) *The New NHS: Modern, Dependable*, London: HMSO.

Department of Health (1999) *National Service Framework for Mental Health: Modern Standards and Service Models*, London: HMSO.

Department of Health (2000) *The NHS Plan: A Plan for Investment, a Plan for Reform*, London: HMSO.

Department of Health (2001) *Shifting the Balance of Power within the NHS: Securing Delivery*, London: HMSO.

Department of Health (2005) *Independent Well-Being and Choice: Our Vision for the Future of Social Care for Adults in England*, London: HMSO.

Department of Health (2006) *Our Health, Our Care, Our Say: A New Direction for Community Services*, London: HMSO.

Department of Health (2009a) *Living Well with Dementia: A National Dementia Strategy*, London: HMSO.

Department of Health (2009b) *Making Policy Count: Developing Performance Indicators for Health and Social Care Partnerships*, London: HMSO.

Department of Health (2010a) *Equity and Excellence: Liberating the NHS,* London: HMSO.

Department of Health (2010b) *Quality Outcomes for People with Dementia: Building on the Work of the National Dementia Strategy*, London: HMSO.

Doran, T.T., Drewer, F., and Whitehead, M. (2003) 'Health of young and elderly informal carers: Analysis of UK census data', *British Medical Journal* 327(7428), available online at **http://www.bmj.com/content/327/7428/1388.full** [accessed 11 July 2011].

Dowling, B., Powell, M., and Glendinning, C. (2004) 'Conceptualising successful partnerships', *Health and Social Care in the Community* 12(4): 309–17.

England, E. and Lester, H. (2005) 'Integrated mental health services in England: A policy paradox?', *International Journal of Integrated Care* 5(3): 1–8.

Fisher, S. and Vaughan-Cole, B. (2003) 'Similarities and differences in clients treated and in medications prescribed by APRNs and psychiatrists in a CMHC', *Psychiatric Nursing* 17(3): 101–7.

Freeman, E., Presley-Cantrell, L., Edwards, V., White-Cooper, S.H., Thompson, K., Sturgis, S., and Croft, J. (2010) 'Garnering partnerships to bridge gaps among mental health, healthcare and public health', *Preventing Chronic Disease* 7(1), available online at **http://www.cdc.**

gov/pcd/issues/2010/jan/09_0127.htm [accessed 16 June 2011].

Giddens, A. (1998) *The Third Way: A Renewal of Social Democracy*, Cambridge: Polity Press.

Gray, R., Parr, A., and Brimblecombe, J. (2005) 'Mental health nurses supplementary prescribing: Mapping progress', *Psychiatric Bulletin* 29: 295–7.

Gray, R., Robson, D., and Berssington, D. (2002) 'Medication management for people with a diagnosis of schizophrenia', *Nursing Times* 98(47): 38–40.

Harvey, D. (2007) *A Brief History of Neoliberalism,* Oxford: Oxford University Press.

Haynes, R., Ackloo, E., Sahota, N., McDonald, H., and Yao, S. (2008) 'Interventions for enhancing medication adherence', *Cochrane Database System Review* 16(2): CD000011.

Hemingway, S. and Ely, V. (2009) 'Prescribing by mental health nurses: The UK perspective', *Perspectives in Psychiatric Care* 45(1): 24–35.

Jones, A. and Jones, M. (2008) 'Choice as an intervention to promote well-being', *Journal of Psychiatric and Mental Health Nursing* 15: 75–81.

Lacro, J., Dunn, L., Dobler, C., Leckband, S., and Jeste, D. (2002) 'Prevalence of and risk factors for medication non-adherence in patients with schizophrenia', *Journal of Clinical Psychiatry* 63(10): 892–909.

Latter, S., Marben, J., Myal, M., Courtenay, M., Young, A., and Dunn, N. (2004) *An Evaluation of Extended Formulary Independent Nurse Prescribing: Final Report*, Southampton: University of Southampton.

Lieberman, J., Stroup, T., McEvoy, M., and Swartz, M. (2005) 'Effects of anti-psychotic drugs in patients with chronic schizophrenia', *The New England Journal of Medicine* 353(12): 1209–23.

Luker, K., Austin, L., Hogg, C., Ferguson, B., and Smith, K. (1998) 'Nurse–patient relationships: The context of nurse prescribing', *Journal of Advanced Nursing* 28: 235–42.

McEvoy, M. (2004) 'Support from our sponsors', *Dermatological Nursing* 3(1): 5–6.

Nolan, P. and Bradley, E.J. (2007) 'The role of the nurse prescriber: The views of mental health and non-mental health nurses', *Journal of Psychiatric and Mental Health Nursing* 14: 258–66.

Norman, I., Coster, S., McCrone, P., Sibley, A., and Whittlesea, C. (2010) 'A comparison of the clinical effectiveness and costs of mental health nurse supplementary prescribing and independent medical prescribing: A post-test control group study', *BMC Health Services Research* 10(4), available online at **http://www.ncbi.nlm.nih.gov/pubmed/20051131** [accessed 16 June 2011].

Norman, I., While, A., Whittlesea, C., Costar, S., Sibley, A., Rosenbloom, K., McCrone, P., Faulkner, A., and Wade, T. (2007) *Evaluation of Mental Health Nurses Supplementary Prescribing*, London: Division of Health and Social Care Research.

Office for National Statistics (2001) '2001 Census output programme: As it happened', available online at **http://www.statistics.gov.uk/census2001/op.asp** [accessed 11 July 2011].

Pawson, R. and Tilley, N. (1997) *Realistic Evaluation*, London: Sage.

Repper, J. and Breeze, J. (2007) 'User and carer involvement in the training and education of health professionals', *International Journal of Nursing Studies* 44(3): 511–19.

Rummery, K. (2009) 'Healthy partnerships, healthy citizens? An international review of partnerships in health and social care and patient/user outcomes', *Social Science and Medicine* 69: 1797–804.

Stenner, K. and Courtenay, M. (2008) 'Benefits of nurse prescribing for patients in pain', *Journal of Advanced Nursing* 63(1): 27–35.

Vermeire, E., Hearnshaw, H., Van Royen, P., and Denekeris, J. (2001) 'Patient adherence to treatment: Three decades of research—A comprehensive review', *Journal of Clinical Pharmacy and Therapeutics* 26: 331–42.

Von Korff, M., Gruman, J., Schaefer, J., Curry, S., and Wagner, E.H. (1997) 'Collaborative management of chronic illness', *Annals of Internal Medicine* 127: 1097–102.

Williams, A. and Jones, M. (2006) 'Patients' assessments of consulting a nurse practitioner', *Journal of Advanced Nursing* 53: 188–95.

Zygmunt, A., Olfson, M., Boyer, C. and Mechanic, D. (2002) 'Interventions to improve medication adherence in schizophrenics', *American Journal of Psychiatry* 159(10): 153–64.

12 Caring in challenging circumstances

KAREN BREESE AND HELEN HAMPSON

Learning outcomes

This chapter will enable you to:

- describe what is meant by the term 'challenging circumstances';
- recognize who may be considered a vulnerable person;
- recognize the differences between safeguarding and protection;
- be aware of the different types of neglect, abuse, and cruelty;
- identify the measures required to protect the vulnerable person;
- reflect on the assumptions made about the way in which vulnerable people communicate when they are in pain or distress; and
- recognize that end-of-life care is difficult for the dying person, their families and friends, and all staff concerned with their care.

Introduction

This chapter is designed to enable you to feel more confident when caring in challenging circumstances. Nurses throughout the course of their practice encounter difficult and challenging situations; these may involve supporting individuals after receiving bad news or those who are dying. These situations can be very hard for nurses to address and manage. This chapter builds on Chapter 2, which provided excellent advice on how to deal with the challenges and opportunities faced in nursing, offering strategies to manage these personally and professionally. This chapter draws on knowledge and skills presented throughout Parts 1 and 2 to enable readers to provide care in challenging situations.

This chapter will consider challenging circumstances, such as working with vulnerable people, breaking bad news, caring for the terminally ill and the dying, and supporting the bereaved. The chapter will demonstrate how you can support patients and their families at vulnerable times, introducing you to what is meant by safeguarding the patient. In addition, the chapter will assist you in recognizing pain and distress in vulnerable patients.

This chapter emphasizes that all patients should be treated as individuals with dignity and respect, upholding their right to privacy and confidentiality. This principle is paramount within codes of ethics and professional conduct for nurses (International Council of Nurses, 2006; Nursing and Midwifery Council, 2008), emphasizing that it is the duty of every nurse to protect vulnerable people in their care. It is important to remember that any individual can be vulnerable at some stage in their life and therefore, may be exposed to a violation of their dignity and, at the extreme, may be subjected to neglect or abuse (The Patients Association, 2009). Having any form of disability, being older or younger, or having a sensory impairment does not necessarily mean that an individual is vulnerable or will experience any form of neglect or abuse; neither will these vulnerable groups necessarily want to be viewed in this way, as the Human Rights Act 1998 explains.

In addition, we all experience points in our life that can make us vulnerable, especially when we or our loved ones receive a bad diagnosis or face terminal illness. There are some situations that are particularly challenging, such as caring for people receiving palliative or end-of-life care. However, the difficulties faced in relation to palliative and end-of-life care are often very complex, and none potentially more so than in the care of people with disabilities who may have multiple co-morbidities, complex pre-existing drug regimes and communication sensory impairments.

The chapter is designed to allow you to reflect on your practice and give you an insight into how you assess each patient with complex needs in a person-centred way.

Case studies within the chapter will enable you to reflect on your own actions when dealing with what can be often very difficult and challenging situations.

Essential knowledge and skills for care

● You must develop a thorough knowledge and understanding of what constitutes a challenging circumstance, recognizing signs of abuse, neglect, and cruelty, and taking reasonable steps to protect individuals from abuse.

● You must recognize the signs and causes of pain, distress, and discomfort in vulnerable patients, and accept the need to work with other healthcare professionals—especially where neglect, cruelty, or abuse are suspected.

● You will use appropriate and relevant communication skills to deal with difficult and challenging circumstances, such as responding to emergencies, unexpected occurrences, saying 'no', dealing with complaints, resolving disputes, de-escalating aggression, and conveying 'unwelcome' news.

● You will work collaboratively with other agencies to develop, implement, and monitor strategies to safeguard and protect individuals and groups who are in vulnerable situations.

Working in challenging situations

As outlined above, nurses work in a wide range of contexts and situations. Some of these situations may be very challenging in terms of the complex needs of the people requiring care and the environments in which nurses find themselves working.

....

Before proceeding with this chapter, we would like you to reflect upon the following question.
What do you understand by the term 'challenging circumstances'?

....

Your responses may have highlighted a number of challenging situations, such as:

● caring for a person with complex physical and psychological needs;
● looking after a confused patient;
● caring for a dying patient and their family;
● having to support patients receiving bad news; and
● been exposed to anger and violence in any environment.

Your list of potential challenging circumstances might be much longer than this and you might have identified several different situations. The point that this exercise reveals is that nurses are exposed to challenging circumstances on a regular basis. There are a wide range of situations that will challenge and test the nurse's knowledge and caring skills. One of these may be recognizing patterns of abuse—perhaps even serial

Box 12.1 Groups of people identified as vulnerable

● Children
● Children with a learning disability
● Older people
● People with mental health problems, including confusion (which may be temporary or permanent), or dementia (which is variable and permanent)
● People with a physical disability
● People with a learning disability
● People with acquired brain damage
● People who misuse substances

abuse, in which individuals are sought and groomed by the perpetrator either sexually or financially.

....

Before proceeding, identify which groups of people may be considered vulnerable.

....

Your reflections may have identified a list of vulnerable groups. Some these may be similar to those presented in **Box 12.1**.

Definition of 'safeguarding'

'Safeguarding' can be defined as the process of protecting vulnerable adults from abuse and neglect, and of ensuring that their safety and well-being is assured and promoted.

Abuse

There are several recent publications and reports revealing that, in some circumstances, nurses are being accused of subjecting their patients to neglectful and cruel treatment and care (Patients Association, 2009; Mid Staffordshire NHS Foundation Trust Inquiry, 2009). Therefore there is a need for all nurses to have a clear understanding of what is meant by the term 'abuse'. The recent Francis Report (2009) highlighted and identified widespread institutional abuse carried out over a number of years. It is evident that, within the organization studied, many of the staff were unaware that they were abusing patients due to a lack of training and knowledge, and an institutional acceptance of bad practice. 'Abuse' is a violation of an individual's human and civil rights by any other person(s) (the alleged abuser). It may consist of a single act or repeated acts; it may be physical, verbal, or psychological; it may be an act of neglect or an omission to act; or it may occur when a vulnerable person is persuaded to enter into a financial or sexual transaction to which he or she has not consented or cannot consent.

No Secrets (Department of Health, 2000) provides guidance and support in helping local statutory agencies and other relevant agencies to come together in a coordinated way to prevent the abuse of vulnerable adults. The prime aim of all agencies is to prevent abuse whenever possible, but if this fails and abuse is suspected or has occurred, then stringent and effective procedures are in place and put into immediate action by the relevant agencies. Institutional abuse involves failure within an organization to provide adequate care or service to vulnerable people. This indicates a failure to ensure that safeguards are either in place and/or effective.

All types of abuse (physical, sexual, psychological, financial, neglect, and discrimination) can occur in a range of institutional settings. The Department of Health (2000) states that institutional abuse can also include repeated instances of poor care, poor professional practice, rigid routines, and an insufficient knowledge base within the service. Unacceptable treatments or programmes that include sanctions or punishment, such as withholding food or drink either intentionally or unintentionally, can be considered abuse. Similarly, the unnecessary and unauthorized use of control and restraint of the patient can also constitute abuse.

Types of abuse

The categories in **Box 12.2** are classed as different types of abuse and are some examples of abuse that you may encounter.

....

Reflect upon these and consider how these may apply to your own practice.

....

Protecting the public and ourselves

Adult protection is everyone's business and we all have a professional responsibility to recognize and take *immediate* action when abuse is either suspected or witnessed. Early recognition is vital in protecting the individual, because other individuals may be at risk.

The referral process must be instigated as soon as a concern is raised. Within the United Kingdom the referrer completes an Adult Protection Form 1 (APF1), which is then sent immediately to the relevant local authority social services, which agency in turn contacts the designated police officers for adult protection. A discussion

Box 12.2 Types of abuse

- **Physical**—including: hitting; slapping; pushing; kicking; scalding or burning; misuse of medication; being locked in a room; the use of inappropriate restraints; inappropriate sanctions; and force feeding
- **Psychological**—including: intimidation; humiliation; extortion; racial abuse; blackmail; deprivation of contact; coercion; harassment; threats of harm or abandonment; rejection; blaming; controlling; indifference; verbal abuse, including shouting or swearing
- **Sexual**—including: sexual assault; unwanted sexual attention; rape; sexual innuendo; sexual acts to which the vulnerable person has not consented or could not consent (if under the age of 16)
- **Financial**—including: theft; fraud; prevention of the appropriate purchase of care; pressure regarding wills or property; the withholding of money or the unauthorized or improper use of a person's money or property (usually to the disadvantage of the person to whom it belongs, such as borrowing money from a patient)
- **Neglect/acts of omission**—including: ignoring medical or physical care needs; a failure to provide access to appropriate health, social care, or educational service; the withholding of the necessities of life, such as medication, adequate nutrition, and heating; a failure to intervene in situations that are dangerous to the person concerned (particularly if that person lacks mental capacity)
- **Discrimination**—including: racism; ageist comments or jokes; comments and jokes based on a person's disability; other forms of harassment; slurs of character; not responding to dietary needs; or not providing spiritual support

then takes place between the two agencies as to which will lead the investigation into the alleged abuse.

If you have concerns that a person in your care is being abused by a colleague, then the referral process remains exactly the same. You should also refer to your organizational 'whistleblowing' policy, introduced under the Public Interest Disclosure Act 1998. The RCN has issued guidance for nurses on whistleblowing and it launched a whistleblowing helpline in May 2009.

We are responsible for protecting the individual in our care; under the 1998 Act, this includes identifying and reporting alleged abuse. The extent of the abuse is often not clear and it is your approach and open communication with the abused person, followed by reporting your concerns, that will begin the process of protecting the individual. Record-keeping and following internal guidelines are essential. Confidential patient information may need to be disclosed in the best interests of the vulnerable person (Department of Health, 1997). Information will only be shared on a need-to-know basis and it is inappropriate to give an absolute assurance of confidentiality (under the Data Protection Act 1998). Confidentiality must not, however, be confused with secrecy (Department of Health, 2000).

Protecting the vulnerable adult

Recognizing abuse and protecting the patient is an extremely challenging and stressful situation in which to be. As health professionals, we are all responsible and accountable for our actions (Dimond, 2005), including the identification and reporting of abuse. Early recognition is vital to ensuring that the patient is protected, especially because other patients/clients may be at risk.

Abuse may be clearly apparent, such as physical injuries that are visible, but it may only be suspected, or something may have occurred or been said or observed that raises concerns, as illustrated by **Practice Example 12.1**.

....

Try to imagine the emotions that an individual is going through when they have been abused.
Can you see this emotion in their face? Or is your intuition telling you something is wrong?
....

There are a range of different emotions that patients can display, many of which you may have identified. These are listed in **Table 12.1**, along with examples of how they may be displayed.

PRACTICE EXAMPLE 12.1

Safeguarding

Rose is a 29-year-old lady admitted to your ward following a fall. She has sustained a fracture of her ankle, which required internal fixation. Rose has a learning disability and mental health problems, but has maintained her independence in the community.

She lives with her older sister, Margaret, and Margaret's family. Margaret is her paid carer. On admission to the ward, Rose appears quite unkempt—particularly in relation to her own personal hygiene—and her clothes are old and worn. She appears very withdrawn and anxious.

Whilst on the ward, Rose is visited daily by her sister. You have asked for her to bring in some toiletries and personal belongings to make Rose's stay in hospital more comfortable. Rose also asks Margaret for some of her own money from home so that she can buy some chocolate. None of this arrives. During afternoon visiting, Margaret is heard shouting at Rose, who appears distraught and upset by this.

As professionals, we all come into contact with the patient's emotions, but to really understand and relate to their situations as individuals, we need to be able to understand and express our own emotions. Raising our own self-awareness and understanding of our own emotion can put us in a far better position to help others (Morrison and Burnard, 1991).

Table 12.1 Emotions that people can display

Emotion	Examples
Anger	Change of behaviour, or outburst of verbal or physical aggression Tense facial expression
Fear	Change of behaviour Anxiety May be triggered by certain people or events
Pain	May be very withdrawn or quiet, or only display a very small change in behaviour Alternatively, may be showing very obvious signs, such as crying and weight loss
Grief	Withdrawal from day-to-day activities Lack of interest in daily life Can see no future
Embarrassment	Change in behaviour May be quiet and unable to communicate, or withdrawn
Disgust	Low self-esteem Can develop into a depression
Sadness	May be demonstrated in facial expression and/or tears May be demonstrated in lack of interest in self or others

··

Reflect on the emotions that you experience and how you may portray them to others.

··

Dementia

Dementia has long been thought to be an inevitable illness affecting the older generation, and it has long been considered that little can be done to help the individual and carer. However, this perception of dementia and ageing is false. The National Dementia Strategy (Department of Health, 2009a) recognizes that this is an extremely vulnerable group of people, including the families and carers, who are often left unsupported.

The strategy outlines three key steps to improve the quality of life for people with dementia and their carers.

1 Ensure better knowledge of dementia, with a clear message that this is not an inevitable consequence of the ageing process and that a great deal can, in fact, be done to help sufferers and also their families/carers, and to improve the quality of their lives. This will involve better education and training for all professionals.

2 A correct and earlier diagnosis of dementia will ensure an earlier intervention, and an improvement in the quality of the lives of sufferers and their families/carers.

3 Develop a range of services for people with dementia and their carers that is accessible throughout the disease process.

See **Practice Example 12.2** for a case study.

As a nurse you will undoubtedly find yourself in similar situations in which you discover that patients in your care have not been diagnosed as suffering from varying degrees of dementia, and that their families or carers are not supported and are struggling to cope. It may well be that you meet the patient with dementia and their carers at a crisis point in their lives.

··

The National Dementia Strategy (Department of Health, 2009a)
Read the executive summary online at **http://www. dh.gov.uk/en/SocialCare/NationalDementia Strategy/index.htm**
How will the National Dementia Strategy promote an increased understanding of dementia, and what difference will it make to suffers and carers?

··

PRACTICE EXAMPLE 12.2

Dementia Care

Mr Price is 76 years old and has been admitted to hospital as an emergency patient suffering with abdominal pain, which the emergency doctor in the community suspects to be possible constipation. Mr Price is married and his wife arrives on the ward with him. On arrival, Mr Price appears particularly unkempt and has a poor standard of personal hygiene. He has, however, a very pleasant demeanour and, initially on admission, he appears to understand the reason why he is in hospital. Mrs Price, meanwhile, appears on edge and very tired.

The admitting nurse can sense Mrs Price's distress and is able to speak to her on her own while Mr Price is being examined by the doctor. Mrs Price admits to being at breaking point as she gives an account of how, over the last two years, her husband has seemed to have a change in personality and becomes aggressive with

her—particularly when she asks him to wash himself properly and change his clothes. He also seems to forget things very easily and this causes him to become very frustrated. At times, he appears low in mood.

Mrs Price has asked her husband to visit their own GP, but so far he has refused. She feels that his symptoms are part of growing old, but would welcome any help, because she feels that the situation is coming to a point at which she can no longer cope on her own.

The doctor examining Mr Price has asked several questions regarding his abdominal pain, and his past medical and social history. It soon becomes apparent that Mr Price is unable to recall some information, and is having difficulty trying to remember his home address and the year in which he was born.

What actions could have been taken prior to admission, during admission, and subsequent discharge?

Communication in difficult circumstances

A major component of care delivery is communication. For the purpose of this chapter, this is defined as an interchange of thoughts, feelings, and opinions among individuals (King, 1971). Chapter 9 gives a full account of communication and care; in this chapter, we specifically address communication in challenging circumstances.

Whether communication is verbal or non-verbal, it occurs during every encounter between a person and a nurse. There is often a general assumption that effective communication is achieved when open, two-way communication takes place, and when patients are informed about the nature of their illness and treatment, and are encouraged to express their anxieties and emotions.

In reality, though, the issue is much more complex and the key for all healthcare professionals is to be able to adapt the way in which they communicate to match the way in which the person communicates and their information needs at that time. In working with vulnerable adults, these challenges may be greater, depending on the cognitive ability, level of distress, and use of non-verbal communication; in palliative care, the expectation is that the healthcare professional will be able to discuss and cope with death and loss (Department of Health, 2010). Vulnerable adults are more likely to disclose their concerns to those who demonstrate that they are prepared to listen to them, and make them feel that what they have is important and that they are valued.

Elements of communication when working with vulnerable people

There are many different elements to communication (Porritt, 1984). When you consider that more than half of people with learning disabilities may present with some form of communication impairment (Kerr et al., 1996), the importance of communicating in a meaningful way becomes clear. This may be very challenging to many health and social care staff and to the families of those with the learning disability. Many people with a profound learning disability are unable to communicate verbally. However, this can also be seen in the general population as people get older: for example, in the effects of a stroke, in long-term conditions (an example would be motor neurone disease), and in terminal disease, such as cancers that affect the head, face, and throat, in dementia, and in the sensory impairments (loss of some hearing and vision) that can arise as people get older.

Many people with a more profound learning disability learn to use different ways of communicating (Granlund and Olsson, 1993; cited in Davies and Evans, 2001), for example through facial expression, head and body movement, and by making noises. We can use different tools to assist with communication for all patients groups: for example, *The Hospital Communication Book*, designed by Clear Communication People Ltd on behalf of Surrey Learning Disability Partnership Board (available online at **http://www.communicationpeople.co.uk/Hospital%20 Book.htm**).

Building a relationship with the person allows us to recognize and detect small changes that are vital to forming the basis of any pain assessments. Healthcare professionals may look at the individual without seeing the problem and attribute any changes in the person as part of their disability, not as evidence of pain or ill health. Accurate history-taking is crucial, and is best achieved by nurses and carers who have meaningful relationships with the people for whom they are caring, because they are skilled at recognizing and interpreting their methods of communication (Davies and Evans, 2001).

Understanding how and on what level the patient communicates is vital for all care. This will allow you to better appreciate their needs, and to build a relationship of trust with both the patient and carers. Sensory impairments can affect a vast majority of the population, as stated above, but are more commonly associated with people with disabilities.

> **PRACTICE TIP**
> Observation of the patient is a key point. Think about how the individual appears and look at their body language.

Points to consider for professionals, family, carers and patients are identified in **Table 12.2**. You may want to think about these when considering the issues arising in **Practice Example 12.3**.

Each situation and each individual will be very different, particularly when abuse has been witnessed or suspected. You should reflect on your actions (Schon, 1983) in order to improve the approach that you take with every patient, developing your skills and raising your self-awareness on how to communicate in all situations (Morrison and Burnard, 1991).

Communication in care situations

In terminal illness—for example, chronic obstructive pulmonary disease or degenerative diseases, such as dementia or motor neurone disease—the process of dying can be lengthy and dying people may find it difficult to talk at length or at all. Neurological damage may have caused impairment to their expression or may otherwise prevent communication. People who have had a stroke, brain tumours, or cancer that has spread to the brain, or who are suffering the effects of medication, may experience difficulties from day to day that may gradually become worse. Patients become frustrated when people assume (because of their illness) that they cannot understand, but, in fact, they can hear and understand, but their illness prevents them from communicating. Other things to be aware of are tracheotomies or patients who have had their tongues removed due to cancer. They may be unable to speak, but their understanding and perception will be retained. It will take you time to build relationships with such patients and to understand how they communicate.

Table 12.2 Points to consider for professionals, family, carers, and patients

Behaviour	Examples
Personal space	If intruded by another, can cause a person to feel uncomfortable Professionals should sit down facing the patient to allow all aspects of the communication to be seen by the patient
Eye contact	Contact indicates that you are listening and connecting with the individual Avoidance of contact can indicate discomfort or disinterest
Gestures and body movement	Illustrates speech and expresses emotion: • more movement can indicate anxiety • limited hand movement can indicate depression
Facial expressions	A great deal of information can be gleaned from the patient's face The patient may display many varied emotions, but do remember that some individuals are able to mask their emotions, for example by smiling and looking pleased to see someone, while thinking that they really do not want to see this person
Body posture and body contact	Shows emotions, attitude, and mood, and complements the words being spoken: • Arms folded and a leg crossed shows a defensive feeling • Touch can help to build trust and develop a caring relationship • Dying patients often feel the need for physical contact with carers NB Remember not to intrude into the personal space of those who are distressed

PRACTICE EXAMPLE 12.3

Communication in difficult circumstances

James is a 25-year-old man living with his parents and two younger siblings. James was born deaf and uses British sign language, Makaton, and gesture to make his needs known. He was referred to the health access team after being assessed at the local learning disability assessment and treatment unit for two weeks for his reluctance to eat and drink.

James has had periods of time in his life during which his behaviour became difficult to manage—particularly at school and college. This was linked to the frustrations that he had with communicating with staff through sign language and gesture. Although these periods had been resolved quickly, his community learning disability nurse and GP felt that a period of assessment at the inpatient unit would be an opportunity to complete a comprehensive assessment on both his health and behaviour.

After two weeks, James was taking almost nothing orally, so was admitted to the medical assessment unit at the local hospital. After investigations, he was found to have a large upper gastro-intestinal tumour. He had a stent and peg fitted. James and his family were told of his diagnosis and prognosis in a six-bedded bay of patients. He died four months later.

What do you think could have been done to improve the experience for James and his family?

At all times, you should create a non-threatening, supportive atmosphere, and ensure that interactions are such that dignity and respect are maintained.

Breaking bad news

Telling someone that they have a new health complication—such as a long-term condition, a terminal illness, or a change in their health—can be traumatic. It is even harder when you are breaking the news to someone who might not fully understand you, for example people with learning disabilities, people with dementia, or children. It is important to assess the patient's understanding and, where necessary, to use other forms of communication (picture, symbols gestures or prompts) to explain what you mean.

The discussions need to be carefully organized in terms of appropriate time set aside, the right venue, and the option of involving family or carers, if appropriate, who may be able to offer valuable support. A quiet setting away from noise and distractions can be a challenge in a ward setting, but remember that screens are not soundproof. The amount of information that you are going to give the patient about their condition may need to be guided by both the verbal and non-verbal cues and clues from the patient. Prior to starting, make sure that you have the right information in the correct format for the patient: in relation to people with cognitive impairment, think about communication aids, hearing devices, language (interpreter), the use of sign language or signs specific to that person, and cultural issues. When working with an individual with a cognitive impairment or varying capacity, you will also need to adhere to the guidance given by the Code of Practice under the Mental Capacity Act 2005.

Why do nurses not want to break bad news?

Many nurses comment that they often do not feel confident to break bad news or to talk to dying patients about their wishes and feelings. They comment that they do not have the right communication skills or the right words; they fear they may upset the patients or, in fact, themselves.

How we avoid breaking bad news

Often, not talking to someone indicates 'bad news', and the patient becomes aware of this from body language or avoidance. Blocking tactics were first identified by Quint (1967); over twenty years later,

Ellershaw and Wilkinson (2003) described a more comprehensive account of behaviours that are still being used to block communication. Many nurses are unaware that they have these behaviours and are using them in their daily practice (ibid).

....

Think about why we find it difficult to talk about dying.

....

These difficulties that we experience when trying to talk about dying derive from different sources, as listed in **Table 12.3**.

The dying process

A 'good death': the challenges

One of the first challenges to enable people to have a 'good death' is to remember that no two people will die in the same way. Therefore there is a need to acknowledge that, when an individual is dying, there is no 'standard' way in which all people will die. A second challenge is to prepare ourselves, and families and carers, for the dying process.

When patients enter the last few hours or days of their lives, there are specific challenges that, if not well addressed, will cause distress to the patient, family, and carers, and the healthcare professional. The Liverpool integrated care pathway for care of the dying patient is a process through which staff can support people who are dying, wherever they chose to do so (Ellershaw and Wilkinson, 2003; Department of Health, 2008).

A 'good death' is the ultimate challenge to every professional, but a very individual thing: what may be a good death to one person may not be to another. However, there is some consensus on what is perceived as a 'good death', as outlined in **Table 12.4**.

Table 12.3 Potential causes of difficulty in talking about dying

Social causes	A century ago, approximately 90 per cent of deaths occurred at home; for the last few decades, they have occurred in hospital or institutions. Increased access to health care has led to people living longer with long-term conditions and people are often not experiencing a death of a close family member until they are in their 40s. Our society is passing through a phase during which the process of death and dying causes fear and anxiety, and carers worry about not being able to cope or to deliver the correct care to a dying loved one.
Psychological causes	The fear of dying is not a single emotion, but can be any or all of many personal fears. How these emotions manifest is unique to each person. Common fears are of: • symptoms (pain, nausea, loss of mobility, side effects of treatments) • not coping (breakdown), dementia • religious/spiritual fear of the moment of death • finances, loss of job, status Caring for people who are dying may be stressful for the professional, involving: • sympathetic pain for the distress of the patent and family/carers • fear of being blamed (for delivering bad news itself or when the patient dies) • feeling unprepared, lacking in skill or confidence to cope with the dying person • not having all of the answers to questions we may be asked by dying patients and their families/carers

Table 12.4 Perceptions of a good death and a bad death

Perceptions of a good death	Perceptions of a bad death
Having family and friends around or choosing to be alone	Dying alone
Having time to say goodbye	Family or carers not getting there in time
Having symptoms controlled	Uncontrolled symptoms
Maintaining control over what is happening	A sudden terminal event, such as haemorrhage, or dying suddenly in a dining room or open area
Understanding the things that might happen during the dying process	Being alone and not understanding the dying process
High-quality care from compassionate staff	Feeling alone and in discomfort, and being inappropriately disturbed for unnecessary washes or interventions
Spiritual or religious preferences being recognized and addressed	Personal beliefs and spiritual preferences being ignored

How to work towards facilitating a good death for patients

When working towards a 'good death' for a patient, you must remember to involve the person, their family, and their carer(s) as much as possible in decision-making about treatments, plan of care, preferences and priorities, and place of death.

You must, however, remember that dying is a unique experience. As a healthcare professional, you are responsible for the care that you give to the patient and your perception of how a patient dies will be very personal to you.

Bereavement

Bereavement is a life event, and has been identified by models and stages through which people go (Kubler-Ross, 1969). The bereaved may pass through these different stages at different rates. The problem with some of the models is that they provide an approach to grieving that is too rigid a framework. They can be prescriptive rather than descriptive, which may lead people to think that this is how they *ought* to feel even if they do not, and they put time limits on people's emotions. The stages/phases identified usually begin with shock and disbelief, and move through to eventual recovery and reorganization.

Strobe and Schut (1998) suggest a dual-process model whereby people can move *across* the phases/stages. This focuses on the coping process, and can be seen as more flexible and appropriate to cultural differences. However, remember that people grieve in different ways, from those who show very few signs of intense grief, to those who are completely incapacitated by it. Some recover in a short space of time and others take much longer; some may go on with their daily lives, but be grieving while outwardly appearing to be living an ordinary life as prior to the bereavement.

Table 12.5 offers some points for supporting the family and carer(s) of a dying patient, or those who have been bereaved.

Table 12.5 Supporting the dying and bereaved

Time	Description
Before death—getting to know family/carers/friends	Make sure that someone is responsible for finding out about these important relationships in a person's life. Doing so will also highlight any special cultural religious or spiritual needs that the patient may have. Often, family/friends will have had a caring role for the patient and it is hard at times to hand over this role to other people; remember to involve them in the care plan and the care of their loved one if you are able to do so. Try to ensure that they have some time to sit and reflect on their feelings away from the patient, and that they are able to approach staff if they need to do so. Keep them informed and involved with all of the changes in the patient's condition—particularly if death is imminent.
At the moment of death	Try to have find out if family/carers/friends want to be present at the time of death: do they want to be called out even at night or do they want to be notified only by a call? If they want a call, do they want it at the time of death (even at night) or would they prefer a call in the morning? Clearly record this in the patient's notes or care of the dying pathway. Refer to information collected about the patient's special needs, religion, culture, or spirituality.
When a person has died	For bereaved family/carers/friends, time with the deceased person may need to be given. Time should be given for others to see the deceased if so desired. Be sensitive to those who do not wish to be with or view the deceased, but retain the living images that they have of that person. Offer time with the key member of staff who has been caring for that person, so that he or she can answer any queries or just talk about the deceased with the family/carers/friends. This will also give them the opportunity to talk about what happens next (death certificate, post mortem, registering the death, funeral planning, issues about property). Check if the bereaved person lives alone and ask if you can contact someone for him or her.

Care of people with a learning disability today

Valuing People: A New Strategy for Learning Disability for the 21st Century (Department of Health, 2001) was the first White Paper on learning disability published since *Better Services for the Mentally Handicapped* (Department of Health and Social Security, 1971). It has since been updated by *Valuing People Now* (Department of Health, 2009), driven by the views of people with learning disabilities, and their families and carers. It is rooted in the overarching aim of providing and delivering public services and support to meet individuals' needs.

Health challenges of vulnerable people with a learning disability

It is estimated that 2 per cent of the population has a learning disability (Kerr et al., 1996). Although people with a learning disability have the same health needs as the rest of the population, they might also have specific health needs, some of which are outlined in **Table 12.6**.

Table 12.6 Specific health needs

Illness	Risk
Respiratory disease	The leading cause of death for vulnerable people with a learning disability. Predominantly found in those more profoundly learning disabled and often linked to swallowing difficulties.
Coronary heart disease	Developing hypertension and obesity risk factors, leading to ischemic heart disease.
Cancer	Currently lower (at 13.6 per cent) than among the rest of the population (26 per cent). However, people with a learning disability have higher rates of gastrointestinal cancer (Gates, 2003).

Most people with a learning disability are now living with parent carers and in community residential settings. Therefore primary care is now the first point of access for these people and their carers. A recent report by Sir Jonathan Michael (Department of Health, 2008) demonstrated that people with learning disabilities do not always receive the standard of health care expected by the rest of the population. This has been found across both primary and secondary care services, and '*it can be seen as a widespread and systematic failure to meet the needs of this particular group*' (Gates, 2003: 28).

The Disability Rights Commission report *Equal Treatment: Closing the Gap* (DRC, 2006) identified inequalities for people with a learning disability and the problems encountered when these people try to access primary care. Conclusions from this report were that there was a lack of training, understanding, and disability awareness amongst healthcare professionals, and that this creates a significant barrier to health care for people with a profound learning disability—especially those who have limited or no verbal communication.

Challenging behaviour in care

Behaviour can be seen as challenging when it is of a level, frequency, or duration that it threatens the quality of life of the person and/or the physical safety of that person or others, and is likely to lead to a response from others around that is restrictive, aversive, or may result in exclusion.

Behaviour that can be viewed as challenging will vary from person to person, as can the reaction to it from health and social care staff. It is important that professionals making treatment decisions are guided by both law and professional guidelines. This is especially important when providing care to people with learning disabilities who present behavioural challenges regularly, and who are often marginalized and excluded from mainstream society, people with dementia, and those suffering a mental illness.

We see anger, verbal, and physical aggression from patients who are experiencing confusion, fear, and anxiety, and we may see acts of extreme violence resulting from emotion, substance misuse, or mental illness. This can test your skills and knowledge around communication with the person and carers.

The actions that can allow you to deliver care in many different types of situation include keeping up to date with legislation, attending mandatory training, and keeping abreast of developments in care through journals and articles. You must use your observation skills to assess people's moods and conditions, and listen and hear what carers are telling you about the person so that reasonable adjustments can be made to accommodate the needs of people who find certain environments and receiving care difficult, as in **Practice Example 12.4**.

PRACTICE EXAMPLE 12.4

Peter is 29 years old, and has a severe learning disability and autism. He lives in his own home, where a number of staff provided him with care 24 hours a day. He has no verbal communication, but will shout and put his head on people or furniture when happy or distressed. Routine and regular staff are of utmost importance to Peter.

1 If this man were presented to you on arrival on shift as an admission for that afternoon, what would you do to prepare for this?
2 What reasonable adjustments would you make for Peter and his carers?

Symptom management in vulnerable adults

Pain and distress in people with a learning disability

It is now widely recognized that how we sense and perceive pain is influenced by many variables. In fact, sense and perception of pain even varies within the same person at different times. Pain assessment in people without disabilities is based on the patient self-reporting the severity of pain (Davies and Evans, 2001). It can be also expressed through some of the behaviours listed in **Table 12.7**, some of which might recall behaviours that we encountered in **Practice Example 12.3**.

Unfortunately, there is very little literature that explores the difficulties of symptom recognition within this group of people. Skelekman and Malloy (1995) found that adult carers instinctively identified cues that corresponded with the common experience of people regarding the recognition of distress, suggesting that this seems to be an implicit rather than explicit act. Theil et al. (1986) 'identify these cues as being pieces of information that can be connected together to form patterns'. This 'pattern recognition' has been the missing step from much of the work to date on distress for people with severe communication difficulties. In palliative care, pattern recognition has been used since 1992 to produce clinical decision flow diagrams and protocols for communicating with patients with advanced diseases—mainly cancer (Reynard and Hockley, 2004). These cues appear to be changes in the usual behaviour observed when they are, or appear to be, content; carers are able to identify these changes, but they can also often disagree about their meaning (Porter et al., 2001).

Table 12.7 Behaviours and indicators

Behaviours	Indicators
A facial and bodily behaviour	Changes in expressions, use of eye contact (more or less, closed eyes), muscle tone, head turning, or banging
Social behaviour	Any change in behaviour, increase in physical movement, or withdrawal from world
An emotion	Crying, anger, fear, anxiety.
Cognition (at least to yourself)	Individuals may know what pain/distress is to them, but may not be able to express it

Identifying pain and distress in vulnerable adults

There are many misconceptions regarding pain and its existence, manifestations, and treatment. This is highlighted in a study by Twycross (2000; cited in Gates, 2003), which shows the limited teaching of pain assessment and management within learning disability pre-registration students. This can also be found in post-registration learning disability nurses and carers, who need to be aware of the variety of ways in which profound and multiple disabilities can generate specific pain experiences, as well as those brought on by ill health.

Pain assessment has long been the focus of attention for the nursing and medical professions, but there is a deficiency in the literature relating to people with disabilities and dementia. A large number of pain assessment tools have been produced (Braillie, 1993; Fuller and Neu, 2000; both cited in Davies and Evans, 2001) and they fall into three categories: self-reporting; behavioural measures; and biological measures. Many of these tools have been used or been designed to be used in relation to children rather than adults. The first category cannot be applied to people with a profound disability. It is also proposed that behavioural and physiological responses differ between adults and children, and likewise between those with or without disabilities (Gates, 2003).

It is often difficult to interpret the cause of distress in people with a learning disability or dementia. An increase of activity while in distress may be misinterpreted as challenging behaviour, whilst reduced activity may be wrongly interpreted as someone being quiet and content.

Often, professional carers find it difficult to estimate the patient's ability to communicate (Banat et al., 2002). Forty per cent of people with a severe learning disability have challenging behaviours (Ashcroft et al., 2001) and up to 45 per cent are on antipsychotic drugs (Ahmed et al., 2000), thus illustrating the importance of identifying and assessing the person's distress. This requires sensitivity to the person, as well as an awareness of ways in which we can manage their needs.

This sensitivity can be highlighted by ensuring that staff know the person with whom they are working. This level of awareness can be gained by liaising directly with the individual's next of kin or primary carer(s) to obtain valuable information about the needs and preferences of the person. It is about working in partnership with others to provide the best possible care. Stress can be identified through the use of a comprehensive assessment recognition tool, such as the DisDAT tool (Manfredi et al., 2003; cited in Regnard et al., 2007). There is also the Abbey pain scale, which can be also be used with people with dementia (Abbey et al., 2004).

....

Now take some time to reflect again on the Practice Examples.

What you would now do within your practice to improve the patients' and carers' experiences?

....

Conclusion

Throughout this chapter, the emphasis has been on vulnerable adults whom nurses meet on a daily basis in many different care settings. It is hoped that you will now be able to recognize different types of abuse and identify when patents are vulnerable. The chapter has also highlighted a number of situations that you may perceive as challenging within the current care environment. We hope that it has empowered you to take action to report any situations that you feel are bad practice. This chapter is only the beginning, and should be a foundation for further reading and training.

Many of the skills required to deal with difficult or challenging situations will come with experience and development throughout one's life. Everyone involved in delivering care has a responsibility to make it the best possible experience that they can for the patient, family, and carers. This, at times, will be a test of skills, resourcefulness, and resilience. The way in which you deal with each situation will remain with that patient, family, and carer for the rest of their lives.

It is also important to look after yourself: when in work, you are under a degree of stress from handling difficult situations, but some of this can be helped by knowing that you are working in an evidenced-based way and delivering best practice—and, most importantly, knowing when to ask for help, guidance, and support.

Further reading

Many employers have a whistleblowing policy—check to see if your employer has one.

RCN whistleblowing guidance
http://www.rcn.org.uk/development/publications/publicationsA-Z RCN members can call 0845 7726 300 if they have serious or immediate concerns about patient safety in their workplace

Elder Abuse
http://www.elderabuse.org.uk/About%20Abuse/What_is_abuse%20define.htm

Macmillan Cancer Support
http://be.macmillan.org.uk

Motor Neurone Disease Association
http://www.mndassociation.org

NHS National End-of-Life Care Programme
http://www.endoflifecareforadults.nhs.uk

National Council for Palliative Care
http://www.ncpc.org.uk

Valuing People Now
http://www.valuingpeoplenow.dh.gov.uk/

References

Abbey, J., Piller, N., De Bellis, A., Esterman, A., Parker, D., Giles, L., and Lowcay, B. (2004) 'The Abbey pain scale: A 1-minute numerical indicator for people with end-stage dementia', *International Journal of Palliative Nursing* 10(1): 6–13.

Ahmed, Z., Fraser, W., Kerr, M.P., Kiernan, C., Emerson, E., Robertson, J., Felce, D., Allen, D., Baxter, H., and Thomas, J. (2000) 'Reducing antipsychotic education in people with learning disability', *British Journal of Psychiatry* 176(1): 42–6.

Ashcroft, R., Fraser, B., Kerr, M., and Ahmed, Z. (2001) 'Are antipsychotic drugs the right treatment for challenging behaviour in learning disability? The place of randomised trials', *Journal of Medical Ethics* 27(5): 338–43.

Banat, D., Summers, S., and Pring, T. (2002) 'An investigation into carers' perception of the verbal comprehension ability of adults with severe learning disabilities', *British Journal of Developmental Disabilities* 30(2): 78–81.

Davies, D. and Evans, L. (2001) 'Assessing pain in people with profound learning disabilities', *British Journal of Nursing* 10(8): 513–16.

Department of Health (1971) *Better Service for Mentally Handicapped People*, London: HMSO.

Department of Health (1997) *Report on the Review of Patient-Identifiable Information*, London: HMSO ('the Caldicott Report').

Department of Health (1998) *The Public Disclosure Act 1998: Whistleblowing in the NHS*, London: HMSO.

Department of Health (2000) *No Secrets: Guidance on Developing and Implementing Multi-Agency Policies and Procedures to Protect Vulnerable Adults from Abuse*, London: HMSO.

Department of Health (2001) *Valuing People: A New Strategy for Learning Disability for the 21st Century*, London: HMSO.

Department of Health (2007) *Promoting Equality: Response from Department of Health to the Disability Rights Commission Report,* Equal Treatment: Closing the Gap—*Information for Practitioners*, London: HMSO.

Department of Health (2008) *End-of-Life Care Strategy: Promoting High Quality Care for all Adults at the End of Life*, London: HMSO.

Department of Health (2009a) *Living Well with Dementia: A National Dementia Strategy*, London: HMSO.

Department of Health (2009b) *Valuing People Now: A New Three-Year Strategy for People with Learning Disabilities—Making it Happen for Everyone*, London: HMSO.

Dimond, B. (2005) *Legal Aspects of Nursing*, 4th edn, London: Pearson Education.

Disability Rights Commission (2006) *Equal Treatment: Closing the Gap—A Formal Investigation into the Physical Health Inequalities Experienced by People with Learning Disabilities and/or Mental Health Problems*, Stratford: DRC.

Ellershaw, E. and Wilkinson, S. (2003) *Care of the Dying: A Pathway to Excellence*, Oxford: Oxford University Press.

Gates, B. (2003) *Towards Inclusion*, 4th edn, London: Churchill Livingstone.

Independent Inquiry into Access to Healthcare for People with Learning Disabilities (2008) *Healthcare for All: Report of the Independent Inquiry into Access to Health-care for People with Learning Disabilities*, available online at **http://www.dh.gov.uk/en/Publicationsandstatistics/Publications/PublicationsPolicyAndGuidance/DH_099255** [accessed 16 June 2011].

International Council of Nurses (2006) *The ICN Code of Ethics for Nurses*, Geneva: ICN.

Kerr, M., Fraser, W., and Felce, D. (1996) 'Primary health-care needs for people with a learning disability', *British Journal of Learning Disabilities* 24: 2–8.

King, I.M. (1971).*Towards a Theory of Nursing*, New York: John Wiley & Sons.

Kubler-Ross, E. (1969) *On Death and Dying*, New York: Macmillan.

Mid Staffordshire NHS Foundation Trust Inquiry (2009) *Independent Inquiry into Care Provided by Mid Staffordshire NHS Foundation Trust January 2005—March 2009, Vols I and II*, London: HMSO (the 'Francis Report').

Morrison, P. and Burnard, P. (1991) *Caring and Communicating: The Interpersonal Relationship in Nursing*, London: Macmillan education Ltd.

Nursing and Midwifery Council (2008) *The Code*, London, NMC.

Nursing and Midwifery Council (2009) *Guidance for the Care of Older People*, London: NMC.

Open University (1994) *Death and Dying: Workbook 4—Bereavement: Private Grief and Collective Responsibility*, Milton Keynes: Open University Press.

Patients Association, The (2009) *Patients ... not Numbers, People ... not Statistics*, available online at **http://www.patients-association.com/DBIMGS/file/Patients%20not%20numbers,%20people%20not%20statistics(1).pdf** [accessed 16 June 2011].

Porritt, L. (1984) *Communication Choices for Nurses*, London: Churchill Livingstone.

Porter, J., Ourvry, C., Morgan, M., and Downes, C. (2001) 'Interpreting the communication of people with profound and multiple intellectual disabilities', *British Journal of Learning Disabilities* 29(1): 12–16.

Quint, J.C. (1967) *The Nurse and the Dying Patient*, New York: Macmillan.

Read, S. (2006) (ed) *Palliative Care for People with Learning Disabilities*, London: Quay Books.

Read, S. and Elliott, D. (2006) 'Care planning in palliative care for people with learning disability', in B. Gates (ed.) *Care Planning and Delivery in Intellectual Disability Nursing*, Oxford: Blackwell Publishing, pp. 195–211.

Regnard, C. and Hockley, J. (2004) (eds) *Guide to Symptom Relief in Palliative Care*, 5th edn, Oxford: Radcliffe Medical Press.

Regnard, C., Reynolds, J., Watson, W., Matthews, D., Gibson, L., and Clarke, C. (2007) 'Understanding distress in people with severe communication difficulties: Developing and assessing the Disability Distress Assessment Tool (DisDat)', *Journal of Intellectual Research* 51(4): 277–92.

Royal College of Nursing (2006) *Meeting the Health Needs of People with Learning Disabilities: Guidance for Nursing Staff*, London: RCN.

Schon, D.A. (1983) *Educating the Reflective Practitioner*, San Francisco, CA: Jossey Bass.

Skelekman, J. and Mallory, E. (1995) 'Difficulties in symptom recognition in infants', *Journal of Paediatric Nursing* 10(2): 89–92.

Strobe, M. and Schut, H. (1998) 'Culture and grief', *Bereavement Care* 17(1): 7–10.

Theil, J., Baltwin, J., Hyde, R., Sloan, B., and Strandquist, G. (1986) 'An investigation of decision theory: What are the effects of teaching cue recognition?', *Journal of Nursing Education* 25: 319–24.

Part 4: Evaluating care

13 Leading, managing, and celebrating care

SAM FOSTER

Learning objectives

This chapter will enable you to:

- review the professional and political drivers behind the importance of leadership in the nursing profession;
- recognize the importance of leadership and management in nursing, which lead to the delivery of quality care;
- review and learn lessons from two high-profile case studies in which poor standards of nursing care were highlighted as contributing to the overall failure of the individual trust to provide quality patient care; and
- recognize the value of celebrating good quality nursing care.

Introduction

This chapter will discuss the key political and professional drivers that have identified the importance of leadership in nursing in order to deliver quality nursing care. It will build on the previous chapter in identifying what the core elements to quality care are, and how they can be driven and led by the nursing community. Two case studies will be used to enable the reader to explore and reflect on elements of care delivery, and on their own ability to lead and manage care, highlighting how this develops towards the point of registration. The chapter will conclude by asking why and how nursing care should be rewarded and celebrated.

Throughout this chapter, the reader will gain an understanding of the importance of leadership at every level of care delivery, by mapping elements of both professional guidance and prerequisites to successful entry as registrants. It will become increasingly evident to the reader that leading and managing care is of fundamental importance in nursing. Leadership and management skills are referenced throughout both the Nursing and Midwifery Council's Code (NMC, 2008), and its *Guidance on Professional Conduct for Nursing and Midwifery Students* (NMC, 2009). There are also

Essential knowledge and skills for care

- You must have an awareness of the importance of using leadership skills to supervise and manage others, and to contribute to planning, designing, delivering, and improving future services.

- You must be prepared to act as an agent of change and to provide leadership through quality improvement and service development to enhance people's well-being and experiences of health care.

- You will have a knowledge and understanding of the need to work with service users, carers, other professionals, and agencies to shape future services, aid recovery, and challenge discrimination and inequality.

- You will be flexible and respond to change, reflecting positively and constructively on practice, for example sharing complaints, compliments, and comments with the team in order to improve and enhance care.

many references identifying nurses' levels of account-ability to their patients. In addition to this, leading and managing care is a clear thread throughout the NMC essential skills clusters (NMC, 2007).

Recent developments

In recent times, nursing has been seen to play a key role in effectively leading, managing, and celebrating care. This chapter will enable you to review the key drivers, along with two damaging national inquiries in the UK that have given new and urgent direction to shaping the National Health Service. These inquiries have shifted the priority from increasing access and capacity, towards the vision set out in a speech made by the Secretary of State for Health in June 2010, who stated that the NHS is now firmly focused on '*The best care for each patient and the best outcome for all patients*' (Lansley, 2010).

In 2008 and 2009, two major reviews of the UK healthcare system and of the nurse's role within this were undertaken. In 2008, the Department of Health published *High Quality Care for All* (Department of Health, 2008a), a review by Lord Darzi, a practicing surgeon, who defined 'quality of care' as clinically effective, personal, and safe. This means protecting patient safety by eradicating healthcare-acquired infections and avoidable accidents. It is about effec-tiveness of care, from the clinical procedure that the patient receives, to their quality of life after treatment. It is also about the patient's entire experience of the NHS and ensuring that they are treated with compas-sion, dignity, and respect in a clean, safe, and well-managed environment. Lord Darzi's review also highlighted the 'centrality of nursing' to improving care.

In March 2010, then Prime Minister Gordon Brown launched the first full-scale review of nursing for nearly forty years. The Prime Minister's Commission on the Future of Nursing and Midwifery in England (2010) was established to explore how both the nursing and mid-wifery professions could be empowered to take a cen-tral role in the design and delivery of twenty-first-century services in England.

You may, at this point, also reflect on what has happened to nursing and midwifery professions globally.

The Commission's terms of reference instructed that it should identify the competencies, skills, and support that front-line nurses and midwives needed to enable them to take a central role in the design and delivery of future services. The Commission was asked to identify any barriers that impede the pivotal role played by ward sisters, charge nurses, and community team leaders (the role of ward leaders will be explored further in this chapter.)

The Darzi Review (Department of Health, 2008a) proposed that all providers of healthcare services should produce a quality account—that is, an annual report to the public about the quality of services deliv-ered. The aim of quality accounts is to strengthen accountability to the public and to further engage the leaders of organizations in their quality improve-ment agenda. The Health Act 2009 then placed the requirement to produce quality accounts on a statu-tory footing, which means that NHS organizations are now required by law to produce quality accounts.

From June 2010, all trust boards were required to publish their quality accounts. The accounts aim to include trust boards' top priorities for improvement and measures describing their quality of care.

Today, every hospital NHS trust has on the trust board a chief nurse or director of nursing who is accountable for providing assurance that quality nurs-ing care is delivered. In a survey by West et al. (2010), more than half of the measures chosen by hospital trusts to demonstrate their quality of care were found to be nursing indicators. West analysed the quality accounts of twenty-five randomly selected acute trusts and found that 55 per cent of the measures of quality chosen by the trusts and 47 per cent of the priorities were strongly related to nursing. In total, the twenty-five trusts set out 133 priorities and 118 measures of quality. The finding suggests the importance of nurs-ing to quality improvement, indicating that this has seized the attention of trust boards. The top six meas-ures are detailed in **Box 13.1**.

Box 13.1 Nurse-related outcome measures commonly chosen by trusts for quality accounts (West et al., 2010)

- Falls—occurrence or prevention
- Infection control and healthcare-associated infection—occurrence
- Incident numbers/reporting rates
- Patient observations/deterioration prevention
- Patient experience/satisfaction measures
- Pressure ulcers—incidence or prevention

What role can nurses play in ensuring that the quality accounts demonstrate quality care?

Political and professional drivers

This section aims to review the drivers that have identified the importance of leadership in the nursing profession. Leadership in nursing has evolved: the role of the matron disappeared from the NHS following a report in 1966 by the Committee on Senior Nurse Staffing Structures (cited in Department of Health, 2002). Further changes in leading and managing care resulted from the introduction of a general management model into the NHS in the 1980s; the introduction of general managers could be viewed as questioning the role of the nurse in leading and managing care.

In the late 1990s, patients and the public were consulted about how the NHS could be improved. One of the strong views was a call for the return of a matron figure—a strong clinical leader with clear authority at ward level. Matrons have also been introduced within community nursing. In response to the public consultation, the NHS Plan (Department of Health, 2000) made a commitment to introduce modern matrons—senior sisters and charge nurses—with the expectation that they would be easily identifiable to patients, and would have the authority and support that they need to make sure that the fundamentals of care are right. Having read through the different chapters in this book, you

will be starting to identify the themes of activities that are recognized to be termed 'basic' or 'fundamental' elements of care. The Royal College of Nursing (RCN) subsequently led an action research study in the 1990s to identify the key factors for high standards of hospital ward nursing care. This study confirmed the role and leadership of the ward sister as absolutely fundamental (Cunningham and Kitson, 2000).

As an outcome of this and other evaluations, the RCN developed a clinical leadership programme, which focused on effective leadership development and support for the ward sister level of nursing. This programme was a welcome development for those individuals who were able to attend, but the role of the ward sister had not, at that time, received the focus and level of professional attention that perhaps it deserved. The findings from these initiatives, while focused on ward-based leadership, have implications for those leading nursing care in diverse care setting.

Why leadership is important

Before proceeding with the remainder of this chapter, reflect on Practice Example 13.1.
What aspects of this situation might have been attributed to poor nursing management and leadership?

Practice Example 13.1 highlights the crucial role that leadership plays in the delivery of nursing care. The lack of management and leadership are central themes in this case study. There seems to be a catalogue of issues that could have been prevented by good nursing management and leadership. For this reason, there is a need to explore how leadership within nursing has evolved and changed within the nursing profession.

Modern matrons

In 2001, a Department of Health, Health Service Circular (2001/010) entitled *Implementing the NHS Plan: Modern Matrons* was issued. It contained guidance for NHS organizations and identified the three main strands of the matron role outlined in **Box 13.2**.

PRACTICE EXAMPLE 13.1

Investigation into outbreaks of Clostridium difficile at Maidstone and Tunbridge Wells NHS Trust, October 2007

The Healthcare Commission (2007) carried out an investigation to look into outbreaks of Clostridium difficile (C. difficile) at Maidstone and Tunbridge Wells NHS Trust and to assess the care provided to patients with this infection. It also considered whether the trust's systems and processes for the identification, prevention, and control of infection were adequate. This followed an unrecognized outbreak during which 150 patients were affected and a number died, for which C. difficile was definitely or probably the main cause of death.

C. difficile typically causes significant loss of fluid and electrolytes, and this can lead to serious complications. The reviewers felt that poor fluid management, for example where there was no evidence of regular assessments and management of fluid and electrolyte losses after diagnosis, was a cause for concern in eighteen out of fifty patients (36 per cent). Most commonly, this was because there was no evidence of regular assessment of fluid and electrolyte status by the doctors in the clinical notes or through blood tests, or because fluid charts could not be found or were not properly completed.

The reviewers used a standardized pro forma to look at the following aspects of the management of C. difficile infection:

- the general management of C. difficile infection, including the involvement of specialists; and
- the prescription of antibiotics.

The fifty cases were selected by random sampling from a list of the 274 people who had a positive laboratory diagnosis of C. difficile, who died in hospital at the trust between April 2004 and June 2006, and who had information on their illnesses. The review considered:

- the management of fluid balance;
- the timeliness of treatment;
- the management of nutritional status;
- the assessment and management of severe C. difficile disease; and
- resuscitation status.

In addition to this, the views of the families on the failure to deliver quality care resulted in the following comments being published.

- 'The patients were left in their excrement for long periods.'
- There was a failure to:
  - 'respond promptly to call bells, to assist patients to go to the toilet or use a commode, to help with patient hygiene';
  - 'respond appropriately, as when instructing patients to go in the bed';
  - 'respect the privacy and dignity of patients';
  - 'give medication promptly and appropriately';
  - 'help with feeding and drinking';
  - 'take proper precautions to prevent spread of infection'.

The twenty-six patients and families who contacted the Healthcare Commission reported some of the same concerns as the reviewers about the care of patients infected with C. difficile; many attributed much of the poor care to the shortage of nurses and talked of seeing exhausted nurses in despair, with their heads in their hands. However, others talked about poor attitude of some staff, including agency nurses. They described instances of nurses shouting at patients, leaving them unattended for hours, and not providing a proper level of care or observation.

Some of the families felt that raising their worries led to no improvement. One family was very concerned that, after the sister on the ward had reprimanded a nurse for a further error in giving medication to their relative, they were seen 'laughing and joking' together five minutes later. This gave the impression that the matter had not been taken seriously by the perceived leader and manager. This example illustrates the importance that good leadership can have on the public's perceptions of care and the overall quality of care provided.

In addition to all of the above, the overwhelming majority of relatives and patients who contacted the Healthcare Commission were not happy with the nursing care received at the trust. Words used by a few included 'despicable', 'sickening', 'appalling', and 'chaotic'.

The Healthcare Commission (2007)

Box 13.2   Top three key deliverables of the matron (Department of Health, 2001)

- Providing leadership to professional and direct care staff in their group of wards to *'secure and assure the highest standards of clinical care'*
- Ensuring the availability of appropriate administrative and support services in their group of wards
- Providing a *'visible, accessible and authoritative presence in ward settings to whom patients and their families can turn for assistance, advice and support'*

Since the NHS Plan (Department of Health, 2000), there have been several policy drivers and consultations focusing on strengthening nurse leadership. In 2002, the Department of Health published a progress report on the introduction of the modern matron, which reported that, by April 2002, there were nearly 1,900 nurses in modern matron posts across the NHS in England (the implementation of the modern matron also applied to other UK countries)—nearly four times as many as originally envisaged (Department of Health, 2002). Over the following years, the NHS embraced the role of the modern matron; publicly, this was viewed as highly successful, but how effective these posts were had not yet been evaluated.

In 2004, Read and Ashman (on behalf of the University of Sheffield School of Nursing and Midwifery), and Scott and Savage (on behalf of the RCN Institute), undertook an evaluation of the modern matron role. They found that the role had essentially been implemented in three styles (Read et al., 2004):

- *the essentially clinical model*—this had some similarities to the 'senior sister' role; involvement in clinical activity may vary, from undertaking rostered duties, to doing occasional 'hands-on' shifts;
- *the essentially managerial mode*—this has some similarities to the 'nursing officer' role and is more remote from the clinical area;
- *the 'mixed mode' model*—this model was associated with the development of a new role, rather than the refashioning or redevelopment of an existing one.

There was no evidence to suggest that any one of these models was the most effective, because there were advantages and disadvantages to all three. Trusts might find it helpful to have these models in mind when planning and establishing matron posts.

The methodology of the research involved two phases:

1 Phase 1 involved 545 questionnaires sent to directors of nursing in all of the NHS trusts, including primary care trusts (PCTs), in England;
2 Phase 2 of the project consisted of ten case studies, which were designed to investigate all aspects of the modern matron role in a sample of NHS trusts and, as far as possible, to evaluate its impact.

The study highlighted significant variability in the ways in which the modern matron role was being implemented. Whilst it was recognized that there were difficulties with evaluating the impact of modern matrons due to the shortage of verifiable information, it was felt that there was enough anecdotal evidence to suggest that individual matrons were having a positive impact on improving standards of nursing care, improving the patient environment, improving skill mix and staff retention, improving staff morale, encouraging staff development, and substantially reducing the number of formal complaints from patients and their families. Other notable achievements were identified, such as that matrons acting collectively had achieved changing the contract for ward cleaning to improve cleanliness (Read et al., 2004).

Matrons and their colleagues indicated that there were some potentially difficult issues that could affect the success of a matron role, including:

- role conflict and tensions;
- lack of clarity and shared understandings about the role;
- fragile sense of authority;
- blurred interface with other organizational roles;
- competing priorities;
- role overload; and
- inequitable grading and responsibilities.

The research team concluded that there were some general recommendations for trusts, including taking a strategic approach to establishing modern matron roles, selection and succession planning, professional development, and the provision of appropriate support. There were three key areas highlighted on which trusts were to focus as opportunities for the matrons to lead and manage care: cleanliness; standards of basic care; and improving patients' experience. The research team concluded that several processes and inputs are necessary to help modern matrons to exert maximum influence over these areas (see **Box 13.3**).

···

Either reflecting on your last clinical placement, or using discussion with your mentor and observation at your next placement, review Box 13.3.

How has your organization chosen to deliver the role of the matron?

To what extent has it progressed in making an impact on the three key areas?

···

In 2006, the Department of Health published *Modernising Nursing Careers*. The aim of the report was to set the direction for nursing careers, including actions that are intended to shape nursing for the future in the context of the government's reform programme. The priorities of the report did focus on the careers of registered nurses, but also identified that nursing teams include more than registered nurses (Department of Health, 2006). Importantly, the report recognized that individual careers take different forms, comparing how some nurses choose to climb an upward ladder of increasing responsibility and higher rewards, while many other nurses choose a more lateral career journey, moving within and between care groups and settings.

Figure 13.1 illustrates the 'visual map' design of careers in nursing (Department of Health, 2009). This map highlights the diversity that exists within nursing,

Box 13.3 Processes and inputs required of the matron role to lead (Read et al., 2004)

Cleanliness and the patient environment
- Matrons should be involved in developing and monitoring cleaning specifications, considering staff views about specific requirements in different clinical areas.
- Whether cleaning services are provided in-house or by external contractors, there should be clear and agreed channels of communication to enable matrons to report concerns about standards.
- Consideration needs to be given to the suitability of the estate and furnishings, to enable effective cleaning to take place and to ensure that adequate financial resources are made available to provide good cleaning services.
- Trusts should ensure that staff responsible for cleaning have appropriate training, especially related to principles of infection control. Staff responsible for cleaning should be seen and function as essential members of the clinical team.
- Trusts should provide regular opportunities for matrons to meet with estates and facilities.

Standards of basic care
- Matrons should be allowed to focus on their ten key responsibilities.

- Matrons should work closely with ward staff to implement systematic approaches to quality improvement, such as 'Essence of Care', with trusts taking account of messages from staff transmitted through matrons about staff numbers, skill mix, and staff capabilities.
- Trusts should provide resources for staff training and education to support matrons in improving patient care.
- Matrons should have regular access to their director of nursing to ensure that their professional concerns about standards of basic care are noted at the highest level.

Improving patients' experience
- Matrons need to be clearly identifiable to patients through the use of appropriate badges, and ward and departmental notice boards.
- Trusts should provide written information for patients on the role and responsibilities of matrons, and how to contact them.
- Trusts should establish clear guidance about the respective roles of matrons and the Patient Advice and Liaison Service (PALS) officers in addressing patient and carer concerns and complaints.

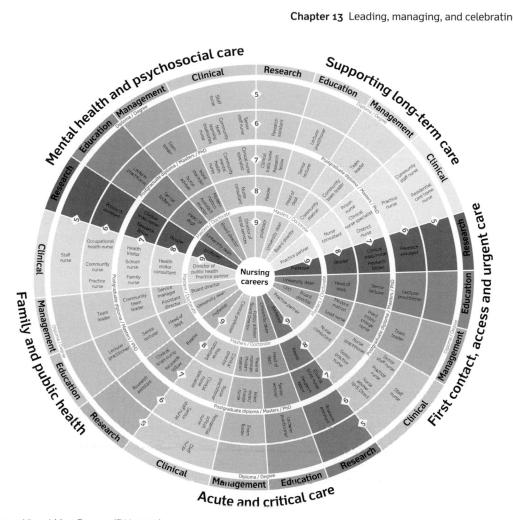

Figure 13.1 Visual Map Design (DH 2009).

indicating that nurses have many options with regards to career development and progression. Nurses can be found leading and managing care in research, education management, and clinical roles. The map illustrates the professional and/or academic qualifications needed by registered nurses to progress to the different bands.

Following *Modernising Nursing Careers*, a national consultation was launched (November 2007–February 2008) (Department of Health, 2008b). The purpose of the consultation was to test the relevance and usefulness of a pathway model to aligning nursing careers with patient and service need and improving the quality of care. It also looked for a steer on nurses' roles and on regulation. Responses suggested that there was an overall support for the main proposals—particularly

the need for clear, academic, and experiential benchmarks to be standardized at thresholds of practice, and to provide a mandate to continue the work. The NHS Next Stage Review gave additional impetus to these issues. The consultation set out options for a new careers framework for post-registration nursing. The results of the consultation were published in 2008 (Department of Health, 2008c).

The consultation proposed aligning nurses' careers in five broad pathways.

1 Acute and critical care
2 Supporting long-term conditions
3 Family and public health
4 Mental health and psychological care
5 First contact, access and urgent care

The report discussed the emerging themes from the findings and outlined next steps.

Ward managers

By 2008, the professional drivers were clearly focused towards re-establishing a clear nursing leadership framework. The role of the matron was becoming embedded across both the acute and community settings, with the aims of the matron being the ability to influence the processes and inputs that were felt to be necessary to lead clinical services. In order to lead effectively, it was felt that matrons should have the appropriate power to influence and empower the ward sister. The benefits of effective ward leaders were highlighted by the Hay Group (2006). Its study of twenty-two ward managers demonstrated that effective ward managers do have an impact on overall performance of the clinical service that they are leading.

···

Identify an inspiring ward leader with whom you have worked in practice.

What do you identify made that person inspiring?

···

The study utilized selected performance indicators over which the ward manager has an influence in order to identify high and low performers across a group:

- patient satisfaction;
- absenteeism rates;
- number and nature of complaints;
- number of drug errors and levels of severity; and
- staff turnover rates.

At a time when there is increasing pressure on resources in health services and a need to demonstrate productivity and efficiency, reducing the usage of agency staff, costs of turnover, and absenteeism showed that effective ward management has a significant impact on resource use, as well as the care-related performance indicators measured. The gap between low-performing and high-performing ward managers was clearly seen in the performance indicators: high-performing ward managers achieved 36 per cent lower staff turnover and a 57 per cent reduction in absenteeism compared with their low-performing peers.

Critically, drug errors were 40 per cent lower under the guidance of high-performing ward managers. Potentially life-threatening drug errors were more than 50 per cent higher for low-performing ward managers. Across the range of indicators, high performers show, on average, a 45 per cent improvement in performance over their low-performing peers.

In 2009, the RCN undertook the largest review of ward leaders. The review examined how the ward sister and charge nurse roles were working across different types of hospital trust in England. The report findings highlighted that work needed to be done to strengthen and support the role for the delivery of high-quality nursing. Entitled *Breaking down Barriers, Driving up Standards: The Role of the Ward Sister and Charge Nurse*, the report recognized that the importance of the ward sister and charge nurse role applies universally, and where the role is supervisory, patient care benefits (RCN, 2009).

The RCN review took place between July and December 2008. The final report was based on a literature review of the research and history of the ward sister role, a re-analysis of RCN annual employment surveys undertaken in 2002 and 2007, and focus groups of ward sisters (approximately ninety) from different types of hospital trust across England. It was another report that raised organizational issues as a potential block to progressing.

Writing in the publication's Foreword, RCN Chief Executive and General Secretary Dr Peter Carter said:

Ward sisters and charge nurses have many roles, but their responsibility is clear—to oversee patient care on a ward.   (RCN, 2009)

The report concluded with a set of recommendations, which can be utilized as a best-practice checklist for organizations.

- The RCN will support nurse directors to promote discussion and a strategy to recognize the importance of the ward sister role for high-quality care in every NHS trust.
- The RCN expects all ward sisters/charge nurses who match the ward sister profile to receive the minimum AfC band 7 salary.

- The RCN recommends that all ward sisters/charge nurses become supervisory to shifts so that ward sisters can: fulfil their ward leadership responsibilities; supervise clinical care; oversee and maintain nursing care standards; teach clinical practice and procedures; be role models for good professional practice and behaviours; oversee the ward environment; and assume high visibility as nurse leader for the ward.
- The RCN therefore recommended that ward sisters and charge nurses assume a title that conveys a clear identity as the nurse leader of the ward. Nurse directors need to review the remit of ward sisters/charge nurses in each NHS trust to ensure that they have the appropriate authority for key issues that underpin care quality—such as ward cleanliness and nutrition—and the appropriate administrative, housekeeping, and human resources support to enable them to manage the ward team and ward environment.

The report identified that the role combines managerial responsibility for the daily delivery of care with managerial responsibility of those who deliver that care, as well as responsibility for the patients who receive care. The ward sister role was therefore recognized as uniquely placed in the hospital system because it is, quite literally, at the centre of, and able to oversee, these different dimensions of service provision. The findings from this report will undoubtedly have a relevance to those leading care across the full health economy

The importance of the ward sister role had been acknowledged over the years. The most recent report to appreciate this was *Front Line Care*, the report by the Prime Minister's Commission on the Future of Nursing and Midwifery in England (2010). This was demonstrated by the Chair of the Commission Anne Keen, the then Secretary of State for Health, who wrote in her chair's letter in the introduction of the report:

One traditional figure, however, should be restored to her former position—the ward sister. I strongly believe that immediate steps must be taken to strengthen this role and enhance its clinical leadership and visible authority, as the guardian of patient safety and the role model for the next generation of nursing students. (ibid: 4)

Later in the report, a whole section is dedicated to nurses and midwives leading services, with a call to action, as outlined in **Box 13.4**.

Potential benefit of nurse-led services

The 2010 report of the Prime Minister's Commission on the Future of Nursing and Midwifery in England acknowledged the opportunities for nurses and midwives to lead services in response to the changing needs of the NHS. With the emphasis on moving care closer to home and the growing need to provide care to people with long-term conditions, more direct access to nurse-led and midwife-led services will improve

Box 13.4 Nurses and midwives leading services: Our call to action

Putting nurses and midwives in the forefront of leading and managing services brings many benefits. They need more development and support to be effective leaders, as well as clearly defined and appropriate accountabilities and roles. Employers, managers and professional colleagues should be fully committed to involving nurses and midwives in making policies and decisions, from the board to the point of care. Leadership from the ward sister and equivalent linchpin roles in midwifery and community settings should be strengthened. Innovative organizational models such as social enterprises led by nurses and midwives also provide important opportunities for improvement and innovation, and should be supported and extended where locally appropriate. These changes should be driven by health policy and guidance, and enabled by appropriate management structures and supportive workplace cultures. Comprehensive development and mentorship programmes must be scaled up to identify and fast-track talented potential leaders.

(Prime Minister's Commission on the Future of Nursing and Midwifery in England, 2010)

cost-effectiveness and health outcomes, and remove system blockages that delay appropriate care.

The benefits of many of the examples of nurse and midwifery-led services were reviewed by Caird et al. (2010). Robust evidence of the benefits of nurse-led services emerged from the systematic socio-economic review, which was funded by the Department of Health. These included improved outcomes in nurse-led in-patient units, such as functional status, psychological well-being, lower readmission rates, and fewer visits to accident and emergency (A&E) departments for people with respiratory conditions. An award-winning, nurse-led paediatric urgent care social enterprise in London enabled service users who would formerly have been admitted via A&E to have their care managed at home with support.

The Caird et al. (2010) report signified a significant change in opportunity for nurses and midwives to lead and develop services. Despite these successes, cultural expectations of the public will still need to be acknowledged: whilst on a countrywide roadshow to test out new ways of working, the team commissioned to write the report suggested that a major barrier to change might be public concerns based on uncertainty or ignorance about the qualifications and competence of nursing and midwifery leaders. While at an event at NHS North West, the team received feedback arguing that:

> **We have to let the public know what nurses are capable of and that they will be taking the lead in services. Our walk-in centre does not have any doctors, which can be a surprise to patients— but it is gradually becoming more and more acceptable; it will filter through that nurses can and will do more and more.**

In Manchester, however, a service user stated:

> **They lead everything anyway! I see them for everything; I was three months in a stroke centre. I didn't realize nurses had the rehabilitation skills before—I didn't see a doctor the whole time. I really got quality of care with the nurses.**   (Caird et al., 2010)

Perhaps tellingly, it was suggested that it was those who had not experienced nurse-led services and interventions who feared that nurses did not have the necessary competence, that they would be exploited to deliver care on the cheap and not have time to do their 'real' job, and that the developments would cause tension with doctors. Although a third of service users' first NHS encounters are with nurses (NHS Information Centre, 2009; cited in Caird et al., 2010) and around 80 per cent of women have direct access to midwives, most members of the public still saw doctors as the gatekeepers to the NHS.

There were two particularly pertinent recommendations from the nursing leadership section as outlined in **Box 13.5**.

Box 13.5 Recommendations for nurses and midwives leading services

Strengthening the role of the ward sister
Immediate steps must be taken to strengthen the linchpin role of the ward sister, charge nurse and equivalent team leader in the midwifery and community settings. These clinical lead roles must have clearly defined authority and lines of accountability, and be appropriately graded. They must drive quality and safety, and provide active and visible clinical leadership and reassurance for service users and staff in all care settings. Organizational hierarchies must be designed to ensure there are no more than two levels between these roles and the director of nursing. Heads of midwifery should report to the board directly or via the director of nursing.

Fast-track leadership development
Regional schemes must be established to develop potential nursing and midwifery leaders, building on existing national work and learning from similar successful schemes in other sectors. They will identify talent, offer training and mentorship, and ensure that successful candidates who reflect the diversity of the workforce are fast-tracked to roles with significant impact on care delivery.

(Prime Minister's Commission on the Future of Nursing and Midwifery in England, 2010)

The final, most pivotal proposal for NHS reform was launched in 2010 in the White Paper *Equity and Excellence: Liberating the NHS* (Department of Health, 2010a), which proposes giving greater autonomy to nurses and midwives to enable them to spend more time with their patients and communities.

The White Paper outlines the plans for achieving this and suggests that because nurses and midwives are the people who have the most day-to-day contact with patients, it is these staff who can ensure that NHS care is guided by the simple mantra 'no decisions about me without me'. The Paper highlights that nurses will be required to build on their strong working relationships across hospitals, primary and community health services, and social care teams to support patients inside and outside the hospital ward. It recognizes that nurses will need to work in partnership with GP consortia, whereby a group of GPs will be responsible for ensuring that the best services are commissioned for patients.

The *Next Stage Review*

The professional drivers that have been highlighted in the chapter thus far all recognize the benefits and ongoing need to strengthen nurse leadership, with an aim to provide a nursing workforce that can effectively take the NHS forward. At the beginning of this chapter, we outlined the important report on the future of the NHS entitled *The Next Stage Review*, led by Lord Darzi (Department of Health, 2008a).

The Darzi Review was led locally by clinicians in each NHS region: seventy-four local clinical working groups, made up of some 2,000 clinicians, looked at the clinical evidence and engaged with their local communities. They developed improved models of care for their regions to ensure that the NHS is up to date with the latest clinical developments, and is able to meet changing needs and expectations.

Overall, the Darzi Review contained many positive messages and recommendations for the nursing profession to lead and improve care. One of the key messages and challenges to nursing was to address the level of variability of care that exists in the NHS. Shortly after its publication, in July 2009, the Secretary of State for Health announced an independent inquiry

into care provided by Mid Staffordshire Foundation Trust. In February 2010, the final report was published (Department of Health, 2010b). The report has had a profound effect on the reputation of the nursing profession and the level of confidence that the public have in nursing care, highlighting a number of significant failings in the quality of nursing care provided that could have been prevented by sound nursing leadership.

There is clear evidence throughout the Darzi Review (Department of Health, 2008a) that effective leadership at all levels has been identified as a key enabler towards putting quality at the heart of everything that we do. As discussed earlier in Chapter 1, caring is a highly theoretical concept to articulate, and a complex and technical skill to deliver in the diverse clinical and non-clinical settings in which care is provided.

The recent political drivers and the recent scandals involving health and social care providers acknowledged concerns from users, patient groups, and in some cases healthcare professionals. This again highlights the need for nursing to refocus on its core caring principles and values, to enable the workforce to recognize the knowledge and skills required to deliver high-quality care.

Defining 'high-quality care'

This section will explore the definition of high-quality care and two high-profile inquiries into failings in care by the NHS—in particular the elements of nursing care that failed, and what should have been in place to enable a high-quality patient environment and a high-quality learning environment to enable learners to grow and develop skills required. The Darzi Review (Department of Health, 2008a), heralded a significant change for the NHS in England, because it has made the quality of care a central organizing principle, alongside access, volume, and cost of health care. This review defined three dimensions of health care quality as:

- *clinically effective*—it is about effectiveness of care, from the clinical procedure the patient receives, to their quality of life after treatment;
- *personal*—it is also about the patient's entire experience of the NHS and ensuring they are treated with compassion, dignity, and respect in a clean, safe, and well-managed environment; and

- *safe*—it is about protecting patient safety, for example by eradicating healthcare-acquired infections and avoidable accidents.

Subsequent communications from NHS Chief Executive David Nicholson to NHS healthcare trusts and strategic health authorities have stressed the rapid pace at which the government expects these dimensions of quality to become core to commissioning and providing NHS services. Some legislative and practical steps are already being put in place to ensure that this happens quickly, including:

- the development of measures or 'metrics' of healthcare quality so that the performance of NHS trusts can be benchmarked and compared to drive forward quality standards; and
- legislation in early 2009 (the Health Act 2009), which made 'quality accounts' of performance by NHS trusts in care quality mandatory, and open to public and patient scrutiny, along with the establishment of a national quality board to oversee implementation of policies that embed quality into the NHS.

There is no doubt that the government is serious about a quality agenda for health services. This agenda will be absolutely essential to the business of every NHS trust, and immensely important to them in terms of performance rating, reputation, and contestability, and their credibility with patients and the public. Nursing is core to this, because it has a demonstrable impact on standards of healthcare quality. Dame Christine Beasley, Chief Nursing Officer for England, published *Framing the Nursing and Midwifery Contribution: Driving up the Quality of Care* (Department of Health, 2008d), which draws together key areas of work that will strengthen the nursing contribution, including:

- the development of measures that identify, quantify, and make visible the impact of the nursing workforce on care quality outcomes, beginning with the publication of an evidence base, state-of-the-art metrics for nursing, a rapid appraisal (Griffiths et al., 2008), and a reaffirmation of the responsibility of nurses for care quality (Maben, 2008);
- the development of a framework of clear roles and responsibilities that makes accountability for the

quality of care, from the point of care to the NHS trust executive boardroom, explicit ('from ward to board'); and
- a strengthening of nurse leadership for care quality performance to oversee and coordinate the different dimensions of service provision to patients.

When high-quality care and leadership is absent

Nationally, by 2009, it was recognized that the role that nurses played in leading professional practice was crucial to the delivery of quality care. It was therefore not surprising when both public and professional regulatory bodies called nursing leaders to account when the failings in care delivery by an acute foundation trust began to emerge.

Practice Example 13.2 highlights the second inquiry into care in this chapter. The inquiry had a strong focus on assessing the delivery of fundamental care at the Mid Staffordshire NHS Foundation Trust. In 2010, Colin Ovington, Mid Staffordshire Foundation Trust's new nursing director, stated that he was adamant that he would not 'let the past re-emerge' and would hold staff to account if they were to fail to meet care standards. Ovington, who joined as nursing director at the beginning of June 2010, stated that the main reasons for previous problems with nursing at the trust were poor leadership and senior management. The Francis Inquiry into events at the trust was particularly critical of the trust's nursing director from February 1998 to July 2006. Ovington said that the past problems at the trust '*demonstrate that leadership is crucial and does have a major influence on an organisation*'.

....

In order to recognize the contribution that you make as an individual to leading and managing care, see NMC (2009) and reflect on the elements of care that nursing failed to provide to patients in the two practice examples.

Self-assess against these skills and reflect upon any gaps in knowledge that you may have in your area of practice or expertise.

Plan how you will gain the knowledge and skills to bridge any gaps.

....

PRACTICE EXAMPLE 13.2

Inquiry into the care delivered at The Mid Staffordshire NHS Foundation Trust

Concerns about mortality and the standard of care provided at the Mid Staffordshire NHS Foundation Trust followed claims that patients were being neglected and deprived of fundamental nursing care. This resulted in an investigation by the Healthcare Commission, which published a highly critical report in March 2009, and a review commissioned by the Department of Health (2010b). These investigations gave rise to widespread public concern and a loss of confidence in the trust, its services, and management.

The areas in which detailed accounts were heard by the inquiry included:

- continence and bladder and bowel care;
- safety;
- personal and oral hygiene;
- nutrition and hydration;
- pressure area care;
- cleanliness and infection control;
- privacy and dignity;
- record keeping;
- diagnosis and treatment;
- communication; and
- discharge management.

Interviews and observations during the inquiry revealed these key area in which care was not delivered and the independent inquiry led to the launch of a public inquiry.

Patients and relatives told us that when patients rang the call bell because they were in pain or needed to go to the toilet, it was often not answered, or not answered in time. Families claimed that tablets or nutritional supplements were not given on time, if at all, and doses of medication were missed. Some relatives claimed that patients were left, sometimes for hours, in wet or soiled sheets, putting them at increased risk of infection and pressure sores. Wards, bathrooms and commodes were not always clean. Nurses often failed to conduct observations and identify that the condition of a patient was deteriorating, or they did not do anything about the results . . .

Many doctors and nurses working in surgery considered that staff on the EAU (Emergency Assessment Unit) and on medical wards did not have the right training and skills to look after surgical patients . . .

For patients who were in hospital for several days, it was clear that fluid charts and summaries of fluid input and output were poorly completed. Even when patients were receiving intravenous or naso-gastric fluids and had a urinary catheter in place, these charts were often incomplete. Transfers from A&E to wards and between wards were also poorly documented in the records, often with no clear handovers recorded in either medical or nursing records.

(Healthcare Commission, 2009)

Skills for leadership

The Darzi Review (Department of Health, 2008a) and the two practice examples in this chapter have identified the need for strong leadership in the NHS. The professional and political drivers discussed in this chapter all conclude that nurses need to take a lead role in the running of local health services. They also suggest that strong leadership is needed at a clinical level. The literature identifies several skills deemed to be essential for clinical leadership, whilst other skills relate to personal traits and qualities.

Pullen (2003) identified four skills for discussion:

- self-knowledge;
- communication skills;
- risk-taking; and
- keeping informed.

It was noted that the way in which these skills are currently developed in the pre-registration nursing curriculum ensures that many opportunities are available to develop these skills in the classroom environment, but that there are many pressures that prevent use of these skills in a practice environment.

In this way, some of these are difficult to achieve through pre-registration nurse education, because they relate to an awareness of the structures and processes of the NHS and the ability to visualize or predict the future.

....

Consider your attributes and attitudes.

Do you feel confident and competent to deliver care at this stage?

Are you aware of any constraints or issues that will prevent this?

....

When quality care is delivered, it leads to the opportunity to celebrate nursing care. The Chief Nursing Officer recognized the contribution of nurses and midwives when she said:

> **We know that nursing and midwifery are fundamental to high quality healthcare. There is hardly an intervention, treatment or healthcare programme in which we do not play a significant part. This means we are in a powerful position to improve the quality of care across the NHS and play a major role in improving health outcomes.**
>
> (Department of Health, 2008d)

No fewer than nine nurses made the 2010 New Year Honours in England, which recognize outstanding achievement and service across the whole of the UK. At a time when the NHS is striving to drive up its quality of service, the impressive number of nurses on the list is cause for celebration. This national recognition is in addition to the many other national awards ceremonies for excellence in practice and innovation, coupled with local staff recognition events, all of which celebrate both individual and team nursing and midwifery contributions.

The *Nursing Roadmap for Quality* (Department of Health, 2010c) set out an explanation of the importance of quality in nursing across health and social care. This document is intended to be used by all nurses as a signposting reference guide to achieving and maintaining quality. It aims to help nurses to understand the quality policy, and the associated tools and techniques that achieve quality outcomes. It suggests innovative methods for nursing teams to report the difference to patients, teams, boards, governors, and regulators. The document suggests that improvements in quality must be recognized and rewarded, because the need to demonstrate quality improvements will be considered a contract between commissioners and providers.

One method of delivering this is through the use of the Commissioning for Quality and Innovation (CQUIN) payment framework. CQUIN makes a proportion of provider income conditional on locally agreed goals around quality improvement and innovation. CQUIN goals are agreed locally between the commissioner and the NHS provider, and will include at least one goal in each of four areas: safety; effectiveness; patient experience; and innovation. The CQUIN framework ensures that both commissioners and NHS providers pay as much attention to the delivery of high-quality care for patients as they do to activity performance.

Conclusion

Throughout this chapter, all of the professional and political drivers reviewed have recognized that the context of nursing is changing; they recognize that health care is changing, and that nurses play a significant role in leading and managing care.

It is clear that nurses care passionately about the care that they give and continually seek ways in which to improve and demonstrate their value. Nurses have embraced the quality agenda as an opportunity to demonstrate continued value and their impact on patient care, wherever that care is delivered. This will become even more important in the current financial context (2010–2015). It also means questioning how we do things, thinking of innovative ways in which to support clinical outcomes, while focusing on promoting and maintaining health and well-being, as well as on prevention.

Quality is always going to be a key priority for nursing; to continue to deliver quality will mean nurses working differently—working across pathways, working with other clinical colleagues, and working in different environments. Nurses are close to patients, so they can see how they can change things to make them better for patients. This also means looking at our everyday processes and seeking to reduce waste from the system.

In terms of leading, managing, and celebrating care, Govier (2009) identified a number of practice points that summarize how transformational leadership approaches can be effective in healthcare settings. Two of these points will conclude this chapter, summing up the importance of effective leading, managing, and celebrating care.

1 Leadership exists at all levels of the organization, especially as people share in a vision that moves them towards achieving the goal of providing safe and quality health care.

2 The core values and principles that underpin nursing and the act of caring provide an internal compass that facilitates authentic and transformation healthcare leadership.

Further reading

Commissioning for Quality and Innovation (CQUIN)
http://tinyurl.com/ylld5v9
National Quality Board **http://tinyurl.com/yhmkagf**
The Quality and Outcomes Framework (QOF)
http://tinyurl.com/6f382t
Releasing Time to Care Series **http://tinyurl.com/ybaqt6xz**

References

Caird, J., Rees, R., Kavanagh, J., Sutcliffe, K., Oliver, K., Dickson, K., Woodman, J., Barnell-Page, E., and Thomas, J. (2010) *The Socioeconomic Value of Nursing and Midwifery: A Rapid Systematic Review of Reviews*, London: EPPI Centre, Social Science Research Unit, Institute of Education, University of London.

Commission for Healthcare Audit and Inspection (2007) *Health Care Commission Investigation into Outbreaks of Clostridium Difficile at Maidstone and Tunbridge Wells NHS Trust*, London: HMSO.

Commission for Healthcare Audit and Inspection (2009) *Health Care Commission Investigation into Mid Staffordshire NHS Foundation Trust*, London: HMSO.

Cunningham, G. and Kitson, A. (2000) 'An evaluation of the RCN clinical leadership development programme: Part 1', *Nursing Standard* 15(2): 34–7.

Department of Health (2000) *NHS Plan 2000*, London: HMSO.

Department of Health (2001) *Implementing the NHS Plan: Modern Matrons*, Health Service Circular 2001/010, London: HMSO.

Department of Health (2002) *Modern Matrons in the NHS: A Progress Report*, London: HMSO.

Department of Health (2006) *Modernising Nursing Careers: Setting the Direction*, London: HMSO.

Department of Health (2008a) *High Quality Care for All: NHS Next Stage Review Final Report*, London: HMSO.

Department of Health (2008b) *Towards a Framework for Post-Registration Nursing Careers: A National Consultation*, London: HMSO.

Department of Health (2008c) *Towards a Framework for Post-Registration Nursing Careers: Consultation Response Report*, London: HMSO.

Department of Health (2008d) *Framing the Nursing and Midwifery Contribution: Driving up the Quality of Care*, London: HMSO.

Department of Health (2009) *Nursing Careers Framework: Developing a Visual Design*, London: HMSO.

Department of Health (2010a) *Equity and Excellence: Liberating the NHS–The White Paper*, London: HMSO.

Department of Health (2010b) *Robert Francis Inquiry Report into Mid Staffordshire NHS Foundation Trust*, London: HMSO.

Department of Health (2010c) *The Nursing Roadmap for Quality*, London: HMSO.

Govier, I. (2009) 'Examining transformational approaches to effective leadership in healthcare settings', *Nursing Times* 105: 18.

Griffiths, P., with Jones, S., Maben, J., and Murrells, T. (2008) *State-of-the-Art Metrics for Nursing: A Rapid Appraisal*, available online at **http://www.kcl.ac.uk/content/1/c6/04/32/19/Metricsfinalreport.pdf** [accessed 16 June 2011].

Hay Group (2006) *Nurse Leadership: Being Nice is not Enough*, available online at **http://www.haygroup.com/downloads/uk/Frontline_leaders.pdf** [accessed 16 June 2011].

Lansley, A. (2010) 'My ambition for patient-centred care', Secretary of State for Health's Speech, 8 June, available online at **http://www.dh.gov.uk/en/MediaCentre/Speeches/DH_116643** [accessed 16 June 2011].

Maben, J. (2008) *Nurses in Society: Starting the Debate*, London: National Nursing Research Centre, Kings College London.

Nursing and Midwifery Council (2007) *Essential Skills Clusters (ESCs) For Pre-registration Nursing Programmes*, Circular 07/2007, Annexe 2, London: NMC.

Nursing and Midwifery Council (2008) *The Code: Standards Performance and Ethics for Nurses and Midwives*, London: NMC.

Nursing and Midwifery Council (2009) *Standards for Pre-Registration Nursing Education*, London: NMC.

Ovington, C. (2010) 'New Mid-Staffs director vows "It will never happen again"', *Nursing Times* 14 August, available online at **http://www.nursingtimes.net/whats-new-in-nursing/acute-care/new-mid-staffs-nurse-director-vows-never-again/5018056.article** [accessed 11 July 2011].

Prime Minister's Commission on the Future of Nursing and Midwifery in England (2010) *Front Line Care: The Future of Nursing and Midwifery in England*, London: HMSO.

Pullen, M. (2003) 'Developing clinical leadership skills in student nurses', *Nurse Education Today* 23(1): 34–9.

Read, S., Ashman, M., Scott, C., and Savage, J. (2004) *Evaluation of the Modern Matron Role in a Sample of NHS Trusts: Final Report to the Department of Health*, Sheffield/London: University of Sheffield School of Nursing and Midwifery/Royal College of Nursing Institute.

Royal College of Nursing (2009) *Breaking down Barriers, Driving up Standards: The Role of the Ward Sister and Charge Nurse*, London: RCN.

West, D., Clews, G., and Taylor, A. (2010) 'NHS boards recognise role of nursing in raising quality', *Nursing Times* 13 July, available online at **http://www.nursingtimes.net/whats-new-in-nursing/news-topics/nursing-quality/nhs-boards-recognise-role-of-nursing-in-raising-quality/5017001.article** [accessed 11 July 2011].

14 When care is absent

JOHN TINGLE AND JEAN McHALE

Learning outcomes

This chapter will enable you to:

- understand the importance of providing care that is safe, legal, and ethical;
- identify factors that have raised patient expectations regarding the nature and delivery of care;
- explore what is meant by the term 'clinical negligence litigation' and its impact on health care;
- appreciate what is meant by a 'just' compensation system; and
- identify strategies that healthcare providers may use to promote the safety of patients.

Introduction

Professional caring practice must be safe, legal, and ethical, and seek to protect patients from harm and wrongdoing. This chapter will explore the legal consequences if patients are exposed to risks and dangers when caring practice is absent.

Today, it is increasingly the case that the actions of healthcare professionals are placed under the spotlight. There are several possible reasons for this. First, expectations have been raised: it seems that virtually on a daily basis new medical developments and treatments at the frontiers of medicine are being portrayed in the media. Patients are assured by government policy statements that they are at the centre of the National Health Service. It is perhaps unsurprising that, over the last decade, patient expectations regarding the nature and delivery of care have risen.

Secondly, we live in a less 'trusting' society; this lack of 'trust' is reflected in responses to healthcare delivery. Today, patients are now less deferential towards healthcare professionals than they once were.

Thirdly, there has been a rise in rights discourse; the NHS also exists within a rights-based culture. The NHS

Essential knowledge and skills for care

- You must act at all times with professionalism and integrity, and work within agreed professional, ethical, and legal frameworks and processes to maintain and improve standards.

- You will demonstrate an understanding of how to work within legal and professional frameworks and local policies to safeguard and protect people—particularly children, young people, and vulnerable adults.

- You will uphold people's legal rights and speak out when these are at risk of being compromised.

- At all times, you will work within relevant legal frameworks when seeking consent, and be able to assess and respond to the needs and wishes of carers and relatives in relation to information and consent.

- You will demonstrate respect for the autonomy and rights of people to withhold consent in relation to treatment within legal frameworks and in relation to people's safety.

- You will understand the need to accept differing cultural traditions and beliefs, UK legal frameworks, and professional ethics when planning care with people, their families, and their carers.

- You will work within ethical and legal frameworks and local policies to deal with complaints, compliments, and concerns.

Constitution (Department of Health, 2010a) explicitly highlights this shift in emphasis:

> **This Constitution establishes the principles and values of the NHS in England. It sets out rights to which patients, public and staff are entitled, and pledges which the NHS is committed to achieve, together with responsibilities which the public, patients and staff owe to one another to ensure that the NHS operates fairly and effectively. All NHS bodies and private and third sector providers supplying NHS services are required by law to take account of this Constitution in their decisions and actions.**

The language of rights has also been strengthened by the enactment of the Human Rights Act 1998 (McHale and Gallagher, 2004). This incorporated part of the European Convention of Human Rights (ECHR) into English law. Litigants can use human rights-based arguments, drawing upon the Convention provision. A number of these provisions are particularly pertinent in relation to healthcare delivery. Article 2 of the ECHR provides respect for the right to life, Article 3 prohibits torture and inhuman and degrading treatment, and Article 8 provides for respect for privacy of home and family life. This last Article has been used to safeguard individual claims to exercise autonomous decision-making. But rights are rarely absolute and thus there is no absolute right to demand medical treatment, for example (*R v Cambridge DHA, ex p B* [1995] 1 WLR 898; *R v North West Lancashire Health Authority, ex p A D and G* [2000] 1 WLR 977). However, today rights do underpin approaches to a range of areas of law, from consent to treatment, to patient confidentiality.

Alongside this rise in expectations over the last few years, controversies over standards of care have been rarely out of the eye of the media. Harold Shipman, the Bristol Royal Infirmary Inquiry (2001), and the consultant Rodney Ledward are but a few examples. Collectively, these factors have all worked to make patients more demanding for medical and nursing accountability, transparency, and governance, and less forgiving should errors occur. It is thus perhaps not surprising

that the trend for litigation has been upwards. Statistics show fairly consistent rises in litigation in health care over the last few decades.

The Chief Medical Officer (Donaldson, 2003) stated:

> **In the late 1970s it was estimated that there were around 700 claims against doctors, dentists and pharmacists each year ... Data on the claims handled by the NHSLA shows a nearly fifteen-fold increase in the number of claims for medical injury arising after 1 April 1995, from 392 in 1996/97 to 5,765 in 2002/03.**

The NHS Litigation Authority quotes more recent figures (NHSLA, 2010):

> **the number of clinical negligence claims reported to the Authority in 2009/10 was 6,652 which represents a 10% increase over 2008/09, which, in turn, recorded an 11% increase over 2007/08. These numbers are particularly disappointing following 3 years of relative stability in claim numbers.**

The amount that these claims are worth reached record levels. Key figures are also quoted in the NHSLA factsheet (NHSLA, 2009):

> **As at March 2009, the NHSLA estimates that it has potential liabilities of £13.51 billion, of which £13.37 billion relate to clinical negligence claims ... This figure represents the estimated value of all known claims, together with an actuarial estimate of those incurred but not yet reported (IBNR), which may settle or be withdrawn over future years.**

Clinical negligence presents a serious challenge for the NHS. It diverts funds away from patient care into defending litigation. It diverts healthcare professionals' attention away from caring patients if they become embroiled in litigation. It can further serve to lower trust in the NHS. But as well as being a problem for the NHS, clinical negligence is also clearly a problem for those patients who suffer harm through inadequate care. The tort compensation system must be fair to both claimants and defendants. The NHS itself needs to be concerned with preventing errors and with the establishment of a patient safety culture in the NHS.

··

Reflect on any recent cases of neglect or poor care that you have read or heard about in the media.

What were the problems and what, if anything, happened as a result?

··

Clinical negligence litigation

If a patient suffers harm as a result of care or treatment, they may decide to bring an action for compensation in the law of tort against a nurse or the employer. To establish an action in the civil courts in the tort of negligence, three elements need to be established: first, there needs to be a duty; second, the claimant needs to show a breach of duty; and third, the claimant needs to show that the breach of duty resulted in harm being caused. Where a healthcare professional treats a patient, there is a duty to act with reasonable care. The standard of care in relation to clinical negligence cases is rooted in the well-known case of *Bolam v Friern Hospital Management Committee* [1957] 2 All ER 118. In this case, McNair J held that, in determining the standard of care:

> **The test is the standard of the ordinary skilled man exercising and professing to have that special skill. A man need not possess the highest expert skill, it is well established law that it is sufficient if he exercises the ordinary skill of an ordinary competent man exercising that particular art …**
>
> **A doctor is not guilty of negligence if he has acted in accordance with a practice accepted as proper by a responsible body of medical men skilled in that particular art … Putting it the other way round, a doctor is not negligent, if he acting in accordance with such a practice, merely because there is a body of opinion that takes the contrary view.** (*Bolam*, at 586, *per* McNair J)

The consequence of this approach was that litigants found difficulty in succeeding in cases. All, in practice, that a health professional needed to do to substantiate their defence was to provide some expert witnesses in support. For decades, the *Bolam* approach to the standard of care in negligence dominated. While there were some cases in which the courts were prepared to scrutinize the views of professional opinion more closely (*Clarke v Adams* (1950) 94 Sol J 599; *Hucks v Cole* (1960) [1994] 4 Med LR 393), orthodoxy was clearly reasserted in the courts in the case of *Maynard v West Midlands H* [1985] 1 All ER 635:

> **a judge's preference for one body of opinion to another is not sufficient to establish negligence in a practitioner whose opinions have received approval, truthfully expressed, honestly held.** (*Maynard*, at 639, *per* Lord Scarman)

In this case, the House of Lords indicated that a judge could not 'cherry-pick' between experts. As long as there was a body of responsible professional opinion supporting the healthcare professional's actions, they would not be found to be negligent. Furthermore, that body of professional opinion need not be large (*DeFreitas v O'Brien* [1995] 6 Med LR 108.)

The *Bolam* test was revisited in the House of Lords in *Bolitho v City & Hackney Health Authority* [1997] 4 All ER 771. In this case, Lord Browne-Wilkinson confirmed the general approach in *Bolam* and the fact that, in the majority of cases, the support of expert opinion would indicate that a body of opinion was reasonable. The court could take the view that experts, in reaching their own view, would have weighed up the relative risks and benefits.

Lord Browne-Wilkinson went on to state that:

> **In particular where there are questions of assessment of the relative risks and benefits of adopting a particular medical practice, a reasonable view necessarily presupposes that the relative risks and benefits have been weighed by the experts in forming their opinions. But if in a rare case, it can be demonstrated that the professional opinion is not capable of**

withstanding logical analysis, the judge is entitled to hold that the body of opinion is not reasonable or responsible. I emphasise that in my view it will be very seldom right for a judge to reach the conclusion that views genuinely held by a competent medical expert are unreasonable. The assessment of medical risks and benefits is a matter of clinical judgement which a judge would not normally be able to make without expert evidence. It would be wrong to allow such an assessment to deteriorate into seeking to persuade the judge to prefer 1 of 2 views both of which are capable of being logically supported. It is only where a judge can be satisfied that the body of professional opinion cannot be logically supported at all that such an opinion will not provide the benchmark by reference to which the defendant's conduct falls to be assessed.

(*Bolitho*, at 778, *per* Lord Browne-Wilkinson)

After *Bolitho*, there was some discussion as to whether this would change the approach of the courts. Some early commentators suggested that this might lead to a judicial sea change in approach, but others were more cautious. Certainly, in the years that have followed there has not been a radical increase in the number of successful negligence actions against healthcare professionals. In many respects, this is unsurprising: the test in *Bolitho* is still rooted in the professional practice based standard in *Bolam*. In the case itself, Lord Browne-Wilkinson does make it clear that it will only be in rare cases that are not capable of logical analysis that a judge will override professional opinion. As Brazier and Miola (2000) comment:

While the medical experts are to be required in rare cases to justify their opinions on logical grounds there still appears to be a prima facie presumption that non-doctors will not be able fully to comprehend the evidence. This leads inexorably to a conclusion that the evidence cannot after all be critically evaluated by a judge.

Nonetheless, what the judgment does illustrate is the need for clinical decisions to be logically supported.

They will need to be rooted in evidence-based medicine. Further uncertainties remain: what if the logic is fine, but the premise is unsound or is not persuasive? *Bolitho* has to be set in the context of other changes in clinical practice. Deference to medical opinion has weakened. Today, healthcare practice is structured through guidance and legislation far more than it was even a decade ago and consequently this constrains the autonomy of professional decision-making (Samanta et al., 2006). Certainly, if healthcare professionals follow professional guidelines, then it is much less likely that they will be ultimately found to be negligent. Since *Bolitho*, there have been some cases in which healthcare professionals have been found negligent and a more *Bolitho*-based approach has been followed. So, for example, in *Marriott v West Midlands Health Authority* [1999] Lloyd's Rep Med 23, it was held that:

It was open to the judge to hold that, in the circumstances as she found them to have been it could not be a reasonable exercise of a general practitioner's discretion to leave a patient at home and not refer him back to hospital.

(*Marriott*, at 27, *per* Belldam J)

Nonetheless, research indicates that such cases are rare (Maclean, 2002). But while cases are not successful, that does not mean that litigation is not increasingly being brought, and defending such cases up to the courtroom is a time-consuming, expensive, and (for the individual) highly stressful process.

The standard of care expected of the nurse is not static. As medicine progresses and with new scientific developments, so the perspective of the responsible body of professional practice will itself therefore change. Moreover, the nurse is expected to keep up to date. This is something that is required both by their professional code of practice and by the law. In the past, the courts were prepared to find a clinician who had not read a particular article in the *Lancet* not negligent (*Crawford v Charing Cross Hospital*, The Times, 8 December 1953). However, as technology changes, thus expectations in relation to keeping up to date with developments in professional practice will change likewise (*Gascoine v Ian Sheridan & Co and Latham* [1994] 5 Med LR 437). This is reflected in the Nursing and Midwifery Council Code, which states that:

- **You must have the knowledge and skills for safe and effective practice when working without direct supervision**
- **You must recognise and work within the limits of your competence**
- **You must keep your knowledge and skills up to date throughout your working life**
- **You must take part in appropriate learning and practice activities that maintain and develop your competence and performance.**

(NMC, 2008)

....

What do you think of as the 'traditional' role of the nurse?

How do you think it has changed in recent decades? What has been the driver for these changes?

....

The fact that a nurse is working in an expanded role will mean that the expectations of them consequently increase. The courts take the view that an expanded role will equate to expanded responsibilities. The nurse is expected to work at the level of a competent professional in the area of practice in which he or she is practising. Indeed, the NMC Code exhorts the nurse to attain the highest standard of professional practice and to '*provide a high standard of practice and care at all time*', and also to '*use the best available evidence*'. It goes on to provide:

- **You must deliver care based on the best available evidence or best practice.**
- **You must ensure any advice you give is evidence based if you are suggesting healthcare products or services.**
- **You must ensure that the use of complementary or alternative therapies is safe and in the best interests of those in your care.**

(NMC, 2008)

The fact that a nurse is inexperienced or working in high-pressure conditions will not alleviate the standard

that is expected of that nurse in law. As was stated in *Wilsher v Essex Area Health Authority* [1988] 3 AC 1074:

... it would be a false step to subordinate the legitimate expectation of the patient that he will receive from each person concerned with his care a degree of skill appropriate to the task which he takes to an understandable wish to minimize the psychological and financial pressures on hard-pressed young doctors.

([281], *per* Mustill LJ)

In defending such an action, what is particularly important is accurate record-keeping, because this will provide some evidence to support a defence. Accurate record-keeping is something that is mandated by the NMC Code, which states that:

- **You must keep clear and accurate records of the discussions you have, the assessments you make, the treatment and medicines you give and how effective these have been**
- **You must complete records as soon as possible after an event has occurred**
- **You must not tamper with original records in any way**
- **You must ensure any entries you make in someone's paper records are clearly and legibly signed, dated and timed**
- **You must ensure any entries you make in someone's electronic records are clearly attributable to you**
- **You must ensure all records are kept securely**

(NMC, 2008)

....

Does your professional body have a code of conduct about record-keeping?

Have you read it and do you understand the consequences of poor record-keeping?

....

Even if the health professional is found to have broken a duty of care, the claimant still faces the difficulty that they have to establish causation. The traditional test is whether, 'but for' the defendant's action, the harm would not have arisen (*Barnett v Chelsea & Kensington Hospital Management Committee* [1969] 1 QB 428).

Proving causation may prove particularly problematic in the case of medical negligence litigations, because frequently there may be a range of possible causes. The treatment is being given to a person who is already ill; the issue then revolves around the issue of probability and whether the negligence has materially increased the risk of harm (*Wilsher v Essex Area Health Authority* [1988] 3 AC 1074).

Subsequently, the courts have taken a somewhat broader approach—namely, whether it has caused or materially contributed to the injury (*Fairchild v Glenhaven Funeral Services* [2002] UKHL 2). On the balance of probabilities, would this harm have resulted? While, in some respects, there has been a broader approach taken, in practice causation is the major stumbling block to litigation. Furthermore, the litigant cannot claim that the actions of the healthcare professionals have led them to lose a chance that they might have recovered (*Gregg v Scott* [2005] 2 AC 176).

The law can be regarded as the ultimate level of professional accountability in nursing if viewed in terms of the sanctions that can be imposed (see **Figure 14.1** on the structure of the courts). The law can deprive a person of their liberty and imprison them. Equally, the law is the ultimate arbiter of what is competent and lawful conduct. The NMC also functions as a mechanism of accountability and its guidance should also be followed. The construct of what is 'professional nursing' is an NMC construct that is explored through its professional codes. These codes would be highly influential to a court if it were asked to determine whether a nurse had been negligent.

A just compensation system?

There has long been a debate as to whether there should be some form of no-fault compensation system introduced into English law. A no-fault scheme enables compensation to be awarded to a claimant who can demonstrate that harm has been caused even though this does not necessarily meant that the individual who has caused the harm has been 'negligent'. It can be seen as justified on policy grounds in enabling compensation while recognizing the difficulties of establishing breach of duty of care. In the 1970s, the Pearson Commission extensively considered, but rejected, such an option (Royal Commission on Civil Liability and Compensation for Personal Injury, 1978).

A limited no-fault system was introduced by the Vaccine Damage Compensation Act 1979, which provides compensation in relation to harm caused through vaccine damage. This Act itself has proved problematic, not least because claimants had to establish that harm was caused through the negligence. Lord Woolf, in 1996, in a wide-ranging review of procedures for civil justice in this country, found that there were severe problems with the system for compensating people for medical or clinical negligence (Woolf, 1996). He singled out medical negligence for an intensive examination during his inquiry and gave his reasons for doing so:

> **The answer is that early in the Inquiry it became increasingly obvious that it was in the area of medical negligence that the civil justice system was failing most conspicuously to meet the needs of litigants in a number of respects.**
>
> a) **The disproportion between costs and damages in medical negligence is particularly excessive, especially in lower value cases.**
> b) **The delay in resolving claims is more often unacceptable**
> c) **Unmeritorious cases are often pursued, and clear-cut claims defended, for too long.**
> d) **The success rate is lower than in other personal injury litigation.**
> e) **The suspicion between the parties is more intense and the lack of co-operation frequently greater than in many other areas of litigation.**   (Woolf, 1996)

The Woolf Report led to some significant reforms being made to civil justice procedure, including the idea of putting the judge in the driving seat in civil cases, judicial case management, and pre-action protocols. The first pre-action protocol to be created was the Pre-Action Protocol for the Resolution of

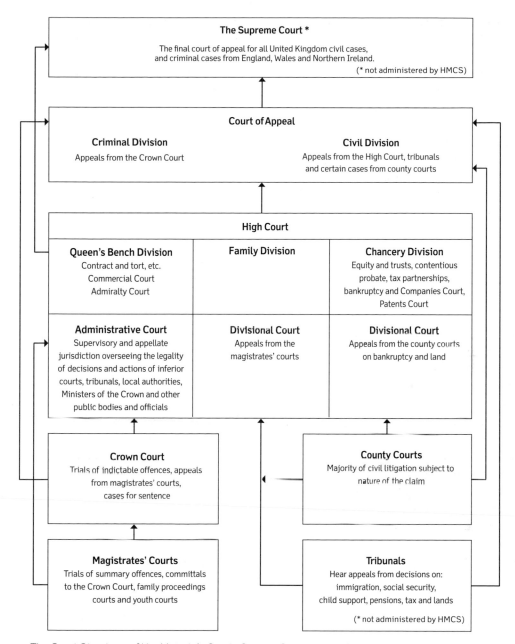

Figure 14.1 The Court Structure of Her Majesty's Courts Service. Crown copyright.

Clinical Disputes. Non-compliance with the protocol can result in sanctions being imposed. The general aims of the protocol are to:

- maintain/restore the patient–healthcare provider relationship; and

- resolve as many disputes as possible without litigation.

Protocols help to streamline the litigation process by specifying clearly the steps to follow pre-action, standardizing relevant information, giving time deadlines, and detailing what records and documents should be disclosed, etc. The civil litigation system is being better managed and there are fewer delays, because the parties have a set number of agreed steps to follow.

Lord Woolf's reforms have speeded up the handling of clinical negligence claims and there are earlier settlements reached without going to court. Lord Woolf's reforms, according to the Chief Medical Officer (Donaldson, 2003), 'are making an impact'. In practice, the majority of cases do not reach the courtroom. As the NHSLA has noted in its annual report:

> **We aim to settle claims as promptly as possible and we encourage NHS organizations to offer patients and staff explanations and apologies. We seek to avoid formal litigation as far as possible and our historical data shows that only about 4 per cent of our cases go to court ...**
> **(NHSLA, 2010)**

But problems still remain. The Chief Medical Officer stated:

> **Legal proceedings for medical injury frequently progress in an atmosphere of confrontation, acrimony, misunderstanding and bitterness. The emphasis is on revealing as little as possible about what went wrong, defending clinical decisions that were taken and only reluctantly releasing information.** **(Donaldson, 2003)**

The report put forward a number of reforms and nineteen recommendations were made, which included an NHS redress scheme. The report considered the no-fault compensation schemes operational in jurisdictions such as New Zealand (Oliphant, 1996; 2007). However, ultimately, this option was rejected. One major concern in moving towards such a system has long been that of cost. The NHS Redress Act 2006 was passed and contains a scheme to deal with low-value tort claims arising out of hospital services, but there are no detailed scheme provisions at the time of writing. There is, however, a government policy statement that does give some structure to the scheme (Department of Health, 2005). This provides that:

> **The NHS Redress Scheme will provide a mechanism for the swift resolution of low monetary value claims in tort arising out of hospital services provided as part of the NHS in England (wherever those services are provided), without the need to go to court. The scheme will only apply to claims in tort in respect of personal injury or loss arising out of a breach of a duty of care and arising as a consequence of any act or omission of a health care professional. The scheme will not, for example, cover liabilities arising from slipping or tripping caused by the act or omission of non-health care professionals such as maintenance staff.**

It has been several years since the legislation was passed, but the law has not yet been brought into force—a fact not gone unnoticed by the Health Committee (2009):

> **We are appalled at the failure of the DH to implement the NHS Redress Scheme three years after Parliament passed the necessary legislation. The DH has explained that it wishes to focus on complaints reform and will consider the matter of redress, 'When the reformed complaints arrangements are embedded'. We find this wholly unsatisfactory.**

The delay has more recently been noted by Lord Young of Graffham in his report to the Prime Minister on health and safety laws and the growth of the compensation culture (Lord Young of Graffham, 2010):

> **The Department of Health has already considered new approaches to the handling of low value clinical negligence claims. The NHS Redress Act 2006 missed an opportunity to improve fundamentally the way that clinical negligence claims are handled. It should have focused on improving the fact-finding phase prior to pursuit of a claim in order to facilitate faster resolution of claims and leaving it to the parties concerned, or ultimately the courts, to determine cases not resolved by the fact-finding. The Department of Health is currently considering ways to improve fact-finding as a means to speed up claims settlement and reduce costs.**

If proposals can be developed along these lines, the Department of Health should also consider how these improvements relate to my recommendation to explore how the Road Traffic Accident Personal Injury Scheme framework could be extended to low value clinical negligence claims.

The earlier and very influential report of the Bristol Royal Infirmary Inquiry (2001) was also critical of the system of clinical negligence, and felt that it was out of step with current initiatives for patient safety and should be abolished:

The system is now out of alignment with other policy initiatives on quality and safety: in fact it serves to undermine those policies and inhibits improvements in the safety of the care received by patients. Ultimately, we take the view that it will not be possible to achieve an environment of full, open reporting within the NHS when, outside it, there exists a litigation system the incentives of which press in the opposite direction. We believe that the way forward lies in the abolition of clinical negligence litigation, taking clinical error out of the courts and the tort system.

If clinical error is taken out of the court system, then this would have the consequence that we would lose a crucial medical and nursing accountability mechanism: the courts. Professionals of all kinds, including doctors and nurses, worry about being sued for negligence in a rights-based society. Professional organizations offer what is termed 'professional indemnity insurance'. The NMC Code advises that nurse obtain such insurance:

The NMC recommends that a registered nurse, midwife or specialist community public health nurse, in advising, treating and caring for patients/clients, has professional indemnity insurance. This is in the interests of clients, patients and registrants in the event of claims of professional negligence.   (NMC, 2008)

As well as being a mechanism of professional accountability and deterrence, the tort-based system also educates through publishing decided cases. But surely an important question to ask is: why should clinical negligence cases be treated differently from those, say, of the negligent solicitor or architect? What makes clinical negligence cases so special?

···

Does your professional body have a disciplinary procedure?
Can you obtain a copy of it and are these cases in the public domain so that other nurses can learn from them?

···

There is the 'one pocket' argument. The NHS (the defendant) provides the care and is probably the only care provider; there is nowhere else for the patient to go. The government owns the NHS and the government would also probably fund the claimant's legal action as well. But is all of this sufficient to warrant a system change? Perhaps not. An argument for retaining the present system can also be based on the need for professionals to be personally responsible for their own actions—that is, 'individual professional accountability'. While nurses are professionally accountable through their professional body, the law of negligence provides an important form of public accountability.

The NHS complaints system has recently been reformed (Department of Health, 2009; The Local Authority Social Services and NHS Complaints (England) Regulations 2009). The focus of the new NHS complaints system is on dealing with complaints locally and not centrally—in a sense, 'bringing complaints home'. This philosophy also applies equally to clinical negligence. The negligent doctor or nurse is always personally liable for their negligence and could be sued personally by the injured patient; this reinforces personal professional accountability, which must practically and ethically be a good thing. In reality, the principle of vicarious liability brings into the frame the employer, who will be held liable if the doctor or nurse was negligent, assuming that he or she was an employee and acting within the course of his or her employment. The employee still remains liable in these circumstances and is not exonerated. He or she could still face disciplinary action. This point should be stressed more by NHS trusts to their staff. The tort-based civil compensation system is still with us for clinical negligence and it should stay with us as an important mechanism of healthcare accountability.

....

Your place of work as a nurse should have a complaints system. Check to see if it has and make sure that you understand how this operates.
How many complaints does your place of work receive every year?

....

Patient safety

As we have seen, the level of litigation has increased, but some of the problems of the tort system, although not all, have been ameliorated. One approach is, of course, that of ensuring that systems of care are safe. Litigation may highlight a problem, but unless the findings of those judicial proceedings are translated into improvements in care, then there is a risk that a failure that is due to an unsafe system, for example, could reoccur in the future. Integral to improving patient care is concern with patient safety, health quality, and clinical governance. It is clear that patients are being avoidably injured in the NHS and that steps must be taken to develop an ingrained patient safety culture. The Healthcare Commission (2009) has commented that:

> **Various studies have been conducted, in the UK and internationally, in an attempt to discover the level of harm done to patients as a consequence of receiving healthcare services. Estimates range from less than 3% to over 16% of patients experiencing an 'adverse event', with around 50 per cent of these being preventable and around 20% being life threatening or fatal'.**

The Commission states in its report that there is patchy NHS trust performance against annual health check safety standards: '*Overall, performance has not improved—only around 50% of NHS trusts met all of the safety standards in each year.*'

The Commission concludes that the governance of safety issues in NHS trusts is '*not all that it could or should be*'. Safety is not always first on everyone's agenda; clearly, it should be. It remains a matter of concern that some evidence suggests that patient safety still requires greater prioritization.

NOTE: The Healthcare Commission, the Commission for Social Care Inspection, and the Mental Health Act Commission all ceased to exist on 31 March 2009, being replaced by the Care Quality Commission (CQC) as the single health and social care regulator for England (**http://www.cqc.org.uk/**).

The National Patient Safety Agency (NPSA; **http://www.npsa.nhs.uk/**) has developed some helpful tools to help NHS trusts in patient safety, including a national reporting and learning service—a reporting system whereby staff report safety incidents, which are then analysed and reports are fed back (NSPA, 2009). There are also helpful publications and root cause analysis training.

....

If you do not work in the UK, is there a similar body to the NPSA in your country?

....

There is some progress being made in making the NHS a safer place, but it is slow, incremental progress. Much depends upon the effective deployment of resources and development of effective structures at NHS trust level by individual NHS healthcare staff, senior managers, and executives.

Healthcare treatment, by definition, is a very risky enterprise, because it depends on human judgement, skills, and complex technology. The NHS is one of the largest organizations in the world, treating over 1 million patients a day, and '*As one of the largest organisations in the world, using a range of technologies, equipment, drugs, skills and expertise, sometimes things do go wrong*' (NPSA, 2005). Errors and mistakes will, to some degree, be an inevitable feature of professional life and practice; the key is to develop clinical risk management strategies to successfully manage the environment of care—to manage risk.

Nonetheless, there is a danger that, in managing risk, we could make doctors and nurses too risk-averse, and defensive medical and nursing practices could creep in. Protocols and guidelines are themselves not the whole answer; there is still an important place for professional judgement and carefully managed risk. There is a delicate balance to be drawn here.

On 26 July 2010, the Department of Health published its review of 'arm's-length bodies', which announced the planned abolition of the NPSA:

We propose to abolish the National Patient Safety Agency. Some National Patient Safety Agency functions will become part of the remit of the NHS Board, while others will be supported to continue in other ways. The following functions will transfer to elsewhere in the wider health system. (Department of Health, 2010b: [3.60])

This is deeply disappointing news: the NHS will greatly miss the NPSA, because it has provided an excellent focal point for patient safety in the NHS. Its publications and risk management tools are excellent, and have been commended both at home and abroad. It remains to be seen whether another equally patient-safety-focused champion will emerge.

Conclusion

The changing nature of nursing practice, with the increased level of specialist roles and the growth of personal autonomy in decision-making, bring with it new challenges, but also new responsibilities. Today, no longer will nurses in law be seen as the 'doctor's handmaidens'. This expanded role of nursing comes at a time when patient expectations have changed and developed. Thus nurses need to be aware of the boundaries of professional responsibility in relation to the NMC Code, and also the legal and ethical issues that arise in the context of nursing practice. It seems very unlikely that, at least in the short term, there will be a dramatic fall in litigation. Nurses must ensure that they maintain their skills, update them as appropriate, and in addition ensure that they

maintain a clear record of their actions. Such a record, while by itself not necessarily being determinative, may prove important as evidence in court. Defensible practice must be safe practice and nurses must work alongside colleagues in the NHS trust to fulfil the requirements of clinical governance, and must be aware of the need to practise a safe system of care.

References

Brazier, M. and Miola, J. (2000) 'Bye-bye *Bolam*: A medical litigation revolution?', *Medical Law Review* 8: 85.

Bristol Royal Infirmary Inquiry (2001) *Learning from Bristol: The Report of the Public Inquiry into Children's Heart Surgery at the Bristol Royal Infirmary 1984–1995*, Cm 5207, London: HMSO, available online at **http://www. bristol-inquiry.org.uk/** [accessed 16 June 2011].

Department of Health (2005) *NHS Redress: Statement of Policy*, London: HMSO.

Department of Health (2009) *Listening, Responding, Improving*, London: HMSO.

Department of Health (2010a) *The NHS Constitution for England,* London: HMSO, available online at **http://www. dh.gov.uk/en/Publicationsandstatistics/Publications/ PublicationsPolicyAndGuidance/DH_113613** [accessed 16 June 2011].

Department of Health (2010b) *Liberating the NHS: Report of the Arms-Length Bodies Review,* London: HMSO, available online at **http://www.dh.gov.uk/ en/Publicationsandstatistics/Publications/ PublicationsPolicyAndGuidance/DH_117691** [accessed 16 June 2011].

Donaldson, L. (2003) *Making Amends: A Consultation Paper Setting out Proposals for Reforming the Approach to Clinical Negligence in the NHS—A Report by the Chief Medical Officer*, London: HMSO, available online at **http:// www.dh.gov.uk/en/Publicationsandstatistics/ Publications/PublicationsPolicyAndGuidance/ DH_4010641** [accessed 16 June 2011].

Healthcare Commission (2009) *Safe in the Knowledge*, London: Healthcare Commission.

Health Committee (2009) *Patient Safety: Sixth Report of the Health Committee*, London: HMSO, available online at **http:// www.publications.parliament.uk/pa/cm200304/cmselect/ cmhealth/696/69602.htm** [accessed 16 June 2011].

Maclean, A. (2002) 'Beyond *Bolam* and *Bolitho*', *Medical Law International* 5: 205.

McHale, J. and Gallagher, A. (2004) *Nursing and Human Rights*, London: Butterworth-Heinemann.

Ministry of Justice (2009) *Pre-Action Protocol for the Resolution of Clinical Disputes*, available online at **http://www.justice.gov.uk/civil/procrules_fin/contents/protocols/prot_rcd.htm#IDAVBJ5B** [accessed 16 June 2011].

National Health Service Litigation Authority (2009) *Factsheet 2: Financial Information*, London: NHSLA.

National Health Service Litigation Authority (2010) *Report and Accounts 2010*, HC 52, London: HMSO, available online at **http://www.nhsla.com/NR/rdonlyres/3F5DFA84–2463–468B-890C-42C0FC16D4D6/0/NHSLAAnnualReportandAccounts2010.pdf** [accessed 16 June 2011].

National Patient Safety Agency (2005) *Building a Memory: Preventing Harm, Reducing Risk and Improving Patient Safety: The First Report of the National Reporting and Learning System and the Patient Safety Observatory*, London: NPSA.

National Patient Safety Agency (2009) 'Practical information, tools and support to improve patient safety in the NHS', available online at **http://www.nrls.npsa.nhs.uk/** [accessed 16 June 2011].

Nursing and Midwifery Council (2008) *The Code*, available online at **http://www.nmc-uk.org/Nurses-and-midwives/The-code/** [accessed 16 June 2011].

Oliphant, K. (1996) 'Defining "medical misadventure": Lessons from New Zealand', *Medical Law Review* 4: 1.

Oliphant, K. (2007) 'Beyond misadventure: Medical injuries in New Zealand', *Medical Law Review* 15: 357.

Royal Commission on Civil Liability and Compensation for Personal Injury (1978) *Report of the Royal Commission on Civil Liability and Compensation for Personal Injury*, Cmnd 7054, London: TSO ('the Pearson Report').

Samanta, A., Mello, M.M., Foster, C., Tingle, J., and Samanta, J. (2006) 'The role of clinical guidelines in medical negligence litigation: A shift from the *Bolam* standard', *Medical Law Review* 14: 321.

Woolf (1996) *Access to Justice: Final Report*, London: HMSO ('the Woolf Report').

Lord Young of Graffham (2010) *Common Sense, Common Safety*, London: HMSO, available online at **http://www.number10.gov.uk/wp-content/uploads/402906_CommonSense_acc.pdf** [accessed 16 June 2011].

Cases

Bolam v. Friern Hospital Management Committee [1957] 2 All ER 118.

Bolitho v. City & Hackney Health Authority [1997] 4 All ER 771.

Clarke v. Adams (1950) 94 Sol J 599.

Crawford v. Charing Cross Hospital, The Times, 8 December 1953.

DeFreitas v. O'Brien [1995] 6 Med LR 108.

Fairchild v. Glenhaven Funeral Services [2002] UKHL 2.

Gascoine v. Ian Sheridan and Co v. Latham [1994] 5 Med LR 437.

Gregg v. Scott [2005] 2 AC 176

Hucks v. Cole (1960) [1994] 4 Med LR 393.

Marriott v. West Midlands Health Authority [1999] Lloyd's Rep Med 23.

Maynard v. West Midlands Regional Health Authority [1984] 1 WLR 634.

Wilsher v. Essex Area Health Authority [1988] 3 AC 1074.

Statutes

Human Rights Act 1998.

NHS Redress Act 2006.

Vaccine Damage Compensation Act 1979.

15 Care to complain

SUSAN HAMER AND STEVE PAGE

Learning outcomes

This chapter will enable you to:

- recognize the importance of learning and improvement from complaints and concerns;
- understand some of the challenges in handling concerns about health services;
- appreciate the importance of leadership and team philosophy to improving the quality of care; and
- critically explore approaches and tools that facilitate learning and improvement.

Introduction

This chapter will consider how feedback from patients and carers can be used to inform healthcare staff learning and improvement in standards of care. It will enable you to reflect on some of the challenges and barriers to learning from these sources, both external to the clinical team and in relation to the team and individual practitioners. The chapter will outline current thinking on dimensions of individual and team ethos and behaviour that can positively influence learning, and this will also provide an opportunity for personal reflection on your own nursing practice. This chapter will also introduce you to some of the practical tools and techniques used to facilitate learning and improvement from complaints and incidents.

Why is learning from complaints important?

As we develop healthcare services, we also improve our understanding of the relationship between clinical quality and the effectiveness of services. However, sometimes the speed of service changes and the availability of different forms of evidence can be challenging, and it can be difficult to know if you are doing the right thing in the right way for the individual in your care. Having the best evidence and the right resources feels like it should be the answer—but, intuitively, we know that it is not always enough.

What is it that makes care high quality for patients?

Most developed health systems spend a lot of time defining the answer to this question in order to both purchase (commission) and supply health services on behalf of patients (see **Box 15.1** for some examples).

Essential knowledge and skills for care

- You must respond appropriately and sensitively when people want to complain, providing assistance and support.

- You will use appropriate and relevant communication skills to deal with difficult and challenging circumstances, for example responding to and dealing with complaints and resolving disputes.

- You will share complaints, compliments, and comments with your team in order to improve care, and to enhance the patient experience and working environment.

- You will work within ethical and legal frameworks and local policies to deal with complaints, compliments, and concerns, acting on findings appropriately.

Box 15.1 Definitions of quality in health services

Examples of UK policy documents that describe clinical quality include:

- *The NHS Constitution* (Department of Health, 2009a);
- *The Essence of Care* (Department of Health, 2001);
- *High-Quality Care for All* (Department of Health, 2008a);
- *NHS Health and Well-Being* (Department of Health, 2009b);
- *NHS Operating Framework 2010–2011* (Department of Health, 2009c); and
- *NHS 2010–2015: From Good to Great* (Department of Health, 2009d).

Indeed, increasingly, patients will be making these choices about quality for themselves.

High Quality Care for All (Department of Health, 2008a) and other recent National Health Service guidance (Department of Health, 2009a; 2009b; 2009c; 2009d) identify three key dimensions of quality:

- safety;
- effectiveness; and
- patient experience.

Patient experience is an important dimension of deciding which health services to purchase and supply, and an area in which health services frequently have the most need for development. When individuals access health services, either as patients or as carers, this is often one of their most stressful life experiences. Patients can often perceive health services as dehumanizing and disempowering, even when they are highly independent and confident in their daily lives.

People generally expect to receive good quality technical care. Whether people feel that they are treated as individuals, with respect for privacy and dignity, and recognition of their cultural and religious needs, is often the factor that differentiates their feelings about the overall quality of care. Poor communication is often cited as one of the main causes for complaint. Good communication from health professionals is key to helping individuals to make effective choices. It can also determine whether and how individuals access

care in the future, and to what extent they are likely to follow healthcare advice.

A focus on the patient's experience is about much more than the finer points of courtesy. It also has a significant impact on success in relation to safety and effectiveness of care. Professionals can sometimes focus heavily on technical guidance, or on processes, without adequate consideration of the circumstances or needs of the individual patient. The best clinical guideline will not be effective if the professional does not relate this to the person's individual circumstances. Patients with long-term conditions often have more expertise in how the illness affects them as individuals than professionals who understand the general issues relating to treatment, but only have a passing knowledge of the individual's needs or reactions to the treatment. Care processes delivered without listening to feedback from patients or carers have also been known to lead to seriously harmful outcomes: for example, the case of Garry Taylor, a person with severe mental illness, who subsequently committed homicide. His mother's urgent and repeated warnings to health professionals when he was in an acute phase of his illness were not heeded, and professionals chose not to initiate further assessment or to increase his level of support. Such action may well have helped to prevent Garry from going on to commit a homicide (NHS North East Strategic Health Authority, 2007).

The National Patient Safety Agency guidance *Being Open* (NPSA, 2009a) addresses the importance of involving patients and carers in their care, and in particular in circumstances in which things have gone seriously wrong. The guidance highlights the need to communicate openly and honestly in such situations, and to provide active feedback about the investigation and follow-up. The guidance also emphasizes the potential contribution of patient and carers as experts in their own care and treatment, and the value of involving service users in the investigation and subsequent solution development.

There is an increasing expectation that healthcare services will be client-focused—responsive both to clients' needs and expectations. The NHS Constitution (Department of Health, 2009a) seeks to enshrine this in an explicit set of written rights and pledges, including statements about:

- access to care;
- quality of care;
- nationally approved treatments, drugs, and programmes;
- respect, consent, and confidentiality;
- informed choice;
- involvement in your health care and in the NHS; and
- complaints and redress.

Key statements include *'You have the right to expect NHS organisations to monitor, and make efforts to improve the quality of healthcare they commission or provide'*, and *'You have the right to know the outcome of any investigation into your complaint'*.

....

Take a look at the NHS Constitution.

Do you agree with its contents?

Do you think this should apply to all health services whoever they are delivered by?

Do you think that all health service staff whom you have seen uphold the Constitution in their practice?

What can we learn from complaints, concerns, and comments from service users and carers?

....

Feedback from people using healthcare services and their carers and families is potentially valuable in many ways. It can help to identify areas for improvement for the individual practitioner, for clinical teams, for an organization, and in some cases for whole health system. The Nursing and Midwifery Council's Code of Professional Conduct (NMC, 2008) features a section that sets out clear standards of professional behaviour in relation to how we should deal with problems (see **Box 15.2**).

Statistical information about formal complaints is published online by the NHS Information Centre for Health and Social Care (2009) (**http://www.ic.nhs.uk/**). According to its collated report, 89,139 written complaints were received by the NHS in 2008–09. These related to all types of NHS service, but the largest categories related to inpatient and outpatient hospital services, mental health services, and community care (see **Box 15.3**). Some 19,111 complaints related to the nursing, midwifery, and health visiting professions.

Box 15.2 *The Code: Standards of Conduct Performance and Ethics for Nurses and Midwives* (NMC, 2008)

Deal with problems

- You must give a constructive and honest response to anyone who complains about the care that they have received.
- You must not allow someone's complaint to prejudice the care that you provide for them.
- You must act immediately to put matters right if someone in your care has suffered harm for any reason.
- You must explain fully and promptly to the person affected what has happened and the likely effects.
- You must cooperate with internal and external investigations.

It can be seen from **Box 15.3** that the complaints relate to all aspects of quality: patient safety; clinical effectiveness; and patient experience. Complaints about clinical treatment are the largest single category, followed by delay or cancelled appointments. Complaints about communication and attitude of staff are major causes of complaint, and it is likely that these issues also underlie many of the issues in other complaint categories.

The Parliamentary and Health Service Ombudsman's annual report reviews cases to share learning from the investigations across the health service. Each year, the ombudsman also publishes a summary of recent complaints, which outlines the issues raised by the complainant and lessons learned from what has gone wrong. In the 2008 report (Parliamentary and Health Service Ombudsman, 2008), twelve cases were highlighted, including the cases of Mr L and Mr W (**Practice Example 15.1**).

These complaints highlight several issues in the patients' care relating to the attitude of individuals and the teams, the effectiveness of communication between team members and across organizations, and the extent to which the care was truly patient-focused. As a result, both the safety and clinical effectiveness of care were adversely affected, and both the patients' and their relatives' experience of the care that they received was undeniably distressing.

Box 15.3 Reasons for formal complaints in the NHS 2008–09

The subjects of the complaints were as follows.

Admission, discharge, and transfer arrangements	4,473
Aids and appliances, equipment, premises (including access)	2,055
Appointments, delay/cancellation (outpatient)	9,738
Appointments, delay/cancellation (inpatient)	2,364
Length of time waiting for a response or to be seen (NHS Direct)	134
Length of time waiting for a response or to be seen (walk-in centres)	255
Attitude of staff	11,332
All aspects of clinical treatment	37,149
Communication/information to patients (written and oral)	8,970
Consent to treatment	238
Complaints-handling	104
Patient's privacy and dignity	1,351
Patient's property and expenses	930
PCT [primary care trust] commissioning (including waiting lists)	1,038
Independent sector services commissioned by PCTs	116
Independent sector services commissioned by trusts	71
Personal records (including medical and/or complaints)	1,047
Failure to follow agreed procedures	820
Patient's status, discrimination (e.g. racial, gender, age)	172
Mortuary and post-mortem arrangements	65
Transport (ambulances and other)	1,450
Policy and commercial decisions of trusts	883
Code of openness—complaints	70
Hotel services (including food)	1,001
Other	3,872
Total	**89,698**

(NHS Information Centre for Health and Social Care, 2009)

The Parliamentary and Health Service Ombudsman is the final arbiter of complaints made against health services in England. There are also public service ombudsman services in Wales (**http://www.ombudsman-wales.org.uk/**), Northern Ireland (**http://www.ni-ombudsman.org.uk/**), and Scotland (**http://www.spso.org.uk/**).

The ombudsman has set out a number of principles of good administration, as follows.

- Getting it right
- Being customer-focused
- Being open and accountable
- Acting fairly and proportionately
- Putting things right
- Seeking continuous improvement

Consider the principles listed above.
(Readers outside of England should consult their local body, but do bear in mind that these *essential principles* inform most complaint services.)
Think about your own practice and the different ways in which you meet these principles in your daily practice.
Do you think that you personally contribute to developing a team culture that supports these principles?
Think of a time when this has not been your experience. What happened to stop best practice occurring? Has it happened more than once? Is it a poor practice habit?

PRACTICE EXAMPLE 15.1

The Parliamentary and Health Service Ombudsman's annual report: Mr L and Mr W

Mr L

Mr L was a patient with Alzheimer's disease (he was not able to communicate) and coeliac disease (needing a gluten-free diet), who lived in a nursing home. He was admitted to a hospital for surgery to remove a skin cancer. The referral letter to the hospital explained about his medical condition, and that he needed help with eating and drinking. The operation was successful and he was discharged back to the home by ambulance eight days later.

The complaint from Mr L's wife related to his discharge arrangements, lack of adherence to dietary requirements, the decision to send him for surgery when she was not present, and inaccuracies in his discharge prescription.

The ombudsman found that Mr L was caused avoidable distress by the failure to ensure that his wife was present when he was taken for surgery and when he was discharged. There was a lack of awareness of his needs arising from the Alzheimer's disease, because he had not been adequately assessed on arrival, there was no individualized care plan, and the hospital team had failed to start discharge planning at an early stage.

The ombudsman also found that the hospital failed to provide a suitable diet, even though it had been advised of his requirements. This resulted in Mrs L bringing food in for her husband, which staff accepted without trying to provide assistance.

The ombudsman also concluded that there was unacceptable confusion over Mr L's medication, which meant that he was given tablets despite his difficulty swallowing and that he was prescribed the wrong medication on discharge, and then did not receive the medication because of an error.

Mr W

In another case, Mr W, a 74-year-old man admitted to hospital for the treatment of an exacerbation of chronic obstructive pulmonary disease, was treated on an intensive care unit (ITU) and subsequently transferred to a respiratory ward. He then had episodes of confusion, difficulty with oxygen intake, and bleeding from his catheter site. He later contracted MRSA, developed diarrhoea, and was found to have Clostridium difficile. Mr W later died in another hospital as a result of respiratory failure.

Whilst the ombudsman concluded that the patient's clinical outcome was probably not affected by the care, there were significant deficiencies in care, including a lack of monitoring whilst Mr W waited to be transferred from ITU, and poor nursing care in relation to care planning, communication, pain management, infection management, patient privacy and dignity, and monitoring fluid intake/output. The ombudsman also found that there was a lack of multi-professional working, poor record-keeping, and poor end-of-life care, with no care plan or discussion with his family about resuscitation and the seriousness of his prognosis.

As part of the final principle, the ombudsman expects services to review policies and procedures regularly to make sure that these are effective, to ask for feedback and use it to improve services and performance, and to ensure that the organization learns lessons from complaints and uses these to improve services and performance.

The ombudsman says:

Part of a remedy may be to ensure that changes are made to policies, procedures and systems, staff training or all of these, to ensure that the maladministration or poor service is not repeated. It is important to ensure that lessons learnt are put into practice.

It is a false economy and poor administrative practice to deal with complaints only as they arise and to fail to correct the cause of the problem. Learning from complaints, and offering timely and effective remedies, gives the best outcome in terms of cost effectiveness and customer service—benefiting the service provider, the complainant and the taxpayer.

The public body should ensure that the person making the complaint receives:

- **An assurance that lessons have been learnt**
- **An explanation of changes made to prevent maladministration or poor service being repeated.**

Quality of service is an important measure of the effectiveness of public bodies. Learning from complaints is a powerful way of helping to develop the public body and increasing trust among the people who use its services.
(Parliamentary and Health Ombudsman, 2009a: 9)

The benefits of complaints

Learning from people's complaints can be of benefit to individual practitioners, healthcare teams, and whole organizations in a number of different ways and at several levels (see **Figure 15.1**).

Learning, for you as *an individual practitioner*, might help you to develop your skills in relation to:

- individualizing care, which achieves dignity and respect (see **Box 15.4**);
- recognizing the importance of viewing the patient as a whole person, rather than in relation to a specific condition;
- assessing the effectiveness of your communication skills with the patient or carer;
- developing technical knowledge and clinical care skills; and
- ensuring a clarity of expectations about care and treatment—for example, during procedures or at the point of discharge from hospital.

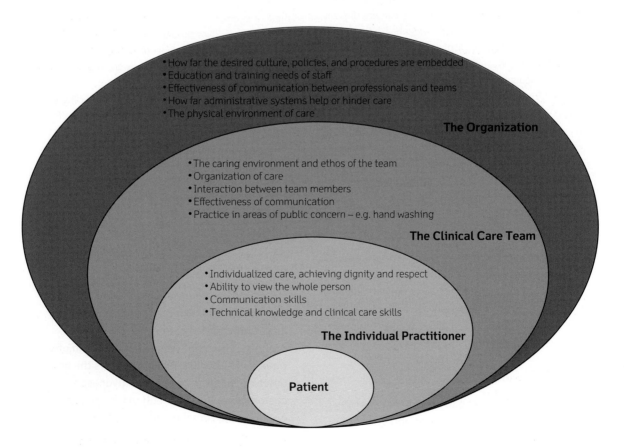

Figure 15.1 The benefits of complaints.

PRACTICE TIP

- Take a step back and look at what is happening with a fresh set of eyes. Try to imagine yourself as someone different, such as a patient, relative, or new employee.
- Just sit and watch: what is *really* happening?
- What are your other senses picking up?
- Do not try to judge, but instead keep an open mind: understanding will come from conversations with others.
- Get people to *show* you what they do rather than tell you.
- Look out for body language and how people have adapted to the work environment.

Box 15.4 Royal College of Nursing campaign: *Dignity at the Heart of Everything We Do*

The Royal College of Nursing campaign *Dignity at the Heart of Everything We Do* (RCN, 2009) focuses on dignity as a key aspect of the patient's experience.

When dignity is absent from care, people feel devalued, lacking control and comfort. They may also lack confidence, be unable to make decisions for themselves and feel humiliated, embarrassed or ashamed.

Providing dignity in care centres on three integral aspects:

- respecting patients' and clients' diversity and cultural needs, their privacy—including protecting it as much as possible—and their decisions;
- being compassionate when a patient or client and/or their relatives needs emotional support, rather than delivering only technical nursing care; and
- demonstrating sensitivity to patients and clients, ensuring their comfort.

The campaign highlights practical actions that nurses can take to meet these needs.

Ensuring a good service to all patients

Even if the approach to care and the supporting systems and processes meet the needs of the majority of patients, they may not be suitable for all. Complaints,

concerns, and other feedback from patients and carers can often also be a valuable source of learning about care for people whose needs are different in some way from those of the majority. This might include, for example, people from minority religious or ethnic groups, refugees or others who have a different first language, or people with a disability. *Six Lives* (Parliamentary and Health Service Ombudsman, 2009b) gives six examples of instances in which health services have not met the needs of people with learning disabilities. One example is that of Mr Cannon, a 30-year-old man with severe learning disabilities (**Practice Example 15.2**).

At the level of clinical care teams, learning from complaints and concerns might relate to:

- the caring environment and ethos of the team;
- organization of care and the ability to focus on the needs of individuals within a busy environment;
- interaction between team members—patients and carers observe health professionals closely and draw confidence or otherwise from their behaviour and the way in which they work together;
- effectiveness of communication between the team members and continuity of care; and
- practice in relation to issues of public concern—for example, cleanliness of the environment and handwashing.

Patient-centred care

In 2009, the Patients Association published its report *Patients ... not Numbers, People ... not Statistics*, in which it highlighted what it felt to be growing failures of fundamental care in hospitals (Patients Association, 2009). The report comprised a collection of stories, developed from a review of the Association's database of patients and relatives who had contacted it about the care that they had received. The majority of the stories centre on nursing care.

The introduction to this report highlights that whilst the national inpatient survey results from 2008 indicated an improvement in the number of patients rating their care as 'excellent', the number rating their care as 'poor' remained at 2 per cent, which was unchanged between 2002 and 2008. The Association estimated that if it were extrapolated to the whole NHS, this

PRACTICE EXAMPLE 15.2

Mr Cannon

Mr Cannon had very little speech, but was able to communicate with his family. He was able to walk unaided, but often needed support when he was feeling unsteady. He was described as having a fine sense of humour and enjoyed social events. He was admitted to hospital after breaking his hip. The bone was repaired and he was discharged home to his mother. However, he was seen by the GP four days later and was readmitted to hospital, because he was in pain and it was difficult to persuade him to eat or drink. He was then discharged again a week later. Over the next two weeks, his condition deteriorated further and he was again admitted to hospital, where he subsequently died.

Mr Cannon's parents complained that their son had been treated less favourably by health and social care agencies because of his learning disabilities, and that this contributed to his death. The ombudsman found many deficiencies in care, including failings in his care

relating to management of pain: his urgent need for pain relief was not met, and assessment and planning for pain management were poor. The assessment, observation, and monitoring of his care in the emergency department were inadequate. Management of his epilepsy was poor, owing to poor monitoring and medication not always being given as prescribed. Discharge arrangements were poor and he was discharged without due concern for his safety, with community healthcare providers not fully aware of his condition or the level of support that he needed. This meant that his mother was left to care for him.

The ombudsman's conclusion was that there were failings in the care and treatment, and that this was at least in part due to his disability. If care had been provided to reasonable accepted standards, the patient's suffering would have been less and he may well have survived. His family would also have suffered less anxiety and distress.

would represent over 1 million patients between 2002 and 2008 who felt that they had received poor care.

The report called to action individual trusts and national agencies in managing and reviewing complaints, and also on key aspects of care: dignity standards; assistance with eating, toileting, and personal hygiene, generally; and in particular in relation to care of older people and end-of-life care.

The first account related to the care of Leslie Kirk, an 86-year-old gentleman, provided by his son Ron Kirk (**Practice Example 15.3**).

....

You may wish to stop and reflect at this point in the chapter on what it is that makes care delivered by one team excellent, whilst that delivered by another team in the same organization so desperately inadequate.

From your own experience, can you list those aspects of a team environment that get the best out of you?

....

For organizations, learning from complaints and concerns might relate to:

- the degree to which the desired culture, policies, and procedures are embedded in everyday practice;

- the education and training needs of staff;
- the effectiveness of inter-professional, inter-departmental, and inter-agency communication, interfaces in care which are frequently the points at which care breaks down, so that the patient does not experience a continuous pathway, but a disjointed series of episodes that can affect both the quality of the experience and, in extreme cases, the safety of the care provided;
- the degree to which administrative systems and processes help or hinder the patient's care—clinical care can be excellent, but if the planning or booking system for appointments or investigations, the referral process for specialist care, or communication between agencies when patients are discharged or transferred are flawed, then the experience will not be a good one;
- the general environment—including cleanliness, organization, quality of food, and other fundamental non-clinical aspects of the patient's experience.

Major inquiries into poor standards of care

There are occasions when care in an organization becomes so poor that it results in a major inquiry.

PRACTICE EXAMPLE 15.3

Leslie Kirk

Leslie Kirk was admitted to hospital after having a stroke. The family was initially greeted on the ward by a nurse who said: 'There is only me and I will get to you when I can.'

The family noted that toilets were not properly cleaned and that they often had to clean the toilet themselves before their father could use it. His swallowing was not safe, but drinks were supplied even when there was an instruction over his bed to the contrary. Soiled linen and dirty food trays were on view, and personal items often went missing. At one point, his personal alarm was removed, making it difficult for him to get help when in severe pain. When challenged, the nurse said that this was because he kept pressing it. His catheter bag was not changed when full, he was not showered or shaved regularly, and he was cold in bed, so his family had to bring a blanket in for him. He was also given no rehabilitation exercises to aid his recovery. The family also witnessed similar problems with the care of other patients. They felt that staff were either off-hand or simply ignored the points raised. They did not feel that anyone cared for the patients and they overheard staff complaining about how long they had been on duty.

Tellingly, the family contrasted this with the excellent care that the patient received when transferred to another ward, which highlighted to them that it was possible for their father to receive the care that he needed.

One such inquiry considered the care given by an organization over a number of years. The report by Robert Francis QC (2010) into the care provided by Mid Staffordshire NHS Foundation Trust between 2005 and 2009 drew on extensive narrative evidence from patients and their families.

A section of the report focuses specifically on the patient experience. This highlights problems relating to:

- continence and bladder and bowel care—for example, one woman describes a situation in which her mother was on the commode, noting that *'everyone could have seen her. That is why I was so distressed because my Mum would have been horrified if she would have known that people were walking past and could see her'*;
- safety—particularly relating to poor assessment and monitoring of patients at risk of falling;
- personal and oral hygiene—for example, *'they left my father with a crusted up mouth, a furred-up tongue, nobody had even gone to wash his mouth or clean his mouth out with a swab or anything'*;
- nutrition and hydration—for example, *'I actually went in that lunchtime to see Mum sitting there looking at a plastic cheese salad that was in a plate at the end of the bed that she could not reach, with an orange that she could not peel'*;

- pressure area care—with examples of patients developing bed sores because they were not moved enough;
- cleanliness and infection control—one side ward was described by a family member as *'absolutely filthy. We cleaned it daily. I had never seen so much dust in all my life'*, while another family commented on clinical waste and blood left lying around on the ward;
- privacy and dignity—patients' needs were described by relatives as being ignored, as though *'it didn't matter if he had been lying there in hours of pain, as long as … in other words, on ward 10 the patients revolved around the staff. If it was inconvenient for staff it wasn't done'*;
- record-keeping—leading, for example, to a lack of consistent care or continuity of communication with the family;
- diagnosis and treatment—arising from poor observation, assessment, and clinical supervision, and a failure to listen to families who had information about the patient;
- communication—including a lack of compassion or sense that staff cared about patients as individuals, lack of involvement of families and patients in decisions, and lack of communication between team members; and

- **discharge management**—without effective assessment of the patient's needs, arrangements or communication.

The report provides examples to illustrate these deficiencies and a number of more detailed vignettes of poor patient care, and it describes the situation as a *'systematic failure of the provision of good care'* (Francis, 2010).

Uncaring attitudes of staff were felt to contribute to the problems, with patients often left struggling to cope for themselves, or with their families having to support them, for example by taking soiled linen home to wash. Inadequately skilled staff and insufficient staff were also found to be contributing factors, with the organization focusing primarily on finance and targets rather than on quality of care. The clinical staff and managers of the organization were described as disengaged from one another, staff morale was low, and there was a lack of openness and acceptance of poor standards. The organization was also described as being isolated from other health services, and in denial about feedback on the care and services.

Clearly, this was an organization that was not focused on using feedback from patients and carers to support learning and improvement at any level. The trust was said to have relied principally on reports from external bodies to give it assurance about the quality of care, rather than direct, 'real-time' information from people using its service or from the clinical staff providing care.

Feedback from patients, carers, and families is highly complementary to learning from other reporting systems and there is often very little overlap between the issues highlighted from the different sources. This suggests that an approach that considers learning from patient feedback alongside that from other systems as a single coherent process is the key to ensuring that important lessons for improvement are not overlooked, and is therefore essential to the provision of safe, high-quality care. Recommendations for organizations arising from the reviews of care such as Mid Staffordshire NHS Foundation Trust emphasize this point, and result in a wide-ranging set of recommendations for all healthcare

organizations arising from this very significant health-care failure.

How can we ensure effective learning and improvement in organizations?

It is essential that organizations have in place effective systems and processes for learning from complaints, concerns, and other service user feedback (see **Figure 15.2**). In order to learn effectively from an individual complaint, we need to look at broader issues.

The absence of such systems and processes has been highlighted in several recent reports as a contributing factor to poor standards of clinical care and patient experience. Newspaper headlines reflect how complaints may be headlined in the media. The Francis Report (2010) highlighted the focus of one NHS trust on finance and targets, and over-reliance on external inspections, without effective processes for collating and learning from patient experiences. As a result, the significant failings in care, which have subsequently been identified through the inquiry based on extensive evidence from patients and carers, were not identified or addressed by the trust.

The Report notes that the investigation of complaints produced:

> **Defensive rather than constructive reports which lacked credibility with complainants … Replies to complaints were often provided too slowly and did not always address all the issues raised. …**
>
> **A particularly disturbing feature of the complaints process was that the Trust often did not apply effective remedial action. This is evidenced by a series of complaints raising similar issues in which the response each time was an action plan which, if implemented, would have avoided a subsequent incident.**   (Francis, 2010)

To ensure effective learning from complaints, organizations need to have a systematic approach and a number of key measures in place (see **Box 15.5**).

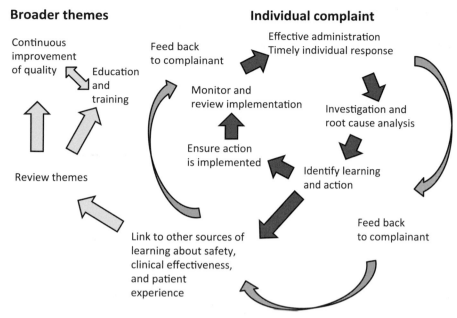

Figure 15.2 The broader issues and an individual complaint.

Box 15.5 Key organizational activities to support learning and improvement

Several key organizational activities have been identified that, if well established, support learning and improvement, as follows.

- There must be clear values and expectations about the primary importance of quality of care within the organization. This needs to be clear at the strategic level—that is, at board level—but communicated and reinforced through action at all levels of leadership in the organization. All leaders need to include a clear expectation that patient feedback will be taken seriously and used to inform learning and improvement.
- Well-defined and effective systems and processes will be used to capture patient and carer feedback, to investigate concerns, and to plan, implement, and monitor any action arising from these investigations. The systems and processes also need to be focused on any patterns of issues that recur across a number of separate complaints or concerns.
- Integrated learning systems and processes will coordinate learning across different reporting systems, so that issues arising from complaints and concerns are considered in the round, along with those from incidents and near misses, claims, and other sources of quality information.
- Effective communication and feedback processes will be in place, so that the complainants and all staff for whom the issues are relevant are aware of the learning and able to apply this to their practice.
- There will be links drawn between learning from complaints and concerns and education and training, so that important learning points can be built into training.
- There will be links made between complaints and concerns and quality audit and improvement processes, to give the organization confidence that learning has been embedded in practice and that the risk of recurrence is minimized.

Simple communication of lessons may not be enough to bring about change in practice. There are many reasons why lessons communicated to clinicians and others across an organization may not be implemented in practice, including competing pressures, systems and processes that do not support change in practice, local culture, and leadership.

Patient-centred teams?

In most situations, healthcare professionals work in teams—often in mixed teams of different professions and supporting roles. The way in which the team as a whole works is a very powerful factor in the quality of care that patients receive. It can support individual practitioners in providing excellent care, or it can actively hinder this.

The philosophy and values of a team help to determine the overall approach to the people in their care. Does the team view patients and carers as the main focus of its work, or is the prevailing view that patients are a nuisance and that patients' expectations of individualized care are unrealistic for such a busy team? Does the team work on the understanding that the professionals know best, or does it recognize that service users can have very different insights and often expertise in their own condition and care needs, based on experiences not available to professionals? Does the team find time to reflect on patient or carer feedback about when things have gone wrong and how these can be improved, or does it shrug these off as 'just one of those things', or react to such feedback defensively and seek to justify practice by blaming external factors? Does the team find time to share and nurture new ideas for improving practice, or are these greeted negatively, because of the extra work that they will entail, or because they have been tried before and failed? Do team members value one another and communicate effectively, or do they work as individuals, communicating only when absolutely necessary? How do individual team members support one another in times of difficulty?

The philosophy and values of the team (often referred to as 'culture', or 'team climate') have a direct impact on the way in which the team members react to patients and carers, and on the quality of care delivered. Studies of team behaviour and patient outcomes by West et al. (2001) have demonstrated that effective, patient-focused teams are far more likely to deliver effective care and to provide a positive patient experience. We also know from complaints that poor attitude and ineffective communication are the most prevalent issues raised in complaints. Poor continuity of care, across shifts, disciplines, or departments, is also a very common issue that is directly affected by poor teamwork.

The responsiveness of a team to its patients and its effectiveness in delivering high-quality care can be positively influenced. Effective leadership to establish the right values and to provide a supportive working environment based on these values is central.

Leadership is insufficient on its own, however. As a nurse, your own contribution to the work of the whole team is as important as the quality of your one-to-one interactions with your patients. For a team to deliver the best quality of care, all of the individuals in the team need to contribute positively to the wider function of the team, and to the processes of learning and development that will enable the team's care to improve continuously over time.

Because of the busy nature of their work, teams can often become immersed in their day-to-day work and environments. They can become constrained by existing processes and bureaucracy, either within the team itself or in the wider organization, or they can be passively accepting of a poor physical environment or support from other departments. Sometimes there is a belief in the team that it is powerless to change these things, either because it has no time or because it does not have the authority and influence. Approaches and toolkits such as the NHS Productive Series, published by the NHS Institute for Innovation and Improvement (2010), are designed to help teams to focus practically on what is important in patient care. The Productive Series provides a framework to help nurses and others to identify those aspects of their work that do not add any value to their care and to manage these more effectively, so that the team can 'release more time to care'. They help nursing teams with practical approaches to their work, which empowers teams to influence the quality of their care.

Developing my own practice?

We can do many things to help to reduce the likelihood of things going wrong, but with busy, complex services, it is always possible that mistakes can happen or that services will not quite match the needs of individual patients. When things go wrong, it is important to acknowledge this, to put things right as quickly as possible, and to learn from the experience.

The new process for managing complaints in the NHS, which was introduced after the *Making Experiences*

Count review (Department of Health, 2008b) emphasizes the importance of a more personal, flexible, and prompt approach to responding to complaints, rather than the previous slow, bureaucratic system. This personal approach underlines the important role of individual nurses and other professionals in responding openly and frankly to concerns and complaints, and in taking action to address issues rather than automatically referring these into a formal complaints department or process.

This helps to give confidence to patients and carers that their concerns are being taken seriously, and often helps to avoid the patient or carer developing a general dissatisfaction or disillusionment with their care, based on an impression that no one is really bothered (Department of Health, 2009e). The review of the complaints system in the NHS in Scotland (NHS Scotland, 2009) included feedback from service users, such as:

I don't really want to complain ... but do not want this to happen to anyone else.

The patient felt so disempowered that they would never complain, or even voice their real concern, because they did not want to make a fuss or draw attention to themselves, or because they worried that their care could be prejudiced in the future.

The report emphasizes the need for active listening to ensure that we can identify and learn from the experiences of service users. This includes:

- encouraging suggestions or comments as opportunities for change;
- ensuring that individuals are given the help that they need to have their voices heard;
- providing staff with the training and support to consistently display sensitivity and understanding to people who are at a vulnerable and stressful part of their lives;
- empowering staff to listen to and act upon the suggestions of the people for whom they care;
- letting people who use services see action being taken to change a negative experience into one that empowers; and
- focusing on partnership between staff and patients that will improve the quality of care for everyone who uses the service.

The report suggests that practitioners should respond positively and appropriately if a patient raises a concern. They should:

- ensure that the patient's immediate health care needs are being met, before dealing with the suggestion or comment rapidly, sensitively, and confidentially;
- discuss the matter of concern with the patient, encouraging them to speak freely;
- provide an honest and objective response—on the spot if possible, or where this is not possible, within a timescale agreed with the patient—which should include an explanation and an apology, where appropriate, and indicate what is being done to avoid the problem happening again (any oral or written response about a clinical matter should be agreed with other appropriate clinicians);
- where a patient has requested it, issue a written response, approved by a clinician or senior member of staff (details of the concern and a copy of the written response should be sent to the organization's complaints officer); and
- consider—based on their assessment of the situation, the nature of the concern, and their knowledge of any previous similar situations—what action is appropriate to share the information and ensure that the organization learns from the process.

Practitioners should also understand that, where they feel unable to respond themselves, they can:

- call on the support of an appropriate senior member of staff; and/or
- offer the patient the option of discussing the matter with someone not directly involved in their care—for example, someone from another ward or department, the practice manager, someone from the organization's complaints staff, or an independent advice and support organization.

Reflection on experience and on the application of knowledge into practice is an important aspect of learning and development for healthcare professionals. Consideration of learning from patient or carer feedback is a central part of this process. It is easy to become defensive when faced with complaints from patients or carers, and to feel that their comments are inaccurate or out of context, but it is important to be self-critical in such circumstances. Often, the patient or carer can see things that professionals overlook when they are busy or simply used to similar situations every day. Even where comments are inaccurate, they are a reflection of the patient or carer's experience of the situation and this is important in itself.

PRACTICE TIP

As a practitioner, it is important to be reflective and to ask questions such as:

- what values and principles do I hold that underpin my practice?
- how far has my practice today reflected those values and principles?
- what have patients and carers told me informally today about the care that I have provided?
- is there anything that I can do to improve my care based on a complaint received from a patient or carer?
- is there anything that I can do to improve my communication with patients and carers based on feedback in a complaint or concern?
- how can I improve continuity of care through my work with other professionals and organizations?
- how can I contribute to creating the right environment within my own team and area of work to support excellent care and treatment?

Conclusion

This chapter has considered the importance of listening to feedback from patients and carers to the provision of safe, high-quality care. Patient and carer feedback can highlight significant factors affecting the safety of care, issues affecting clinical effectiveness of treatments, and also aspects of attitude, environment, or interpersonal and physical care affecting the dignity and well-being of vulnerable individuals.

As an individual nurse, you can choose whether to care about the patient or carer's complaints or concerns. You can also choose how you respond and act on such concerns. Your organization and immediate team can support or hinder you as an individual professional, but equally you have a key role to play in making and contributing to an effective team with the right patient-focused ethos. Above all, you have a professional duty to care and to raise concerns yourself if standards are not as they should be.

We hope that this chapter has provided some insights into the importance of complaints, concerns, and other feedback to your understanding of the quality of care being delivered, and that it has helped you to develop your approach to using this feedback constructively to continuously improve your practice.

Further reading

National Health Service Institute for Innovation and Improvement

NHS Institute for Innovation and Improvement (2010) *The Productive Series,* Warwick: NHSI, available online at **http://www.institute.nhs.uk** [accessed 16 June 2011]

National Patient Safety Agency

National Patient Safety Agency (2009a) *Being Open: Communicating Patient Safety Incidents with Patients, their Families and Carers,* available online at **http://www.nrls.npsa.nhs.uk/beingopen/?entryid45=65077** [accessed 16 June 2011]

National Patient Safety Agency (2009) *Ombudsman's Principles of Good Complaint Handling,* available online at **http://www.ombudsman.org.uk/improving_services/principles/index.html** [accessed 16 June 2011]

Royal College of Nursing

RCN (2009) 'Dignity at the heart of everything we do', available online at **http://www.rcn.org.uk/newsevents/campaigns/dignity** [accessed 16 June 2011]

The Patients Association

The Patients Association (2009) *Patients ... not Numbers, People ... not Statistics,* available online at **http://www.patients-association.com/DBIMGS/file/Patients%20not%20numbers,%20people%20not%20statistics.pdf** [accessed 16 June 2011]

References

Department of Health (2001) *The Essence of Care: Patient-Focused Benchmarking for Health Care Practitioners*, London: HMSO.

Department of Health (2008a) *High Quality Care for All: NHS Next Stage Review—Final Report*, Cm 7432, London: HMSO.

Department of Health (2008b) *Making Experiences Count: The Proposed New Arrangements for Managing Health and Social Care Complaints—Response to Consultation*, London: HMSO.

Department of Health (2009a) *The NHS Constitution for England*, London: HMSO.

Department of Health (2009b) *NHS Health and Well-being: Final Report*, London: HMSO.

Department of Health (2009c) *The Operating Framework for the NHS England 2010–2011*, London: HMSO.

Department of Health (2009d) *NHS 2010–2015: From Good to Great*, Cm 7775, London: HMSO.

Department of Health (2009e) *Listening, Responding, Improving: A Guide to Better Customer Care*, London: HMSO.

Francis, R. (2010) *Independent Inquiry into Care Provided by Mid Staffordshire NHS Foundation Trust, January 2002– March 2009: Vol. 1*, London: HMSO.

National Patient Safety Agency (2009a) *Being Open: Communicating Patient Safety Incidents with Patients, their Families and Carers*, available online at **http://www.nrls.npsa.nhs.uk/beingopen/?entryid45=65077** [accessed 16 June 2011].

NHS Information Centre for Health and Social Care (2009) *Data on Written Complaints in the NHS 2008–09*, available online at **http://www.ic.nhs.uk/statistics-and-data-collections/audits-and-performance/complaints/data-on-written-complaints-in-the-nhs-2008-09** [accessed 5 July 2011].

NHS Institute for Innovation and Improvement (2010) *The Productive Series*, Warwick: NHSI, available online at **http://www.institute.nhs.uk** [accessed 16 June 2011].

NHS Scotland (2009) *Can I Help You? Learning from Comments, Concerns and Complaints*, Edinburgh: NHS Scotland.

North East Strategic Health Authority (2007) *Report to the North East Strategic Health Authority of the Independent Inquiry into the Health Care and treatment of Garry Taylor*, available online at **http://www.northeast.nhs.uk/_assets/media/pdf/inquiries/Garry_Taylor_Independent_Inquiry_report_-_14_Decem.pdf** [accessed 16 June 2011].

Nursing and Midwifery Council (2008) *The Code: Standards of Conduct Performance and Ethics for Nurses and Midwives*, London: NMC.

Parliamentary and Health Service Ombudsman (2008) *Remedy in the NHS: Summaries of Recent Cases*, London: HMSO.

Parliamentary and Health Service Ombudsman (2009a) *Principles for Remedy*, available online at **http://www.ombudsman.org.uk/__data/assets/pdf_file/0009/1035/Principles-for-Remedy.pdf** [accessed 5 July 2011].

Parliamentary and Health Service Ombudsman (2009b) *Six Lives: The Provision of Public Services to People with Learning Disabilities*, London: HMSO.

Patients Association, The (2009) *Patients ... not Numbers, People ... not Statistics*, available online at **http://www.patients-association.com/DBIMGS/file/Patients%20not%20numbers,%20people%20not%20statistics.pdf** [accessed 16 June 2011].

Royal College of Nursing (2009) 'Dignity at the heart of everything we do', available online at **http://www.rcn.org.uk/newsevents/campaigns/dignity** [accessed 16 June 2011].

West, B.A., Borrill, C., and Unsworth, K.L. (2001) 'Team and effectiveness in organisations', in C.L. Cooper and I.T. Robertson (eds) *Organisational Psychology and Development*, Chichester: John Wiley & Sons, pp. 150–96

16 So you think you've cared

SALLY BREARLEY AND PETER GRIFFITHS

Learning outcomes

This chapter will enable you to:

- understand what is meant by 'quality of care' in the context of this chapter;
- explore some of the techniques and tools commonly used for measuring quality of care;
- begin to evaluate the quality of your own care-giving;
- begin to develop skills in questioning care;
- begin to develop informed and critical practice; and
- consider how to use feedback and evaluation to improve the quality of care.

Introduction

We can only be sure to improve what we can actually measure.

(Department of Health, 2008)

Chapter 3 introduced the subject of quality and considered the question: How do you know you are giving good quality care? Chapter 15 examined how complaints and media reports sometimes highlight bad or inadequate care given by nurses, and stressed the importance of learning from these events and using them to bring about positive change. One lesson to be learned is that nurses cannot feel truly confident in the quality of the care that they deliver and demonstrate it to others unless they are able to measure and evaluate its quality. This chapter explores the measurement and evaluation of care, and the ways in which this can increase nurses' confidence in their caring skills and competencies.

> **Essential knowledge and skills for care**
>
> - You must be responsible and accountable for keeping your knowledge and skills up to date through continuing professional development (CPD), aim to improve your performance and to enhance the safety and quality of care through evaluation, supervision, and appraisal.
>
> - You will continuously evaluate your care to improve clinical decision-making, quality, and outcomes, using a range of methods, amending the plan of care, where necessary, and communicating changes to others.
>
> - You will be prepared to act as an agent of change and to provide leadership through quality improvement and service development to enhance people's well-being and experiences of health care.
>
> - You will be aware of the need to systematically evaluate care and ensure that findings are used to help to improve people's experience and care outcomes, and to shape future services.

In recent years, nurses have started to develop ways in which to measure objectively the outcomes of the care that they give; we will refer to this as the 'clinical effectiveness of care'. There is a slightly longer history of asking patients to express their level of satisfaction with the care that they receive or to describe their experience of that care. Patients and their carers also need to know that they are being cared for by competent professionals and in an environment that will do them no harm, so patient safety is another element of quality of care. It is worth remembering that one of Florence Nightingale's most important contributions to health care was the use of mortality statistics to demonstrate how unsafe care in hospitals was at the time and the development of nurse training to ensure that nurses were properly qualified to provide safe care. Taken together, measures of patient safety, patient satisfaction or patient experience, and the clinical effectiveness of care can give us a good picture of the overall quality of care that we are giving. But what tools are available to measure these three dimensions of quality?

This chapter will look at some of the tools and techniques for measuring care, and consider how useful they are. Some of the tools can be used by nurses 'at the front line' of everyday care-giving. Others are used at a unit, organizational, or national level to give a broader picture of quality of care. How can we use each of these tools to develop a picture of the quality of care that we give? It is equally important to consider how we can use measurement and evaluation to *improve* the care that we give to patients. Are there ways in which we can build measurement, feedback, and evaluation into our day-to-day practice and use this to improve our care-giving?

It can be hard to measure ourselves and find that we are less than perfect. And it can be difficult to hear criticism from colleagues, our patients, or their carers—particularly if we feel that we are doing our best, perhaps under difficult or trying circumstances. We will discuss the importance of being open to a process of measurement, evaluation, and improvement from the very start of a nursing career. Nursing and other health service leaders acknowledge that nurses need support to maintain this process of critical reflection; resources and support are also needed to bring about improvements in care. We will mention some sources of the support on which nurses can draw as they develop both personally and professionally.

What do we mean by 'quality of care'?

∙∙

Think about care that you gave recently (for example, the final day of your most recent placement or another day that you can remember well).
What do you think about the quality of the care that you gave? Was it good, bad, or indifferent?

How do you know? For example, did you feel good about it? Did it have a good outcome for your patient? Did someone tell you that you had done a good job?
If someone had asked, 'How well have you cared today?', would there have been anything to which you could have pointed to answer this question?
∙∙

The definition of 'quality' that we will be using in this chapter is that given in *High Quality Care for All* (Department of Health, 2008), which was the outcome of the Next Stage Review of the National Health Service in England, conducted by Lord Ara Darzi ('the Darzi Review'). This defined quality for the English NHS in terms of patient safety, clinical effectiveness, and the experience of patients (see **Figure 16.1**).

In May 2010, a new British government was elected, the Secretary of State for Health in which has indicated that he approves of this three-part definition of quality and will not replace it (Department of Health, 2010a).

The Next Stage Review also highlighted the importance of measurement to support improvements in the quality of services. The quotation at the start of this chapter is taken from *High Quality Care for All*:

> **We can only be sure to improve what we can actually measure.**
>
> (Department of Health, 2008)

Again, the new government has endorsed the importance of quality measurement, but is keen to shift the focus from measuring 'processes' to measuring 'outcomes' (Department of Health, 2010b). In other words, we should concentrate on measuring the results of care-giving rather than on how we deliver care; for example measuring how many of our patients develop pressure sores rather than recording how many risk assessments we have carried out on them.

Measurement for Quality Improvement: The Approach (NHS Information Centre, 2009) sets out the Department of Health's intentions for the development and use of indicators of quality at all levels of the system. This will include:

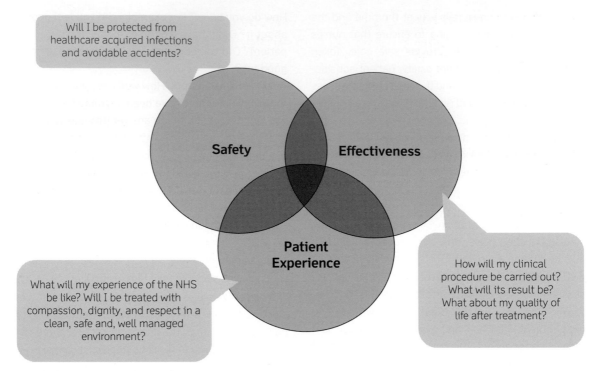

Figure 16.1 A definition of quality from Lord Darzi's review of the NHS 'High Quality Care for All' (Department of Health, 2008). Crown copyright.

- clinical teams using local measures for benchmarking and monitoring the care given day to day;
- organizations that provide NHS services to report on quality to their local population through quality accounts;
- those commissioning services using information on quality in their contracts through the Commissioning for Quality and Innovation (CQUIN) payment scheme;
- strategic health authorities and regional quality observatories supporting local measurement and driving improvements; and
- a national quality board to determine national priorities, coordinate quality improvement initiatives, and benchmark performance against other countries.

The dramatic worsening of the country's financial situation since that publication of the Darzi Review has led to a focus on increased productivity and efficiency across the NHS, the establishment of the Quality,

Innovation, Productivity and Prevention (QIPP) initiative, and the launch of a campaign to implement 'high-impact changes' for nursing and midwifery. The changing structure of the NHS and social care under the coalition government will present new challenges, the nature and extent of which are difficult to anticipate at the time of writing. These changes include the shift to GP commissioning and the likely abolition of primary care trusts and strategic health authorities in England. However, one thing is certain: there will be an increasing need to demonstrate the value of services in terms of both quality and productivity if they are to go on being paid for and delivered, and if nurses are to continue being employed in them.

Government policy and Department of Health initiatives can seem very far away from the day-to-day work that nurses do and those for whom they are caring. What we *can* do on a daily basis is capture what is important to service users and patients, seeking to measure this in a practical way and finding ways in which to make care better.

What do we mean by 'measurement' and 'evaluation'?

The *Shorter Oxford English Dictionary* gives several definitions of 'measure'. Those that we will be using here are:

To ascertain the spatial magnitude or quantity of something.

To appraise by a certain standard or rule, or by comparison with something else.

Before proceeding, consider how often we come across some form of measurement in everyday life.

You might, for example, think about when we weigh ourselves or cooking ingredients, or the marks or grades that we obtain in examinations or assignments.

'Evaluation' is defined as:

To work out the value of something.

Think of the measurements that you listed above. You will find that, whenever we measure, we tend to make evaluations as well. For example, are we the right weight? Have we got the amount of flour specified in the recipe? Did we do as well in the exam as our friend?

In everyday nursing practice, we routinely use measurement and evaluation. For example, we weigh and measure patients, we take their blood pressure and temperatures, we assess their fluid balance, and we ask them how they feel. With all these measurements we also evaluate. For example, we ask ourselves—and perhaps seek advice—to answer the question: is this normal in the circumstances, depending on the clinical situation, and for the individual concerned? Vital as these measurements and evaluations are to the work of the nurse, they are not the ones on which we will be focusing in this chapter. Instead, we shall look at measurement and evaluation that allows us to stand back a little from delivering care and our interactions with patients, and which helps us to answer the question: how well have we cared?

Theory, rationale, and evidence base

In the healthcare system as a whole, there are very many organizations and initiatives that have something to say about the quality of care, including nursing care. This section gives an overview of the most important of these, starting with national quality monitoring, then focusing on recent developments in nursing measurement, and ending with some tools that nurses can use with their own patients to improve quality of care.

We shall look in turn at:

- inspection and monitoring by outside organizations;
- peer review and benchmarking;
- patient satisfaction and patient experience;
- patient surveys and other ways of gathering feedback;
- patient-reported outcome measures (PROMs);
- nursing metrics and indicators;
- patient stories and experience-based design; and
- psychological aspects of measurement and evaluation.

Inspection and monitoring by outside organizations

A whole range of organizations inspect and monitor performance in the NHS. At the time of writing, these include the Audit Commission, the Health and Safety Executive (HSE), patient environment action teams (PEATs), and the National Patient Safety Agency (NPSA). However, for the NHS and social care in England, the main regulator for quality is the Care Quality Commission (CQC). CQC is a fairly new organization, having taken over from the Healthcare Commission (HCC) in 2009. It is perhaps best known for its sometimes high-profile inspections of services when problems have been identified with the quality of care being received by patients, for example Maidstone and Tunbridge Wells NHS Trust in 2007 and Mid Staffordshire NHS Foundation Trust in 2008. In addition to these occasional inspections, the CQC carries out a vast amount of measurement and inspection, and produces regular reports on all health and social care providers.

From 2010, a new registration system means that health and adult social care providers must be registered with CQC to show that they meet a wide range of essential, common quality standards. These standards are aimed to make the system fairer and more transparent, and to make it easier for one provider to be compared with another.

CQC also has the job of making sure that providers continue to meet its essential, common quality standards after registration. It does this by analysing and inspecting services, by asking providers to assess themselves, and by collecting information to help it to monitor how they are performing. If there is evidence of a serious and urgent problem that is putting people at risk, CQC promises that it will investigate and take immediate action where necessary.

CQC encourages everyone, whether a patient or staff member, to let it know through its website of any concerns that they have about quality of care in organizations providing NHS or social care services.

....

Visit http://www.cqc.org.uk and see what it has to say about an NHS organization in which you have worked, or in which you or a relative have been treated as a patient.

Ask members of staff with whom you work with if they have been involved in an HCC or CQC inspection and, if so, what it felt like.

In England, all independent clinics and hospitals that provide cosmetic surgery must be licensed with CQC. Next time you see an advertisement for cosmetic surgery, look for evidence that the organization is licensed.

....

Peer review and benchmarking

Hopefully, you will be familiar with the concept of 'peer review', whereby nurses review the work or performance of other nurses in order to maintain or enhance quality. This large and important topic will not be explored further here, except to issue a note of slight caution: feedback from our peers can definitely help us to improve the quality of care that we give, but we should not exclude the patient's perspective.

Sometimes, other nurses are better placed than the patient to know what care we could and should have provided, or how we could have improved its objective quality. For example, patients may not realize that they have been exposed to a risk to their safety. However, when nurses are reviewing each other's performance, they should check whether patients got the care that was important to them, which usually involves asking patients and carers about this in some way.

A 'benchmark' is a standard by which something can be measured or judged. Benchmarking can be very useful, because it enables us to compare our performance against that of other individuals, teams, or organizations. However, it is sometimes difficult to find the appropriate benchmarks and, ideally, benchmarking information needs to provide not only a comparison, but also some indication of what 'acceptable', 'good', and 'excellent' look like in relation to what is being measured. It is no good being told that we are delivering care as well as the next team if we do not know what quality of care we should be aiming to deliver and how we might bring about improvements to achieve this.

For nursing, one important benchmarking tool, which has been around for some time now, is the Essence of Care (EoC). EoC came about because of unacceptable variations in standards of care across the UK and was first launched in 2001. It has been updated several times since then and a new version appeared in October 2010 (Department of Health, 2010c). It uses best practice to structure a patient-focused approach to care and contributes to the process of clinical governance, which is the umbrella term for everything that helps to maintain and improve high standards of patient care.

In its present form, EoC has twelve benchmarks, which are fundamental aspects of care that were identified by patients and carers as being important to their experience of health care.

1 Bladder, bowel and continence care
2 Care environment

3 Communication

4 Food and drink

5 Prevention and management of pain

6 Personal hygiene

7 Prevention and management of pressure ulcers

8 Promoting health and well-being

9 Record-keeping

10 Respect and dignity

11 Safety

12 Self-care

Each of the benchmarks has a number of areas that must be addressed: for example, food and nutrition includes such topics as identifying patients' needs, assessing whether they need help when eating, and monitoring what they eat.

....

If you are not familiar with the EoC, ask your tutors or mentor about it.

When you are on placements, ask how it is used where you are working.

....

Patient satisfaction and patient experience

Many people talk about measuring patient *satisfaction*. For example, *From Good to Great* (Department of Health, 2009a) states:

> **Over the coming years we will greatly expand the measurement of patient satisfaction on a service-by-service basis within each hospital.**
>
> (ibid: 31)

However, there are widely acknowledged problems with using simple measures of patient satisfaction. For example, satisfaction can be influenced by aspects not related to direct experience of services, including personal expectations and demographic factors. We have probably all come across people who are very grateful for the care that they receive and are reluctant to say they are dissatisfied, even when we and they know that their experience has not really been very good. Also, measures of patient satisfaction alone often do not provide information that can be acted on to achieve change. If we simply ask someone, 'Were you satisfied with your care?' and they tick a box saying 'No', we will need to ask more questions to find out exactly what went wrong and what we might do to improve the situation.

Concern about the problems with patient satisfaction surveys has led to an emphasis on measuring patients' experience, rather than satisfaction. Instead of asking patients to rate their care using general categories (for example, 'excellent', 'very good', 'good', 'fair', 'poor'), they are asked to report in detail about their experiences of a particular service. The questions ask people to report on whether certain processes or events occurred rather than ask for the patient's evaluation of what occurred (Coulter et al., 2009).

Some of the large-scale surveys in the NHS (see next section) focus mainly on patient experience—what actually happened to the patient from their point of view—although they do also contain an element asking for a rating of overall satisfaction. Analysis of the survey responses can show how overall satisfaction relates to various components of experience. This provides information on where attention could be focused to improve general satisfaction. For example, one question about experience that is included in the National Inpatient Survey asks former patients if doctors or nurses talked in front of them as if they were not there. Politicians, in particular, are understandably interested in how to make people more satisfied with the health service as a whole. (If you would like to know more about the distinction between patient satisfaction and patient experience, see the further reading listed at the end of this chapter.)

Another reason for concentrating on patient experience rather than satisfaction is because professional and patient concerns about the state of nursing often centre on perceptions of a loss of compassion and expressions of caring (Corbin, 2008). Asking patients about their experiences of care and communication is, potentially, a useful indicator of the quality of nursing care (Griffiths et al., 2008).

Patient surveys

In recent years, the main way in which patient satisfaction and experience have been measured at organizational and national levels is through patient surveys.

Large-scale surveys of hospital patients began in the USA in the early 1990s. In England, annual postal surveys of hospital patients have been conducted since 1997, and since 2004 the results have been reported to the HCC (and now to the CQC). There is also a range of other national surveys, such as the GP Patient Survey and the National Patient Choice Survey.

It is perfectly possible to run small-scale patient surveys, and many people have used this technique to measure aspects of patient experience for groups of patients at service, unit, and ward levels. However, to make this an effective use of staff and patient time, those running the survey need to know what they are doing:

> **The world is full of well-meaning people who believe that anyone who can write plain English and has a modicum of common sense can produce a questionnaire.**   (Oppenheim, 1966)

In this quote from the preface to the first edition of an influential book on questionnaire design, the author implies that those well-meaning people are mostly wrong! Designing a good questionnaire is not as easy as it may seem. Fortunately for those on the receiving end of surveys, most people who start out to write a questionnaire quite quickly realize this. A considerable degree of training and skill is involved in every aspect of survey design and implementation: for example, testing that the questions make sense to those completing the survey, selecting the respondents, collecting and analysing the results, and ensuring the results are valid and reliable, and that they are useful for service improvement. You may already have this knowledge and skill, or you may acquire it during your course. If not, you are advised to seek help if you are considering conducting a patient survey, even a small one, so as not to waste everyone's time—including your own.

There are also ethical considerations to be addressed when surveying, or indeed gathering any feedback from, patients and carers. Patient surveys focusing on the quality of services received (service evaluation) are not usually viewed as research and should not require consent from the local ethics committee. However, this does not remove the need for the ethics to be considered. The questions used must be sensible (so as not to waste people's time) and sensitive (so as not to cause distress). If you use only questions from the National Patient Survey Programme or the Chief Nursing Officer's measures for dignity and compassion, you are unlikely to encounter significant ethical issues (Department of Health, 2009b). Nevertheless, it is always wise to check with your local research ethics committee. Also, there may be a particular procedure to follow for projects being conducted as part of an academic course. Your lecturers will be able to advise you.

Other methods of gathering patient feedback

Apart from patient surveys, large or small, there is a whole range of ways of gathering patient and service user feedback, including:

- feedback sheets, suggestion boxes, comment cards, and focus groups;
- handheld electronic patient feedback devices;
- membership panels, websites, and mystery shopper programmes; and
- comments made to the Patient Advice and Liaison Service (PALS), community engagement events, patient forums, or volunteers speaking to patients on wards or in waiting areas.

All of these ways of gathering feedback need skilled and careful handling, but can be very informative.

Patient-reported outcome measures (PROMs)

Feedback about patients' experience of care is not the same as PROMs. PROMs have a very specific meaning, as described by Coulter et al. (2009). They are standardized, validated instruments (question sets) to measure patients' perceptions of their health status (impairment), their functional status (disability), and their health-related quality of life (well-being). There are many sets of PROMs around, and they are usually applied before and after a course of treatment to measure any changes due to the treatment, and to assess whether the outcome is beneficial.

The Department of Health has implemented a new programme for routine PROMs measurement throughout the NHS, starting with hip and knee replacements, hernia repair, and varicose vein surgery. The idea is to provide a reliable measure of clinical quality of care as perceived by patients themselves. The plan is then to extend the collection of PROMs to other conditions and to link this to financial incentives given to organizations providing NHS services.

....

If you are working in one of the areas mentioned above, see if you can find out how PROMs data is gathered and the sort of questions that patients are asked.
Do you think that nursing care can contribute to the answers that patients will give to the PROMs questions, or not?
Wherever you work, see if you can think of some simple questions that you might ask patients at the beginning and end of your care-giving, which would help to evaluate the difference that you had made to their well-being. These do not have to be part of a written survey—simply something that you might ask your patients informally.

....

If you would like further information about PROMs, see the list of further reading at the end of this chapter.

Nursing metrics and indicators

Nursing has not stood still whilst these developments in quality and quality measurement have been going on. We have already mentioned the EoC, but some other initiatives are under way. A paper from the National Nursing Research Unit, *Nurses in Society: Starting the Debate* (Maben and Griffiths, 2008) discusses the recent NHS quality initiatives and suggests that there are two important elements to driving up the quality of care with which nurses must engage. First, they should identify a set of metrics (measurements) for nurses that can be included in national indicator development, so that the nursing contribution is made visible. Second, nurses need to embrace a model of service management that defines responsibility and accountability for care quality, from the point of care, to the board level in the organization, using metrics as a tool.

A second paper from the National Nursing Research Unit, *State-of-the-Art Metrics for Nursing: A Rapid Appraisal* (Griffiths et al., 2008) discusses the 'state of the art' of nursing measurement and looks at metrics that provide indicators for the quality of nursing care. This report showed the vast number of outcomes and indicators of quality that have been proposed as measures of nursing quality. The most promising indicators for development are identified in the report as follows.

- Safety
  - Failure to rescue (death among patients with treatable complications)
  - Healthcare-associated pneumonia
  - Healthcare-associated infection
  - Pressure ulcers
  - Falls
- Effectiveness
  - Staffing levels and patterns
  - Staff satisfaction
  - Staff perception of the practice environment
- Compassion
  - Experience of care (patient-reported)
  - Communication (patient-reported)

Some of these indicators have been taken forward by the Department of Health for testing and further development. Over the course of time, nurses can expect to see a whole new range of indicators for quality improvement (IQIs). The quality 'landscape' for nursing is well described in *The Nursing Roadmap for Quality: A Signposting Map for Nursing* (Department of Health, 2010d). As part of this initiative, the Royal College of Nursing, commissioned by the Department of Health, is producing practice standards for nursing. Practice standards will describe the characteristics underpinning good practice for all nursing care in every healthcare setting.

The use of indicators and metrics may not provide a complete solution to improving quality, but they can provide a powerful way of encouraging it. For example, *From Good to Great* (Department of Health, 2009a) sets out an ambition to eliminate all avoidable pressure ulcers in NHS-provided care. Achieving this ambition obviously rests on reliable measurement of the numbers of pressure ulcers occurring, together with accurate assessment of whether or not they are avoidable.

Griffiths et al. (2008) acknowledge that the overall contribution of nursing can be difficult to measure, and that the identification and use of indicators are by no means straightforward. However, many, if not all, of the areas identified for measurement are things that nursing managers and clinical nurses should know about their own performance. While it might appear to be an added burden on ward staff to collect information on pressure sore incidence, it is hard to argue that nurses do not need to know and should not gather the data. It is harder to ask nurses to collect information solely for the purposes of quality monitoring, and so it is important that the additional burden of compiling information for reports is kept to a minimum and is clearly going to be of use in improving care. Much further work is needed to realize the potential of measurement in nursing.

Patient stories

We must not forget that nurses have other important opportunities to assess quality of care, through their '*access to stories people tell*' (Maben and Griffiths, 2008). Across many settings, in the community and in hospital, nurses are often providers of the greater part of direct care and are ideally placed to ask people for direct feedback on how they, or their loved ones, have been cared for. Some may argue that this is not 'measurement', but it is useful information that will enable you to reflect on your day-to-day practice, and perhaps modify it, in ways that a patient survey may not.

Some schools of nursing ask students to obtain feedback from patients or carers on the care that the student has given during placements. Sometimes mentors or clinical teachers will seek feedback from patients on the student's care-giving and use it to inform their assessment of the student. However, this approach has not been adopted everywhere and it has to be admitted that there complications with asking for direct feedback from patients whilst they are receiving care, or face-to-face immediately before discharge, including the following.

- Patients or carers may feel that if they give negative feedback, it will affect their relationship with the nurse, or even that they will be treated less favourably.
- Patients might give positive feedback because they do not want to hurt the nurse's feelings or cause difficulties for him or her. They may appreciate a nurse's good intentions even if the care received has been less than perfect.
- Some patients find it troubling to reflect on what might be a less-than-perfect experience of care, and would rather just forget it and get on with their lives.
- Patients might need time to reflect on their experience and make a meaningful story out of it.
- Some people might prefer to put their feedback in writing rather than express it face-to-face.

Nevertheless, if done sensitively, the immediacy of this approach makes it one of the best ways in which to gather feedback, improve professional practice, and, hopefully, quickly put right deficiencies in the quality of care—if not for the patient giving the feedback, then for future patients.

> **PRACTICE TIP**
>
> At the end of an episode of care (one day or longer), try asking a patient and/or their carer if they are present: 'Can you please tell me one thing that I have done particularly well in caring for you/your relative) today and one thing that I could perhaps have done better?' You can choose words with which you are more comfortable, or perhaps write the questions on a piece of paper with a space for reply. You might want to give the patient time to think about it. Do not challenge what the patient says, but thank them for their feedback and reflect on it. Is there anything of which you will do more in the future and anything that you will try to change?

Experience-based design

Experience-based design (EBD) is an approach that uses patient stories, but allows staff to tell their stories too (Bate and Robert, 2007). It focuses on designing better experiences and starts with helping patients, carers, and staff to tell the story of their experience in their own way. These stories help to uncover not only the care journey, but also the *emotional* journey people experience when they come into contact with a particular pathway or part of the healthcare service. This makes EBD an approach well suited to the type of caring that we have been discussing throughout this book.

There are four aspects to the EBD approach, as follows.

1 Capture the experience.
2 Understand the experience.
3 Improve the experience.
4 Measure the experience.

The NHS Institute for Innovation and Improvement has developed tools and practical tips for each of these aspects. For example, imaginative ways in which experience can be captured include interviews, diaries, photographs and photo journals, observation and shadowing, conversation cards, focus groups and 'listening labs', and compliments and complaints.

Ways of measuring improvement are divided into:

- *subjective outcomes*—for example, the way the patient feels (the experience); and
- *objective outcomes*—for example, reduced waiting times, fewer critical incidents, and improved performance, safety, and reliability.

For more on the EBD approach, see the list of further reading at the end of this chapter.

Use one of the EBD practical tips for capturing experience by taking a step back and looking at what is happening around you in the clinical situation with fresh eyes.
Try to imagine that you are a patient, a visitor, or a child. What do you notice and how would you feel? The next time that you are a patient, whether at your GP surgery, the dentist, or in a hospital, think what your feedback would be about the experience if someone were to come up to ask you. Whilst you are there, look for any way in which you could provide

this feedback: is there a suggestion box or survey form available, or a poster inviting comments? Have you any suggestions for improving the service? When you get home, look at some of the websites listed at the end of this chapter, such as Patient Opinion or I Want Great Care, and try to submit your feedback on the service that you have experienced.

Psychological aspects of measurement and evaluation

Find some patient feedback about an organization in which you have had a placement.
Ask the placement area if it has any patient feedback that you can see, or use the tools at the end of the chapter to find some feedback from patients or carers on one of the patient opinion websites listed—preferably about a care situation in which you have worked. Ask yourself the following questions.
Do I recognize what the feedback says from my knowledge of that area or organization?
How does it make me feel to read feedback from patients?
How would I have responded if patients had made these comments directly to me?
If I had been caring for the patient or patients concerned, could I have done anything to make the situation better, or—if the feedback was good—even better?
If something goes wrong, does the fault ever lie with the patient?
Do you think that patients ever expect too much, or too little, from those caring for them?

It is not always easy to expose ourselves to criticism, or even praise, from those for whom we care. In Chapter 2, you looked at therapeutic relationships and how a nurse must be self-aware. The chapter also discussed reflective practice and being open to criticism.

You may wish to review these aspects of Chapter 2 at this point.

Conclusion

We are at the start of an exciting era for nursing, in which its unique contribution is better recognized, nurses accept the challenge of learning how to measure and evaluate the care that they give, and they then use this knowledge to improve the quality of care for patients and their carers.

In a time of financial hardship, it becomes more important than ever to be able to demonstrate the value of what we do, both in terms of outcomes and in terms of a positive experience for patients.

Our professional and personal development as nurses requires us to reflect upon what we do for patients, to remain open to hearing their feedback, and to assessing the effectiveness and safety of our care-giving.

....

Near the beginning of the chapter, you were asked to list ways in which you might measure the care that you give. Now, take a few minutes to think about this question again.

Is your list longer this time?

What measurements can you start using right away?

Be on the lookout for new tools and techniques that you can use to measure, evaluate, and improve your care.

....

In this chapter, you have heard about some of the policy drivers for measuring and evaluating the care that you give. You have learned about work going on to develop metrics and indicators for nursing, and looked at the pros and cons of some of the commonly used tools for measuring quality. Hopefully, you have tried out some of the exercises to obtain and respond to feedback from patients, and thought about incorporating this into your everyday practice. You should be aware of some of difficulties of remaining open and responsive to patient experience feedback in many working environments, and recognize that you have a right to be supported to give high-quality care to patients and their carers. Finally, you also need to remember what you have learned in Chapter 14: if care is absent, as a nurse you have a duty to act.

Further reading

Care Quality Commission
The main regulator of health and social care in England, offering information about quality of care in all NHS providers http://www.cqc.org.uk

Cure the NHS
Website run by carers of patients harmed at Mid Staffordshire NHS Foundation Trust http://www.curethenhs.co.uk

Dr Foster Intelligence
Publishes information on measurement and quality in the NHS http://www.drfosterintelligence.co.uk

GP Patient Survey
Information for the public about the national GP Patient Survey http://www.gp-patient.co.uk

I Want Great Care
Rate your healthcare professional and see how other people have rated him or her http://www.iwantgreatcare.org

NHS Choices
Information for the public on all aspects of the NHS, including information for choice http://www.nhs.uk

NHS Institute for Innovation and Improvement
User-friendly tools and support for measuring and improving care http://www.institute.nhs.uk

For experience-based design (EBD), see: http://www.institute.nhs.uk/quality_and_value/experienced_based_design/the_ebd_approach_%28experience_based_design%29 [accessed 16 June 2011]

Patient Opinion
Patients tell their stories of care and get a reply from the providers http://www.patientopinion.org.uk

Patient Reported Outcome Measures Group
Resources and readings from some of the leading academics in the field of PROMs http://phi.uhce.ox.ac.uk/

Patient satisfaction
J. Sitzia and N. Wood (1998) 'Patient satisfaction: A review of issues and concepts', *Social Science and Medicine* 45(12): 1829–43

Picker Institute
A large, not-for-profit research organization responsible for running many of the national patient surveys and championing the use of patient experience to improve services http://www.pickereurope.org

References

Bate, S.P. and Robert, G. (2007) *Bringing User Experience to Healthcare Improvement: The Concepts, Methods and Practices of Experience-Based Design*, Oxford: Radcliffe Publishing.

Corbin, J. (2008) 'Is caring a lost art in nursing?', *International Journal of Nursing Studies* 45(2):163.

Coulter, C., Fitzpatrick, R., and Cornwell, A. (2009) *The Point of Care Measures of Patients' Experience in Hospital: Purpose, Methods and Uses*, London: The King's Fund.

Department of Health (2008) *High Quality Care for All: NHS Next Stage Review Final Report*, London: HMSO, available online at **http://www.dh.gov.uk/ en/publicationsandstatistics/publications/ publicationspolicyandguidance/DH_085825** [accessed 16 June 2011].

Department of Health (2009a) *NHS 2010–2015: From Good to Great—Preventative, People-Centred, Productive*, London: HMSO, available online at **http://www.dh.gov. uk/en/Publicationsandstatistics/Publications/ PublicationsPolicyAndGuidance/DH_109876** [accessed 16 June 2011].

Department of Health (2009b) *Understanding What Matters: A Guide to Using Patient Feedback to Transform Services*, London: HMSO, available online at **http://www. dh.gov.uk/en/Publicationsandstatistics/Publications/ PublicationsPolicyAndGuidance/DH_099780** [accessed 16 June 2011].

Department of Health (2010a) *Equity and Excellence: Liberating the NHS*, London: HMSO, available online at **http:// www.dh.gov.uk/en/Publicationsandstatistics/Publica-tions/PublicationsPolicyAndGuidance/DH_117353** [accessed 16 June 2011].

Department of Health (2010b) *Transparency in Outcomes— A Framework for the NHS*, London: HMSO, available online at **http://www.dh.gov.uk/en/Consultations/Live consultations/DH_117583** [accessed 16 June 2011].

Department of Health (2010c) *Essence of Care 2010*, London: HMSO, available online at **http://www.dh.gov. uk/en/Publicationsandstatistics/Publications/ PublicationsPolicyAndGuidance/DH_119969** [accessed 16 June 2011].

Department of Health (2010d) *The Nursing Roadmap for Quality: A Signposting Map for Nursing*, London: HMSO, available online at **http://www.dh.gov.uk/en/Publi cationsandstatistics/Publications/PublicationsPolicy AndGuidance/DH_113450** [accessed 16 June 2011].

Griffiths, P., Jones, S., Maben, J., and Murrells, T. (2008) *State of the Art Metrics for Nursing: A Rapid Appraisal*, London: National Nursing Research Unit, King's College London, available online at **http://www.kcl.ac.uk/ content/1/c6/04/32/19/Metricsfinalreport.pdf** [accessed 16 June 2011].

Maben, J. and Griffiths, P. (2008) *Nurses in Society: Starting the Debate*, London: National Nursing Research Unit, King's College London, available online at **http:// www.kcl.ac.uk/content/1/c6/04/32/16/ NursesinsocietyFinalreport.pdf** [accessed 16 June 2011].

National Health Service Information Centre (2009) *High Quality Care for All: Measuring for Quality Improvement— The Approach*, available online at **http://www.ic.nhs. uk/webfiles/Work%20with%20us/consultations/ CQI/MeasuringforQualityImprovement%20_2_.pdf** [accessed 16 June 2011].

Oppenheim, A.N. (1966) *Questionnaire Design, Interviewing and Attitude Measurement*, New York: Basic Books Inc.

Shorter Oxford English Dictionary, Sixth Edition (2007), Oxford: Oxford University Press.

Part 5: The cost of care

17 Cost of care and resource allocation

JOANNE GRAY

Learning outcomes

This chapter will enable you to:

- outline the drivers for the increasing costs of care;
- understand the need for choices in resource allocation;
- define what we mean by 'efficiency' in resource allocation;
- detail contemporary methods for resource allocation;
- explore how to measure quality of life; and
- detail the importance of the National Institute for Health and Clinical Excellence (NICE) and its impact on nursing care.

Introduction

Health care, and in particular nursing care, is something that touches all of our lives at some stage, whether it be a visit from a health visitor shortly after birth, a visit to see a practice nurse at the local GP surgery, or through care provided as a result of an admission to hospital. It is therefore imperative that nurses can appreciate the costs of care and the implications for making choices regarding care, thus ultimately allocating resources. This chapter addresses some fundamental questions: what are the drivers for increasing costs of care? How do you know that you are making choices and allocating healthcare resources efficiently? What economic methods are used for healthcare resource allocation? How does the policy context and the role of the National Institute for Health and Clinical

Excellence (NICE) impact on nursing care? Reflective questions and case studies will be used to encourage you to reflect on clinical situations and, in turn, to help you to reflect positively and constructively upon your *own* nursing practice. These reflections will enable you to build up a comprehensive knowledge, understanding, and confidence to support you in the provision of nursing care that is effective and efficient.

The fundamental economic problem in health care

Health care is subject to a fundamental economic problem—that is, 'scarcity'—which comprises two elements.

1 Human wants and desires are infinite,
2 Resources to meet these wants or desires are limited.

Essential knowledge and skills for care

- You must understand how socioeconomic and other factors in the care environment and its location can affect health, illness, health outcomes, and public health priorities, and take these into account in planning and delivering care.

- All nurses must be able to appreciate the need to identify priorities and manage resources effectively to ensure that quality of care is maintained or enhanced.

What are the implications of this for health care? We will examine each element of scarcity in turn.

The wants

People want, and therefore demand, health care because they want to be healthy. This desire to remain healthy has led to a continuous growth in demand for care and has been a major cause of escalating costs of providing care in developed countries. There are a number of specific reasons why demand for health care and the associated costs of providing it have expanded so dramatically over the last fifty years:

- Demographic changes

  Changes in the age structure of the population have increased the demand for health care. The UK and countries like it have an ageing population. In other words, people are living longer and therefore the numbers of people who are 65 years old and older are increasing.

  The National Service Framework (NSF) for Older People (Department of Health, 2001) states that:

  Since the 1930s the number of people aged over 65 has more than doubled and a fifth of the population is over 60. Between 1995 and 2025 the number of people over the age of 80 is set to increase by almost a half and the number of people over 90 will double.

  Older people tend to have much greater need for health care than do the young, so this has serious implications for increasing demands on any health system and associated costs. For example, the National Health Service spent around 40 per cent of its total budget—£10 billion—on people over the age of 65 in 1998–99 even though they comprised only 16 per cent of the total population.

- Increasing expectations

  People's expectations of health care continue to increase as they get richer in real terms and have greater access to health information regarding health due to the Internet. People are no longer willing to put up with pain, suffering, and discomfort, and as a consequence put increasing demands on services.

- Advancements in medical technology

  Technological advancements have meant a continuous increase in the range of care and treatments that are possible. Examples include increased diagnostic radiology techniques, such as computed tomography (CT) and magnetic resonance imaging (MRI) scanning, or new medicines allowing us to treat long-term conditions more effectively.

The resources

The other element of the scarcity problem relates to the finite nature of resources. Resources can be thought of as all inputs used to produce any good or service, including health services. Economists often refer to these as 'factors of production' and categorize them as follows:

- *land*—the physical resources of the planet and all of its natural derivatives, such as oil and gas;
- *labour*—the workforce as a human resource; and
- *capital*—resources created by humans to aid the production of any good or service, such as medical equipment and computers.

All of these factors are relevant for the production of health care. Given that there is a fixed quantity of these, it therefore follows that there is some maximum amount of health care that can be produced at any one time.

· ·

Think of a hypothetical economy in which all available factors of production are utilized to produce only two types of service: education and health.
If we were to redirect all factors of production, and thus resources, to the health service such that we ceased to produce an education service, would this solve the fundamental economic problem regarding scarcity?

· ·

The answer to the above reflective question is 'no'. As additional resources were redirected to the health service, although we would produce more in the health service, demand would once again increase due to changing demographics, increasing expectations, and advances in technology.

Choices and resource allocation

Taken together, the two elements of scarcity—that needs and wants are infinite relative to the finite resources used to produce goods and services—pose the fundamental economic problem. This means that choices have to be made in deciding how resources are utilized or allocated—that is, given scarcity, choices have to be made regarding how budgets and resources for health care are used. These choices have to be made because we cannot produce everything that is demanded and neither can we produce everything that is possible.

Another way in which to think about this is that we need to make choices and allocate resources such that decisions are made regarding:

- what health services should be produced;
- how we should produce them; and
- who should receive them.

....

Imagine that you are a ward manager on an acute medical ward. You have been allocated an increase in budget from the previous year, which you can use _either_ by employing more healthcare assistants _or_ by employing more qualified nurses.

What factors would you take into account when making your decision regarding how to allocate the budget and thus resources?

....

Rationing

Scarcity of resources means that some degree of rationing is inevitable. Rationing is a process of priority setting, of making choices between alternative courses of action and different kinds of health services, packages of care, or interventions. Rationing is a concept that the caring professions, such as nursing, face with unease. However, rationing has been evident within the NHS for most of its history: for example, GPs act as gatekeepers to services and waiting lists have been traditionally used to prioritize patients for access to secondary care.

Opportunity costs

Making decisions regarding resource allocation and thus making choices involve sacrifices in the form of benefits that would have been generated had some other service been provided using the same resources. Economists refer to this as 'opportunity cost' and the ideal is that these sacrifices or benefits forgone should be minimized by allocating resources to the services that maximize health or, more generally, well-being. In order to do this, information is required regarding the relationship between costs and outcomes of different health services. It is this relationship that economists call 'efficiency'.

....

Think about the opportunity costs of the following.
Nursing time spent conducting paperwork instead of direct contact time with the patient
Preventative community nursing programmes for patients with coronary heart disease (CHD) rather than patients attending GP appointments

....

There is a sacrifice or opportunity cost involved in any activity regardless of whether resources required to provide a particular service involve financial costs. For example, the opportunity cost of a family caring for a patient in the home is the benefit that would have arisen had their time been used elsewhere, such as in employment or leisure. Thus, regardless of financial costs, the use of resources does have an opportunity cost in terms of the benefit that the resources would have accrued in their best alternative use. Thus opportunity cost, unlike financial (or accounting) cost, represents the true economic cost of resource allocation in providing a particular service.

Efficiency and resource allocation

Given that scarcity forces us to make choices regarding how resources are allocated in the NHS, it would therefore seem logical that we allocate those resources in such a way that maximizes benefit or welfare of the population as a whole. In other words, resources should be allocated and decisions should be made in order to maximize efficiency.

Decision-makers do, however, face different types of choice that require more specific definitions of efficiency. A decision-maker may be faced with choice of treating obese patients with medication or a lifestyle education programme. This is a 'technical efficiency' issue: the most efficient way of achieving a given objective—in this case, reduction in obesity. A measure of technical efficiency would be the cost per patient of reducing levels of obesity for the two treatment modalities.

Alternatively, a decision-maker may be faced with a broader issue of whether to invest and allocate more resources to hyper-acute stroke beds in secondary care or to improve access to psychological services in the community for patients with mild-to-moderate depression. This is an issue of 'allocative efficiency', which relates to the question of whether treatments are worthwhile per se across a range or clinical areas. Allocative efficiency involves the relationship between costs and benefits, in which benefits may relate to a range of different objectives.

Regardless of whether we are concerned with technical or allocative efficiency, both issues of resource allocation require information regarding the relationship between costs and benefits of services, interventions, or programmes of care.

Contemporary methods for evaluation of efficiency: economic evaluation

From the discussion above, it is evident that simply measuring the costs of an intervention will not tell us anything about efficiency. A cheap intervention or programme of care may represent poor value for money because it may have little effect on benefits or patient outcomes. Evaluation of efficiency of healthcare programmes or interventions is more commonly known as 'economic evaluation'. Economic evalu-

ation can be defined as '*the comparative analysis of alternative courses of action in terms of both their costs and consequences*' (Drummond at al., 2005).

An economic evaluation involves two essential features: both costs and outcomes must be analysed; and more than one alternative strategy must be compared.

- Costs

  The measurement of costs is similar regardless of the type of intervention. They can be divided or categorized in a number of ways—most commonly:
  - costs to the NHS (staff, hotel services, medical equipment);
  - costs to the patient and family (loss of income, travel expenses); and
  - costs to the rest of society (social services).

- Benefits

  The benefits of an intervention are usually measured by health improvement, which can be measured in a number of ways, including:
  - health effects, such as cases of disease averted, life years gained, or some notion of health outcome that is captured by a reliable and valid outcome metric, such as the Beck Depression Scale (Beck et al., 1961); and
  - the value of health improvement or quality or life.

Types of economic evaluation

There are several types of economic evaluation. It is the measurement of outcome that largely determines what type of economic evaluation is performed:

Cost-minimization analysis

Cost-minimization analysis is used when the outcomes of interest of the two procedures being compared are proven to be the same (for example, day case versus inpatient stay for the treatment of hernias and haemorrhoids). The aim of this is to find the lowest cost programme.

Cost-effectiveness analysis

Cost-effectiveness analysis is one of the most widely used methods of economic evaluation and is fundamental to resource allocation decisions related to technical efficiency—that is, given that it has been decided that this type of health care will be provided, what is the best way of doing so? This type of analysis is used when alternative programmes have differential successes in outcome, as well as differential costs. The outcomes tend to be measured in unidirectional natural units, such as life years saved, blood pressure reduction, or change in score on a disease-specific outcome, such as pain or anxiety and depression.

Cost-effectiveness analysis is normally expressed as a cost per unit of effect, which helps to determine which strategy or programme maximizes a given objective, such as improving levels of anxiety and depression, with the lowest cost. This is a useful technique for comparing alternative treatment programmes, the effects of which are measured in the same units (technical efficiency), and hence cannot be used to compare programmes the effects of which differ (allocative efficiency). However, when comparing two alternative treatment programmes for a given objective, it is rarely the case that a particular programme is both more effective and cheaper than its comparator (often referred to as 'dominant'). A more likely scenario is a treatment programme that will be both more effective and more costly (in other words, 'non-dominant').

Cost-effectiveness analysis can help decision-making in this latter case by presenting the results as an incremental cost effectiveness ratio (ICER):

$$ICER = \frac{(\text{Cost of programme A} - \text{Cost of programme B})}{(\text{Outcomes of programme A} - \text{Outcomes of programme B})}$$

This tells us how much extra we must pay for an additional unit of outcome and allows decision-makers to consider whether alternative uses of the same resources would generate more health benefits.

Cost–utility analysis

Cost–utility analysis is the method of choice when quality of life is the outcome measure, or when an intervention or treatment programme affects morbidity and mortality, or when treatments have a wide range of different outcomes and a common unit is required. For cost–utility analysis, the outcomes of health interventions are measured in units of health outcome that combine quality and quantity of life. The most well-known example of a measure of health utility is the quality-adjusted life year (QALY) (Briggs and Gray, 2000). 'Utility' is a term used by health economists to refer to the subjective level of well-being that people experience in different health states. Quality of life is measured on a scale from '0' to '1', where '0' equates to death and '1' equates to perfect health. QALYs are then calculated as follows:

> QALY = Quality of life × Time period in quality-adjusted state (usually measured in years)

See **Practice Example 17.1**.

Cost–utility analysis is useful in that it can be used to aid resource allocation decision-making for both technical and allocative efficiency issues.

Cost–benefit analysis

Cost–benefit analysis refers to a method of analysis in which both costs and benefits of health interventions are valued in monetary units. Because both costs and benefits are measured using the same units, they can be compared directly. However, measuring benefits in monetary units presents substantial methodological difficulties and thus is relatively less commonly used than other methods in health care.

The National Institute for Health and Clinical Excellence (NICE), economic evaluation, and the impact for nursing care

Health systems in most developed countries face the same fundamental challenges when it comes to improving quality, fostering innovation, and ensuring value for money. The UK government has attempted to address these issues in part with the creation in 1999

PRACTICE EXAMPLE 17.1

A comparison of drug treatments and quality of life in the treatment of bowel cancer

As a registered general nurse, midwife, or student nurse, you attend a multidisciplinary meeting at which a debate emerges between the consultant gastroenterologist and principle pharmacist about the cost of medications and impact on the quality of life for the treatment of bowel cancer. The cost and effectiveness of treatment can be illustrated as follows.

Suppose that two drug treatments (A and B) are being compared for the treatment of bowel cancer. Drug A costs £20,000 per annum per patient and gives patients are quality of life assessment of 0.9 over a life span of twenty years. Drug B costs £15,000 per annum per patient and gives patients a quality of life assess-

ment of 0.7 over a life span of thirty years. The QALY calculations are as follows:

$$\text{QALYs Drug A} = 0.9 \times 20 = 18$$
$$\text{QALYs Drug B} = 0.7 \times 30 = 21$$

Cost–utility analysis is usually presented as a cost per QALY gained if an intervention is dominant or, in the case of non-dominance, an ICER. Using the example above, given that Drug B is both cheaper and more effective in terms of QALYs gained, the cost per QALY gained for each intervention is calculated as follows:

$$\text{Drug A} = \text{Costs} \div \text{Outcomes} = 20,000 \div 18$$
$$= £1,111 \text{ per QALY gained}$$
$$\text{Drug B} = \text{Costs} \div \text{Outcomes} = 15,000 \div 21$$
$$= £714 \text{ per QALY gained}$$

---

of the National Institute for Health and Clinical Excellence (NICE), a special health authority for England and Wales. Economic evaluation of health care is a core component of the work of NICE. Its role is to provide patients, health professionals, and the public with authoritative, robust, and reliable guidance on current best practice in order to help the NHS to meet three continuing objectives (Department of Health, 1998):

  (i) to improve continually the overall standards of care;
 (ii) to reduce unacceptable variation in clinical practice; and
(iii) to ensure the best use of resources so that patients receive the greatest benefit.

NICE was established against a policy rhetoric in which there was growing concern regarding rising healthcare costs, and variations in quality of care and the range of care received, which was largely determined by postcode or where a person lived (known as the 'postcode lottery').

In order to meet its objectives, NICE produces national guidance on four distinct programmes (Pearson and Rawlins, 2005):

  (i) individual technologies, or classes of health technology, such as pharmaceuticals, diagnostic methods, devices, or procedures (appraisals);
 (ii) the management of specific conditions (clinical guidelines);
(iii) the safety and efficacy of interventional procedures (both diagnostic and therapeutic); and
 (iv) public health initiatives and implementation.

All programmes of work by the Institute—with the exception of the safety and efficacy of interventional procedures—are underpinned by appraisal and assessment of clinical and cost effectiveness.

NICE responds to requests by the Department of Health for guidance on the use of new and established technologies in the NHS. The Department selects technologies for assessment using four criteria: possible health benefit; links to health-related policies; impact on NHS resources; and the added value of NICE guidance (Department of Health, 1999).

Guidelines regarding new and existing technologies are produced as a result of robust and relatively lengthy appraisal processes. The NICE process concludes with a judgement as to whether an intervention can be recommended as a cost-effective use of NHS resources (Sculpher et al., 2001). This involves the use of cost-effectiveness analysis, the primary outcome of which is the cost per QALY or the incremental cost-effectiveness ratio (ICER), which is calculated as:

$$ICER = \frac{(Cost\ of\ intervention\ A - Cost\ of\ intervention\ B)}{(QALYs\ of\ intervention\ A - QALYs\ of\ intervention\ B)}$$

NICE's use of QALYs is one example of its commitment to making consistent decisions across different technologies over a range of clinical areas (Walker et al., 2007). The decision on whether an intervention is considered cost-effective hinges on the threshold ICER, determined by the Institute to represent an efficient use of resources. If an intervention or programme's ICER is lower than the threshold value, it should be adopted and would be deemed cost-effective.

As a result of these processes, at its most definitive, NICE guidance will either recommend the routine use of the technology in all appropriate clinical situations or recommend that the NHS does not adopt the technology. Alternatively, guidance will recommend restricted use, for example in certain patient categories only or as part of ongoing research (Williams et al., 2008). Three examples of technology appraisal topics and their related judgements are given in **Table 17.1**. In one case, NICE gave a blanket approval for use of the technology (alteplase for acute ischaemic stroke); in another, NICE recommended that the therapy not be used in the NHS (pemetrexed for non-small cell lung cancer); and in the last, use of a drug was limited to patient subgroups likely to receive higher levels of benefit (donepezil for Alzheimer's disease).

NICE guidance to change clinical practice

In April 2009, NICE Chairman Sir Michael Rawlins reported that, since its inception, NICE has published more than 550 guidance reports, including 169 appraisals of health technologies, 88 clinical guidelines for the management of specific diseases and conditions, 289 guidelines for interventional procedures, and 18 public health guidelines (Rawlins, 2009). Despite this impressive volume of guidance material, the critical question is whether guidance is adopted and implemented: has NICE brought change in clinical practice and thus had impact on patient outcomes?

Initially, NICE was expected to play no part in the implementation of its guidance, but it soon became apparent that production of guidance did not ensure universal implementation. For example, a study by Sheldon et al. (2004), covering the first years of the Institute's existence, noted that implementation of guidance was variable.

In response to concerns about lack of uptake of its guidance, NICE established its own implementation programme, with the aim of supporting the uptake and the use of its guidance by the NHS. This programme is designed to have an impact at national, organizational, and individual levels (NICE, 2008). Furthermore, although NICE guidance is not mandatory in a legal sense (the National Health Service Act 1948 stipulates that the NHS cannot interfere with how individual clinicians practise medicine), 2003 saw a directive for primary care trusts in the NHS (that is, the budget holders) to make funds available to pay for technology appraisal guidance from NICE within three months of publication. This process mechanism essentially mandates the technology appraisal part of NICE guidance. However, it does not extend to other of the Institute's programmes.

Additional governance mechanisms have also been put in place to support and monitor the implementation of NICE guidance with the existence of the Care Quality Commission (CQC), an independent regulator of all health and adult social care in England (**http://www.cqc.org.uk**). The CQC requires organizations to be able to demonstrate that they are implementing technology appraisals within the three-month time frame, that they are compliant with interventional procedure guidance, and that they are working towards achieving standards set in NICE clinical and public health guidelines.

Within the context of these relatively recent implementation initiatives, it is perhaps not surprising that current evidence regarding uptake of guidance is more encouraging. Furthermore, a change of government in 2010 saw reform proposals for the NHS with

Table 17.1 Examples of NICE technology appraisals

	Donepezil for the treatment of Alzheimer's disease	Pemetrexed for the treatment of non-small-cell lung cancer	Alteplase for the treatment of acute ischaemic stroke
Policy question	The use of donepezil for the treatment of mild to moderately severe Alzheimer's disease	The use of pemetrexed for the treatment of non-small-cell lung cancer	The use of alteplase for the treatment of acute ischaemic stroke
Findings from the evidence	*Clinical effectiveness* In terms of impact on cognitive functioning, donepezil is beneficial in treating Alzheimer's disease. Its effect on quality of life and behavioral symptoms is less clear. Subgroup analysis based on severity of cognitive impairment suggests greater benefit for more severely impaired patients. *Cost effectiveness* For mild patients: cost/QALY ranged from £61,000 to £81,000 For moderate patients: cost/QALY ranged from £ 39,000 to £46,000 For moderate to moderately severe patients: cost/QALY ranged from £31,000 to £38,000	*Clinical effectiveness* Pemetrexed was not clinically effective compared with docetaxel. The clinical effectiveness of pemetrexed compared to best supportive care (BSC) has not been established. *Cost effectiveness* For pemetrexed versus docetaxel, cost/QALY up to £1.8 million For pemetrexed compared with BSC, cost/QALY of £60,000	*Clinical effectiveness* Alteplase is beneficial for the treatment of acute ischaemic stroke *Cost effectiveness* Less than £20,000 per QALY gained
Guidance	Donepezil is recommended as an option in the management of patients with Alzheimer's disease of moderate severity only.	Pemetrexed is not recommended as an option for the treatment of locally advanced or metastic non-small-cell lung cancer.	Alteplase is recommended for the treatment of acute ischaemic stroke.

PRACTICE TIP

As a registered general nurse, midwife, or student nurse, remember that the CQC involves an annual inspection of healthcare providers against a set of standards known as *Standards for Better Health* (Department of Health, 2004). These standards incorporate NICE's technology appraisals and interventional procedures as 'core standards', and clinical guidelines and public health guidance as 'developmental standards'.

the publication of the White Paper *Equity and Excellence: Liberating the NHS* (Department of Health, 2010a). This set out a vision of an NHS that achieves among the best outcomes of any health service.

To help achieve this, a new NHS Outcomes Framework was published (Department of Health, 2010b) to provide national accountability for the outcomes that the NHS delivers and the care that is commissioned. At the heart of this are quality standards that have been, or will be, developed by NICE, the role of which generally has, arguably, been extended. NICE will develop quality standards that will set out the evidenced-based characteristics (in terms of clinical and cost effectiveness) of a high-quality service for a particular pathway or condition. Eventually, a broad library of 150 NICE quality standards will be available that cover the majority of NHS care. Drawing on these quality standards, commissioners of care will be held to account for their contribution to improving outcomes. Thus it is ever more pertinent that healthcare professionals have an awareness and understanding of these standards, and of their implications in terms of providing clinically and cost-effective care.

Conclusion

The high and rising cost of health care is a near universal problem (Pauly, 2003, 2004; Aaron, 2004; Garber, 2004), which manifests itself in different ways in different countries, depending on how countries structure their health care financing. In the USA, which relies heavily on private insurance, it is seen in rising health insurance premiums, increasing direct payments by insured individuals, cutbacks in public programmes, and growth in the number of uninsured (Jost, 2003; Garber, 2004). In the UK and other countries with predominantly tax-financed health insurance systems, the pressure of increasing healthcare costs reveals itself through a growing frustration with constraints on access to some high-cost modern health care and restrictions on rapid access to health care generally (Jost, 2005).

The introduction of new healthcare technologies (that is, drugs, devices, and medical procedures) is a major factor contributing to health expenditure growth in developed countries. Governments must therefore respond by making decisions regarding whether the costs of these interventions should be reimbursed or covered. In other words, it involves setting limits on the healthcare services that can be accessed or provided (Daniels and Sabin, 2002).

Increasingly, we see limit-setting decisions being made explicitly in the UK by NICE. The context is a healthcare system predominately financed through the taxpayer, with explicit 'cash constraints'; setting limits is part of the territory.

The policy context surrounding NICE suggests that nursing practice—particularly in terms of types of care packages offered to patients—will undoubtedly be affected. Guidelines and standards regarding cost effective pathways of care are very much integral to the future of all healthcare professions. An understanding of conceptual issues such as efficiency and value for money, and the methodologies that underpin these, is therefore essential for the caring professions practising in any health care system, not only the NHS. We face an era in which it is impossible to practise without acknowledgement and understanding of the economic and policy contexts of health care. All professional groups and their practice within health are increasingly being affected by these. Surely it is better to educate and train our clinical staff in such issues in order that they enter practice with their eyes wide open?

Further reading

Care Quality Commission **http://www.cqc.org.uk**

National Institute for Health and Clinical Excellence **http://www.nice.org.uk**

References

Aaron, H.J. (2004) 'Should public policy seek to control the growth of health care spending?', *Health Affairs* Web exclusive, 31 March: 28–36.

Beck, A.T., Ward, C.H., Mendelssohn, M.J., and Erbaugh, J. (1961) 'An inventory for measuring depression', *Archives of General Psychiatry* 4: 561–71.

Briggs, A. and Gray, A. (2000) 'Using cost effectiveness information', *British Medical Journal* 320(7229): 246.

Daniels, N. and Sabin, J.E. (2002) *Setting Limits Fairly*, New York: Oxford University Press.

Department of Health (1998) *A First Class Service: Quality in the New NHS*, London: HMSO.

Department of Health (1999) *Faster Access to Modern Treatment: How NICE Appraisal Will Work*, London: HMSO.

Department of Health (2001) *National Service Framework for Older People*, London: HMSO.

Department of Health (2004) *Standards for Better Health*, London: HMSO, available online at **http://www.dh.gov. uk/en/Publicationsandstatistics/Publications/ PublicationsPolicyAndGuidance/DH_4086665** [accessed 16 June 2011].

Department of Health (2010a) *Equity and Excellence: Liberating the NHS*, Cm 7881, London: HMSO.

Department of Health (2010b) *The NHS Outcomes Framework 2011–12*, London: HMSO, available online at **http://www.dh.gov.uk/en/Publicationsandstatistics/ Publications/PublicationsPolicyAndGuidance/ DH_122944** [accessed 16 June 2011].

Drummond, M.F., Sculpher, M.J., Torrance, G.W., O'Brien, B.J., and Stoddart, G.L. (2005) *Methods for the Economic Evaluation of Health Care Programmes*, Oxford: Oxford University Press.

Garber, A.M. (2004) 'Cost-effectiveness and evidence evaluation as criteria for coverage policy', *Health Affairs* Web exclusive, 19 May: 284–96.

Jost, T.S. (2003) *Disentitlement? The Threats Facing Our Public Health-Care Programs and a Rights-Based Response*, New York: Oxford University Press.

Jost, T.S. (2005) 'The Medicare coverage determination process in the United States', in T.S. Jost, *Health Care Coverage Determinations: An International Comparative Study*, Maidenhead: Open University Press, pp. 207–35.

National Institute for Health and Clinical Excellence (2008) *How to Put NICE Guidance into Practice: A Guide to Implementation for Organisations*, available online at **http://www.nice.org.uk/media/848/D0/ HowtoputNICEguidanceintopracticeFINAL.pdf** [accessed 16 June 2011].

Pauly, M.V. (2003) 'Should we be worried about high real medical spending growth in the United States?', Health Affairs Web exclusive, 8 January: 15–27.

Pauly, M.V. (2004) 'What if technology never stops improving? Medicare's future under continuous cost increases', *Washington and Lee Law Review* 60:1233–50.

Pearson, S.D. and Rawlins, M.D. (2005) 'Quality, innovation, and value for money: NICE and the British National Health Service', *Journal of the American Medical Association* 294(20): 2618–22.

Rawlins, M.D. (2009) 'The decade of NICE', *The Lancet* 374: 351–2.

Sculpher, M., Drummond, M., and O'Brien, B. (2001) 'Effectiveness, efficiency and NICE', *British Medical Journal* 322: 943–4.

Sheldon, T.A., Callum, N., Dawson, D., Lankshear, A., Lowson, K., Watt, I., West, P., Wright, D., and Wright, J. (2004) 'What's the evidence that NICE guidance has been implemented? Results from a national evaluation using time series analysis, audit of patients notes, and interviews', *British Medical Journal* 329: 999.

Walker, S., Palmer, S., and Sculpher, M. (2007) 'The role of NICE technology appraisal in NHS rationing', *British Medical Bulletin* 81/82: 51–64.

Williams, I., McIver, S., Moore, D., and Bryan, S. (2008) 'The use of economic evaluations in NHS decision-making: A review and empirical investigation', *International Journal of Health Technology Assessment* 12(7): 1–175.

Index

Page numbers in *italic* indicate boxes, figures, and tables.

A

Abbey pain scale 186
abreaction 100
abuse 174–6
acceptance 111
ACCESS model 69–74
access to health care 89, 90
accountability, *see* professional
   accountability
Acheson Report 90
acting, deep and surface 24
activities of daily living (ADLs) 56,
   70, 124
acts of omission *175*
addressing patients 53–4
adherence issues 164
adolescence 107
adult protection 174–6
Adult Protection Form 1 (APF1)
   174
affective caring 6–7
ageism 72
agency 64, 88
allocative efficiency 252
alteplase therapy for stroke *256*
alternative treatments 109
American Nurses Association 35
anger 111, *176*
anorexia nervosa 101
anti-discriminatory practice 69
anxiety 90
appraisal and stress 21
assessment 69–70
associative learning 102
asylum seekers 91
attending 139, 144–5
attending posture 145
attitude
   promoting respect 52

quality nursing care 37
social attitudes to care provision
   83–4
authenticity 137–8, 139
availability of health care 89, 90

B

bargaining 111
basic care 4
Beck, A. 99, 103
behaviour
   challenging behaviour in care 184
   challenging colleagues' behaviour
    54
   communicating care 141
   conforming 87
   indicator of pain and distress *185*
   quality nursing care 37
   risky behaviour 90
   social behaviours 86
   Type A 20, 110
behaviour modification techniques
   103
behaviourism *98*, 101–3
beliefs
   health beliefs 108
   holistic care 56
   illness beliefs 70
   personal beliefs and nursing
    practice 128–9
   respecting individuals 48
   self-care 19–20
benchmarking 43, 238–9
benefits of interventions 252
bereavement 110–12, 182, *183*
'Big Society' 83, 161
biological approaches in
   psychology *98*
biological determinism 87

biological dimension of the individual
   53, *119*
biological factors in emotion 105
Black Report 90
blocking communication 180–1
blushing 105
body language 145, *179*
Bolam test 154, 209
Bolitho v City & Hackney Health
   Authority [1997] 209–10
breaking bad news 180–1
Briggs Report 4
burnout 23–4

C

Cannon, Mr 225, 226
carative factors 8
care and caring; *see also* self-care
   affective aspects 6–7
   behaviours communicating care
    141
   caring about 6, 11
   caring for 6, 11
   communicating care with patients
    137–8, 143–6
   dimensions 10–11
   essential skills and knowledge 3,
    16, 33, 47, 61, 82, 96, 117, 135,
    150, 159, 173, 191, 207, 219,
    234, 249
   has it left nursing? 3–4
   instrumental aspects 6–7
   investigating 9–10
   meanings 5–6
   measuring and evaluating 43–4,
    235–6, 237–43
   natural reaction 113
   nurse's views of 12
   outcome 6, 7

care and caring (*continued*)
  patients' perceptions 12
  place in nursing 8, 14
  psychosocial dimension 10–11,
    12
  research into 9–10
  returning to the centre of
    nursing 3
  students' perception of 11–12
  styles of 140
  technical and professional
    dimension 10–11, 12
  theories 7–9, 136
  traits *8*
care assistants 13–14
care partnerships, *see* partnerships
    of care
care pathways 150–8
  alternative names for 150, 152–3
  basic criteria 151
  benefits 153–5
  core elements 151
  defining 150–1
  evaluation 155–6
  evidence-based care 154
  implementation 153, 154
  legal issues 154–5
  origins 152–3
  outcomes 151
  patient-centred care 153
  professional accountability 154–5
  safety 151
  variance within 151
Care-Q 9
Care Quality Commission 162, 237–8,
    255, 257
career development 196–7
carers
  informal 83, 160–1
  involving in partnerships of care
    165–7
caring, *see* care and caring
Caring Behaviours Inventory 9
Caring Dimensions Inventory 9, *10*
catastrophizing 28
causation 211–12
celebrating nursing care 204
celebrity culture 86

change
  self-care 19
  social change 85–6
charge nurses 198–9
chemotherapy, anticipatory nausea
    102
childhood experiences 97, 101
choice and resource allocation 251
chronic disease, increasing preva-
    lence 162
client-centred therapy 104
clinical governance 42–3
clinical leadership programme
    (RCN) 193
clinical negligence 208, 209–12
Clostridium difficile, Maidstone and
    Tunbridge Wells NHS Trust
    outbreaks 194
cognitive approaches *98*
cognitive-behavioural approaches
    29, 103
cognitive-behavioural therapy
    (CBT) 28, 103
colleagues
  challenging their behaviour 54
  suspicion of abuse by 175
comfort strategies 140
comforting interaction–relationship
    model 140–1
commissioning 162
Commissioning for Quality and
    Innovation (CQUIN) framework
    204
commitment 12
communication
  barriers to 146–7
  basic skills 144
  blocking tactics 180–1
  breaking bad news 180–1
  challenging care situations 179–81
  comforting interaction–relationship
    model 140–1
  communicating care with patients
    137–8, 143–6
  complaints about 220
  difficult circumstances 178–81
  diversity 70–2
  explanatory model 143, *144*

family-focused 137
  filters 147
  knowing your limitations 139–40
  non-verbal 145
  nurse–patient relationship 138–9,
    147
  nurse prescribing 165
  nursing-focused 136–7, 140, 143
  one-way 140
  patient-centred 136, 137, 138,
    140, 143
  person-centred care 139
  quality care 37, 220
  referrals 140
  respect for patients 52
  self-awareness 139, 141–2
  sensitivity 73
  therapeutic communication 143
  vulnerable people 178–9
communities
  defining 82
  inequalities in health and health
    care 89–92, 184
  professional role in caring 81–2
  social change 85–6
  social context of health care 82–4
  social factor and health 89–91
community-based health care
    providers 83
comparative benchmarking 43
compensation systems 212–16
complaints
  benefits of *224*
  learning from 219–24, 225,
    226, 228–32
  NHS complaints system 215
  personal approach in dealing with
    231
  positive and appropriate response
    to 231
  reasons for 221, *222*
  statistical information about 221
confidentiality in safeguarding 175
conflict 87
conforming 87
congruence 105
consensus 87
control 19–20, 107–9

coronary heart disease 90, 110
corporate ideology 141
cost-benefit analysis 253
cost-effectiveness analysis 253, 255
cost-minimization analysis 252
cost per unit of effect 253
cost–utility analysis 253
costs
    clinical negligence 208
    economic evaluation 252
    fundamental economic problem
        249–51
    pressure ulcers 155
counselling 100, 104–5
court service structure 213
CQUIN framework 204
critical disability theorists 64
cultural diversity 66–8
cultural negotiation and compromise
    61, 73
cultural safety 61, 73 4
culture-specific (sensitive) nursing
    66, 67

D
Darzi Review 35, 192, 201, 236
death and dying 57, 124, 181–2
deep acting 24
defence mechanisms 98, 100
demand for health care 250
dementia care 166, 177–8
demographic changes 250
denial
    loss 111
    psychodynamic theory 98, 100
Department of Health 36, 41, 43–4
depression 90, 105, 108, 111
diabetes treatment 162
diet 29
dignity 47–51, 225
dimensions of caring 10–11
disability
    caring for disabled people 63–5
    health outcomes 90
    individual model 63–4
    medical approach 63–4
    personal tragedy approach 63, 64
    social model 65

discrimination 63, 74, 120–1, 175
DisDAT tool 186
disgust 176
displacement 98
display rules 106
distress, identifying in vulnerable
        groups 185–6
diversity 61–77
    ACCESS model 69–74
    cultural 66–8
    diversity management 62–3
    ethnic 66–8
    hidden 61
    managing diversity 62–3
    putting in action 68–9
    theory, research, and evidence
        base 61–3
    visible 61
documenting standards of care 43–4;
        see also record-keeping
dominant treatment 253
Donabedian, Avedis 41
donepezil therapy, Alzheimer's dis-
        ease 256
dream analysis 100
drives 97
dying, see death and dying

E
e-medicine 83
eating habits 29
economic evaluation 252–3
    NICE 253, 254, 255
education of nurses 4–5, 9, 66
effectiveness 36, 37
efficiency
    allocative efficiency 252
    core element of quality care 36, 37
    evaluation of 252–3
    resource allocation 251–2
    technical efficiency 252
Ellis, A. 99, 103
embarrassment 106, 176
emotional intelligence 24
emotional labour 24–5
emotions
    abused individuals 175, 176
    associative learning 102

defined 105
    psychology of 105–6
    self and 106–9
    universal 106
empathy 105, 143
employment security 90
empowerment 36, 37, 63, 69, 120
enrolled nurses 13
environmental factors and learning
        102
equality 62
Erikson, E. 99, 107
Essence of Care (EoC) 238–9
essential care 4
ethical issues
    authenticity and human-ness 139
    patient surveys 240
    spiritual care 120
ethnic minorities 91
ethnicity 66–8
evaluation
    care pathways 155–6
    efficiency 252–3
    partnerships of care 163
    quality of care 237–43
evidence 9
evidence-based care
    care pathways 154
    partnerships of care 167, 168
evolutionary psychologists 113
exercise 29
expectancies 19
expectations 107, 250
experience-based design 242–3
experience of patients 220, 239
explanatory model
    of communication 143, 144
    of illness 70
external locus of control 19, 108
eye contact 70, 179

F
facial expressions 179
factors of production 250
family-focused communication 137
fear 102, 176
feedback 221, 228, 239–40, 242
filters 147

financial abuse *175*
financial support 161
five 'C's 68
folk systems 67
Forrest, D. 9
Francis Report 34, 84, 174, 201, 202, 203, 227–8
free association 100
Freud, S. 97–8, *99*, 100–1
Freudian slip 97–8
functional incapacity 63
fundamental economic problem 249–51

G

gate control theory 109
Gaut, D. A. 9
gender 70–1, 90
General Medical Council 51
gestures *179*
Gibbs's model of reflection 137
going the extra mile 141
good death 181–2
governance
    clinical governance 42–3
    partnerships of care 162–3
grief *176*

H

happiness 112
hardy personality 23–4
health
    impact of work on nurses' health 17–18
    inequalities in 89–91, 92
    NHS workers 17
    social factors 89–91
    wealth and 90
    see also mental health, physical health
Health and Safety at Work Act (1999) 25
health belief models 108
health care
    access and availability 89, 90
    demand for 250
    fundamental economic problem 249–51

inequalities 91, 184
    providers 83
    settings 82–3
    social context 82–4
    wants 250
health inequalities 89–91, 92
health policy 121
Health Professions Council 51
health promotion 88
health status 89, 90
high-quality care 201–2, 219–24
holistic care 54–6, 118–19
    core element of quality care 36, 37
    nature and key dimensions 52–4
    spiritual care component 119–20, 124–5
homeless 91
human-ness 139
Human Rights Act (1998) 51, 208
humanistic nursing theories 57
humanistic psychology *98*, 104–5
hypnosis 100

I

idealism 11
identity
    patient's loss of identity 51
    social identity and stigma 87
ill-health, NHS workers 17
illness beliefs 70
implementation
    care pathways 153, 154
    NICE guidance 255
inclusivity 61, 62, 68–9
income levels and health 90
incremental cost effectiveness ratio (ICER) 253, 255
independent peer review 43
individual model of disability 63–4
individual–organization interface 23
individuality 51
individualized care, nature and key dimensions 52–4
individuals
    dimensions 53, 119
    providers of health care 83
    stress identification and management 22–3, 25

inequalities in health and health care 89–92, 184
informal carers 83, 160–1
information technology 83
inspection 237–8
instincts 97
institutional abuse 174
instrumental caring 6–7
insurance, professional indemnity 215
integrated care 126
integrated teamwork 36, 37
integrity 138
interacting with patients 37, 145
internal locus of control 19, 108
International Council of Nurses (ICN) 34, 35, 51, 121
international directives 121
Internet 83
interpersonal skills 52
interpretations 87, 103
interpreters 70
interviews 5
intimate tasks 106
inventories 9
inverse care law 91

J

'Jade Goody' effect 86
job strain model 21
job type and health 90, *91*
judgemental comments 54
Jung C. G. 100–1

K

keeping up-to-date 210–11
Kennedy Inquiry 84
King's College London National Nursing Research Unit 35
Kirk, L. 227
knowledge and respect 52
Kübler-Ross, E. 111

L

L, Mr 223
language 63, 70, 71, *72*
leadership 191–2, 198–9
    fast-track leadership development *200*

importance of 193
political and professional drivers
193
skills for 203–4
transformational 205
learned helplessness 20, 108
learning disabilities 57–8, 178, 183–4,
185–6, 225
leg ulceration 88
legal issues
care pathways 154–5
clinical negligence 208, 209–12
compensation systems 214
court service structure 213
discrimination 120–1
health and safety at work 25
human rights 51, 208
keeping up-to-date 210
quality care 202
safeguarding 175
spiritual care 120–1
vaccine damage compensation
212
Leininger, M. 9
LGBT 74
life change models 110
life stages 107
listening 37, 139, 144
Little Albert 102
Liverpool integrated care pathway
181
local involvement network (LINk) 162
locations of health care 83
locus of control 19–20, 108
loss 110–12, 182, 183

M
macro perspective 87
management skills 191–2
Marmot Review 90, 92
matrons 193–6
measures of quality care 43–4, 235–6,
237–43
media coverage 3–4, 34
medical approach to disability 63–4
medical errors, emotional impact on
staff 24–5
medical model of care 56, 124

mental health
gender 90
partnerships of care 163, 164
sense of control 108
micro perspective 87
mid-life crisis 100
Mid Staffordshire NHS Foundation
Trust Inquiry (Francis Report) 34,
84, 174, 201, 202, 203, 227–8
midwife-led services 199–201
mind-reading 29
mindfulness training 30
mixed economy 83
MMR vaccine 86
models of nursing care 56–7
modern matrons 193–6
modern societies 86
monitoring performance 237–8
moral values in spiritual care 120
mortality rate and social grouping
90, 91
motivation and self-care 18
multi-agency care 162

N
National Dementia Strategy 177
National Institute for Health and
Clinical Excellence (NICE) 162,
253–7
National Patient Safety Agency 216, 217
needs
meeting patients' needs 52
spiritual needs 126–7
neglect 175
neurotransmitters 105
New Labour 160
newspaper stories 3–4, 34
NHS complaints system 215
NHS Constitution 51, 120
NHS Outcomes Framework 256
NHS Productive Series 230
NHS Redress Scheme 214
Nightingale, Florence 7
no-fault compensation 212, 214
No Secrets (DoH) 174
non-adherence 164
non-dominant treatment 253
non-judgemental stance 54

non-medical prescribing 163–5
non-verbal communication 145
nurse-focused communication 136–7,
140, 143
nurse-led services 199–201
nurse–patient interactions
37, 145
nurse–patient relationship
communication 138–9, 147
holistic care 54–5
knowing your limitations
139–40
rapport 73
self-awareness 139, 141
therapeutic relationship 142
nurse prescribing role 163–5
nurses
impact of work on health 17–18
views of caring 12
what makes a suitable nurse 7
nursing
career development 196–7
caring in 8, 14
celebrating 204
defining 35
education 4–5, 9, 66
metrics and indicators 241–2
nursing actions 140
Nursing and Midwifery Council's
Code 34, 38, 40, 51, 81–2, 121,
154, 211, 215, 221
nursing auxiliaries 13
nursing care 6; see also care and
caring
nursing care models 56–7
nursing patterns of relating 140–1
Nursing Roadmap for Quality:
A Signposting Map for Nursing
(DoH) 43, 204

O
occupation and health 90, 91
occupational health psychology
25, 26
older people
ageism 72
demand for health care 250
positive outcome 107

ombudsman services 221–4
'one pocket' argument 215
opportunity costs 251
oppression 64, 65
organizational level
    learning from complaints 228–32
    stress management 23, 25
'other' 62, 72, 73
outcomes
    care and caring 6, 7
    care pathways 151
    partnerships of care 163
    poor health outcomes in disabled 90
    positive outcome in old age 107
    quality assurance 41, 42
overgeneralizing 28
Ovington, C. 202

P

pain
    abused individuals *176*
    assessment 109–10, 185, 186
    coping with 109–10
    identifying in vulnerable groups
        185–6
palliative care 185
panic attacks 103
Parliamentary and Health Service
    Ombudsman 221–4
partnerships of care 159–71
    benefits 164–5
    carer involvement 165–7
    defining 161–2
    evaluation 163
    evidence 167, 168
    governance 162–3
    making them work 167–8
    outcomes 163
    public and private partnerships
        159–60
    service user involvement 165–7
    third way 160–1
pathways of care, *see* care pathways
patient-centred care 153, 225–6
patient-centred care model 57
patient-centred communication
    136–7, 138, 140, 143
patient-centred teams 230

patient-reported outcome measures
    (PROMs) 240–1
patients
    addressing 53–4
    empowerment 36, 37
    experience of 220, 239
    feedback from 221, 228, 239–40,
        242
    loss of identity 51
    meeting their needs 52
    perceptions of caring 12
    safety 36, 37, 73–4, 151, 216–17
    satisfaction 239
    stories 242
    surveys 239–40
Patients' Association 84, 124
pattern recognition 185
patterns of relating 141
peer influences 107
peer review 238
pemetrexed therapy, lung
    cancer *256*
perceptions of caring 11–12
performance 20–1
person-centred approach 37, 54
person-centred care 125, 139, 163
personal beliefs, *see* beliefs
personal control 20
personal space *179*
personal tragedy approach 63, 64
personality
    hardy personality 23–4
    Type A 20, 110
personalized models of care 164
personalizing 28
Petrie, C. 128
physical abuse *175*
physical dimension of individuals
    54, 55, 56, 119
physical exercise 29
physical health
    self-care 29
    sense of control 108
    social support 112
pity 143
planning self-care 27–8
policy issues in holistic care 121
political issues

leadership 193
    public/private sector provision 160
    spiritual care 120–1
poor care 34
possibilities 27–8
post-modern societies 86
practice standards 241
prayer 128–9
pre-action protocols 212–13
preferred name 53–4
presence 113
press coverage 3–4, 34
pressure 18, 20, 22; *see also* stress
pressure ulcers 155–6
primary interventions 23
Prime Minister's Commission on the
    Future of Nursing and Midwifery
    in England (2010) 34, 37, 44, 85,
    129, 192, 199, 200
private sector provision 159–60
problems to possibilities 27–8
process 41, 42
professional accountability
    care pathways 154–5
    core element of quality care 36, 37
professional distancing 140
professional drivers of leadership 193
professional indemnity insurance 215
Project 2000 4–5
protection issues 174–6
providers of health care 83
psychoanalysis 97, 100–1
psychodynamic approach *98*
psychological abuse *175*
psychological dimension of
    individuals 53, 54, 55, 56, 119
psychological flexibility 30
psychological issues
    emotion 105
    exposure to nursing 11
    healthcare staff 17
    measurement and evaluation of
        care 243
    talking about dying *181*
psychology
    approaches in 97, *98*
    emotions 105–6
    key theories 97–101

psychosocial dimension of caring 10–11, 12
public health 163
public sector provision 159–60
punishment 102

Q

qualitative research 9
quality accounts 192, *193*, 202
quality-adjusted life year (QALY) 253
quality care processes 38, 40–3
quality care systems 38, 40–3
Quality, Innovation, Productivity and Prevention (QIPP) 236
quality nursing care 33–46
  accessing support 44
  checklist *38, 39–40*
  core elements 35–6
  definition 34–8, 235–6
  dimensions 220
  documenting 43–4
  drivers of 34
  highlighting 44
  legislation 202
  measuring 43–4, 235–6, 237–43
  NICE standards 257
  seven steps to 44
  systems and processes 38, 40–3
quantitative research 9
questioning 146
questionnaires 9

R

rapport 73
rationalization 98, 100
rationing 251
record-keeping
  NMC Code 211
  safeguarding 175
Redfern Report 84
reductionism 125
referral
  communication 140
  safeguarding 174–5
reflection 137, 232
reframing 28, 29, 103
reinforcement 102

religion
  part of spiritual care 68
  personal and professional relationship 128–9
religious care 118
repression 98
research into caring 9–10
resilience 30, 112
resource allocation
  choice 251
  efficiency 251–2
resources
  coping with nursing work 17–18
  production of health care 250
respect
  communicating care 145
  definition 47–51
  establishing 73
  for individuals in nursing practice 51–2
responding 37
responsibility
  for own health 88
  range of individuals responsible for caring 83
  safeguarding 175
  stress identification and management 23, 25
reward 102–3
Reynolds Empathy Scale 143
rights 51, 207–8
risk management 216–17
risk-taking behaviour 90
Rogers, C. *99*, 104–5
role models 86, 107
Royal College of Nursing 35, 193

S

sadness *176*
safeguarding 174–6
safety of patients 36, 37, 73–4, 151, 216–17
scarcity 249–50
science 87
screening 108
secondary interventions 23
selection process 5
self

interrelated aspects 141–2
  sense of 106–9
self-awareness
  communication 139, 141–2
  developing 142
  respecting individuals 52
  spiritual care 127–8
self-care 16–32
  definition 18
  key elements 18–20
  physical health 29
  planning 27–8
  relevance 16–17
  resilience 30
  responsibility 25
  thought-traps 28–9
self-determination 20
self-efficacy 20, 88, 109
self-help groups 112
self-sacrifice 11, 12
Seligman, M. *99*
sensitivity 73
serotonin 105
service exclusion 91
service users, involving in partnerships of care 165–7
seven steps to quality 44
sex 71
sexist language 71
sexual abuse *175*
sexuality 57, 74, 124
shell shock 100
Shipman Inquiry Final Report 84
sick role 86–7
sickness absences 17
skills and respect 52
Skinner, B. F. *99*, 102
sleep 29
social action 87, 88–9
social approaches in psychology 98
social attitudes to care provision 83–4
social behaviours 86
Social Care Institute for Excellence 162
social change 85–6
social constructionism 87

social context
    emotions 105–6
    health care 82–4
social determinants of health 89
social dimension of the individual
        53, 54, 55, 56, 119
social divisions 86, 87
social gradient of health 90
social identity 87
social inequality 89–92
social issues
    emotion 105
    health 89–91
    talking about dying 181
social model of disability 65
social policy 85
social processes 86
social research approach 88
social roles 86–7
social stratification 86, 87
social structures 86
social support
    burnout 24
    job strain 21
    physical health 112
    resilience 112
socially constructed 'other' 62, 72,
        73
societal change 120
sociological imagination 85
sociology
    definition 85
    focus and scope 86–7
    key debates 87–8
    relevance in nursing education
        84–5
    social change 85–6
    social policy 85
spiritual care
    challenges 127–8
    definition 118
    drivers of 120–1
    holistic nursing practice 119–20,
        124–5
    religious dimension 68
    self-awareness 127–8
spiritual dimension of individuals 53,
        54, 55, 56, 119

spiritual needs 126–7
spirituality
    definition 118, 121–4
    dignity 50
    historical aspects 123–4
    health and well-being link 57
    resilience 30
stereotyping 62, 67, 107
stigma 87
stimulation 19
stress
    burnout 23–4
    causes 17
    emotional labour 24–5
    job strain model 21
    long-term effects 17
    management 20, 22–3, 25, 110
    physiological response 110
    sense of control 20
    signs 17
    student nurses 11
    theories 20–1
    transactional model 21
stroke 90
structure
    ageism 72
    quality assurance 41, 42
    social action 88–9
    sociological sense 87
student nurses, perception of caring
        11–12
styles of care 140
surface acting 24
surveys of patient satisfaction and
        experience 239–40
sympathy 143
systematic desensitization 102

T
talking 71
Taylor, G. 220
team climate 230
team culture 230
team working 36, 37, 230
technical and professional dimension
        of caring 10–11, 12
technical efficiency 252
technological advancements 250

tertiary interventions 23
therapeutic communication 143
therapeutic relationship 142
'third sector' 83
third way 160–1
thoughts
    self-care 19–20
    thought-traps 28–9
    see also beliefs
training
    of nurses 4
    stress management 22
traits of caring 8
transactional model of stress 21
transcultural nursing 66–7
transformational leadership 205
triple bookkeeping 107
trust 207
Type A 20, 110

U
unconditional positive regard 52,
        105
unconscious 97, 101
undressing patients 106
unemployment 91
university education 4, 5
utility 253

V
Vaccine Damage Compensation Act
        (1979) 212
values 48, 56, 128–9
variance form 151
vicarious liability 215
visual analogue scales 110
vulnerable groups 172–3
    communicating with 178–9
    groups identified as vulnerable 173
    health challenges 183–4
    identifying pain and distress 185–6
    safeguarding 174–6
    symptom management 185–6

W
W, Mr 223
wants 250
ward managers 198–9

ward sisters 198–9, *200*
washing patients 106
Watson, J. B. *99*, 102
Watson, Jean 8
wealth and health 90

welfare benefits 161
well-being
    pressure 22
    spirituality 57
whistleblowing policy 175

Wodaabe tribe 71
Woolf Report 212–14
work satisfaction 108–9
World Health Organization 121
Wundt, W. *97, 99*